Primary Care of Musculoskeletal Problems in the Outpatient Setting

Edward J. Shahady, MD
Tallahassee, FL, USA

Editor

Primary Care of Musculoskeletal Problems in the Outpatient Setting

With 207 Illustrations

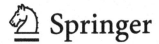 Springer

Edward J. Shahady
3085 Obrien Drive
Tallahassee, FL 32309
USA

ISBN-10: 1-4939-0212-1
ISBN-13: 978-1-4939-0212-5

Printed on acid-free paper.

9 8 7 6 5 4 3 2 1

springer.com

This book is dedicated to my lovely wife Sandra,
our six beautiful and gifted children, their wonderful
spouses and our ten lovely and talented grandchildren.
Through them I have learned the real joy
and meaning of life.

Contents

Contributors ix

PART I. GENERAL TOPICS

1 Key Principles of Outpatient Musculoskeletal Medicine 3
   Edward J. Shahady

2 Exercise as Medication 13
   Edward J. Shahady

3 Nutrition for Active People 28
   Eugene Trowers

4 Altitude, Heat, and Cold Problems 35
   Edward J. Shahady

PART II. UPPER EXTREMITY

5 Shoulder Problems 51
   Edward J. Shahady, Jason Buseman, and Aaron Nordgren

6 Elbow Problems 93
   Edward J. Shahady

7 Wrist Problems 118
   Edward J. Shahady

8 Hand Problems 136
   Edward J. Shahady

PART III. SPINE

9 Neck Problems 159
   Edward J. Shahady

10   Back Problems   178
     Edward J. Shahady

PART IV. LOWER EXTREMITY

11   Hip and Thigh Problems   203
     Edward J. Shahady

12   Knee Problems   228
     Jocelyn R. Gravlee and Edward J. Shahady

13   Lower Leg Problems   268
     Edward J. Shahady

14   Ankle Problems   289
     Edward J. Shahady

15   Foot Problems   310
     Mike Petrizzi and Edward J. Shahady

Index   343

Contributors

Jason Buseman, MS, BS
Senior Medical Student, Florida State University College of Medicine, Tallahassee, FL, USA.

Jocelyn R. Gravlee, MD
Assistant Professor, Department of Family Medicine and Rural Health, Florida State University College of Medicine, Tallahassee, FL, USA.

Aaron Nordgren, BS
Fourth Year Medical Student, Florida State University College of Medicine, Tallahassee, FL, USA.

Mike Petrizzi, MD
Associate Clinical Professor, Department of Family Medicine, Virginia Commonwealth University School of Medicine, Richmond, VA, USA.

Edward Shahady, MD
Clinical Professor, Department of Family Medicine and Community Health, University of Miami; Adjunct Professor, Department of Family Medicine, University of North Carolina; Associate Faculty Family Practice Residency Tallahassee Memorial Hospital, Tallahassee, FL, USA.

Eugene Trowers MD, MPH, FACP
Assistant Dean, Department of Clinical Sciences, Florida State University College of Medicine, Tallahassee, FL, USA.

Part I

General Topics

1

Key Principles of Outpatient Musculoskeletal Medicine

Edward J. Shahady

Musculoskeletal (MS) problems are common in primary care. Up to 15% of diagnoses made in primary care are MS. These diagnoses may be the primary reason for the patients' visit or an associated diagnosis or complaint. The complaints are common in the physically active especially the *weekend warrior* who is too busy during the week to be active and overextends himself or herself on the weekend. Unfortunately, many patients do not receive effective care for MS problems. In order to provide effective care there are key principles that should be followed:

1. Knowledge of the anatomy of the area involved is critical to diagnoses and treatment. Devoting a few extra minutes to rediscovering the anatomy will facilitate a more accurate diagnosis and prescription of effective treatment.
2. A focused history and examination that includes the mechanism of injury is 95% accurate in making the diagnosis of MS problems.
3. Imaging for MS problems is sometimes overordered and used as a substitute for the physical examination and history.
4. Rehabilitation for an injury begins with rest, ice, compression, and elevation (RICE). The next phase of rehabilitation includes stretching, strengthening, heat, ultrasound, and stimulation. Medications have a role but only a temporary one. Medications should never be used alone with MS problems.
5. Treatment always includes a reduction of training errors and use of orthotics if needed.
6. Older patients, especially those with chronic disease, will have minor MS problems that will lead to major disability if not properly addressed.
7. Exercise is an excellent medication for many chronic diseases. Understanding how to motivate patients and yourself to prescribe exercise is difficult and may require a change in clinician and practice attitude.
8. Exercise can induce MS problems if the potential for training errors and anatomic risks are not properly accessed and addressed.
9. Medications for relief of pain and inflammation are helpful but can also have negative effects especially in the elderly.
10. The place where physical activity occurs can represent a risk. High and low altitudes as well as heat and cold are environments that can lead to

problems. The most important role for the primary care clinician is prevention and early recognition of these problems.

11. When does being sick limit physical activity? An upper respiratory infection (URI) or infection of any type should not necessarily limit physical activity. Infectious mononucleosis (MONO) is not necessarily a contraindication to physical activity.

1. Principle 1

Each chapter of this book stresses some aspect of the anatomy of the MS problems of that chapter. The anatomy stressed is not the total anatomy of the area but the key anatomy most often involved in the diagnosis and treatment of MS problems. For example, Chapter 5 describes the importance of the difference between the shoulder joint and the hip joint. This difference allows for more movement of the shoulder than the hip. The hip is not as movable because the head of the femur fits into a socket from the pelvis, so bone aids in preventing it from dislocation and excessive movement. The head of the humerus fits on a flat glenoid process that covers only 1/3 of the surface of the humerus. A rim of cartilage (labrum) ligaments and rotator cuff muscles provide the rest of the stability for the shoulder. This anatomical arrangement permits the shoulder to move the arm in multiple directions. Many of the activities of daily living are possible because of this flexibility. Unfortunately, this anatomical arrangement places the shoulder at greater risk of dislocation, making it the most commonly dislocated joint in the body.

Knowledge of the shoulder anatomy also helps with rehabilitation. The rotator cuff muscles originate on different parts of the scapula and insert on the humeral head in different sites. Knowledge of the origin and insertion aids in understanding the exercises that need to be prescribed. Review the shoulder exercises to help you understand this principle. For example, the infraspinatus muscle originates on the posterior scapula and inserts on the humeral head. Look at the exercise for strengthening this muscle and you will see the anatomy in action.

2. Principle 2

The history helps the clinician not only make the diagnosis but better understand the risks for injury and the mechanism that led to the injury. Many of the cases presented in the different chapters highlight this importance. For example, the boy with leg pain in Chapter 13 was not in shape over the summer so he was not well conditioned at the start of practice. His shoes were 2 years old and had been used by his brother for a full season. They provided minimal support medially and the cleats were worn out on the medial side. This information helped with both diagnosis and treatment of his condition.

The physical examination helps confirm the history and make the diagnosis. Knowledge of the anatomy helps the clinician perform the examination. For example, in Chapter 15 in the case of the 36-year-old man with foot pain, examination revealed pain upon palpation of the left heel over the medical tubercle of the calcaneus. The plantar fascia attaches at this site. The pain was aggravated by dorsiflexion of the great toe and standing on the tips of his toes. Both of these maneuvers stretch the plantar fascia. Dorsiflexion of the left foot was decreased, indicating tightness in the posterior calf muscles. Tapping over the area posterior to the medial malleolus does not produce any numbness or tingling (negative Tinel's sign). This helps the clinician rule out other causes of the foot pain. The examination confirmed the history, and the patient was diagnosed with plantar fasciitis. Treatment was instituted and the patient improved. The patient's history and examination were all that was needed to make the diagnosis and start treatment.

3. Principle 3

The advent of computerized tomography (CT) scan and magnetic resonance imaging (MRI) has increased our ability to diagnose many MS problems. But CT and MRI have not replaced history and physical examination. Unfortunately, many clinicians have learned to rely on CT and MRI and lost confidence in their ability to make a diagnosis by history and examination. One popular reason stated for imaging is the need to protect the clinician from malpractice. There are no data to support this notion. In fact, one small study discovered that ordering images was a function of physician knowledge about that disease or problem. The less they knew about the clinical entity the more they ordered images. Plantar fasciitis (PF) is a good example. Some clinicians order an X-ray looking for a heel spur. Heel spurs do not cause PF. Many patients with heel spurs do not have heel pain and many patients with PF do not have heel spurs. Removal of heel spurs in PF has been shown to be harmful and not helpful for PF.

4. Principle 4

Treatment of MS problems follows a logical sequence. Chronic problems are treated differently than acute problems but many of the treatment strategies are similar. The foundation for chronic problem treatment is stretching and strengthening. Most patients with chronic MS problems do not understand this. This is especially true of patients with osteoarthritis (OA). Osteoarthritis usually begins as a mild discomfort that the patient self-treats with a nonsteroidal anti-inflammatory drug (NSAID). If the pain is mentioned in the early stages, it is an afterthought and not the primary reason for the complaint and NSAIDs are usually prescribed. In an effort to protect the osteoarthritic joint, patients decrease joint movement. This leads to muscle atrophy and decreased strength and flexibility. Osteoarthritis of the knee is a good example. Knee extension is decreased in order to reduce the discomfort in the knee. The decreased extension leads to atrophy and weakness of the quadriceps. Weakness of the quadriceps reduces the patient's ability to perform activities of daily living like rising from a chair. This places more stress on the knee joint and increases pain and disability. This could have been prevented if quadriceps-strengthening exercises were the initial treatment strategy employed when the patient was first seen. Exercises given at the end of most chapters can be used to prevent and treat the problems discussed.

If it is an acute problem, the treatment will depend on the phase of tissue injury. The first 48 to 72 h is the acute or the first phase. Control of pain and edema decreases the associated inflammatory process in this phase. RICE is the mainstay of treatment at this point. Ice reduces the release of inflammatory chemicals at the injury site. Application of ice for 15 min decreases pain and inflammation. Elevation of the extremity above the heart and compression also aid in reduction of the swelling. Immobilization can be employed depending on the extent of the injury. Immobilization can include casting, splinting (air, rigid, etc.), orthotics, taping, crutches, and bracing. Prolonged immobilization can cause muscle atrophy, weakness, and loss of range of motion (ROM). The R in RICE may mean immobilization and/or protection of the injured part but does not mean stopping all activities. Non-weight-bearing movement is encouraged to decrease stiffness. Some strengthening exercises can be performed in this phase in order to prevent atrophy. An example is an isometric contraction of the quadriceps. The patient fully contracts the quadriceps muscle while the limb is supported on a bed or floor. The knee joint does not move during this exercise.

Beyond 72 h is considered the recovery or tissue-healing or the second phase. It may last for days to weeks. Stretching techniques are instituted in this phase. Stretching can decrease pain and reduce loss of ROM and flexibility. For example, in ankle injury, towel stretching and non-weight-bearing movement increases the ability to dorsiflex and plantar-flex the foot. Stretching also reduces the incidence of reinjury. Once pain-free weight bearing is achieved, strengthening exercises should be initiated. Examples include both closed kinetic chain (CKC) and open kinetic chain (OKC) exercises. Closed kinetic chain exercises are those in which the distal end of the limb is fixed on a surface. A standing squat where the foot is planted is an example of a CKC exercise for quadriceps strengthening. Closed kinetic chain exercises are less stressful for the knee joint because the distal limb is not moving. Closed kinetic chain exercises are started before OKC exercises. Use of a leg extension machine or placing a weight on the ankle and extending the knee against resistance is an example of an OKC exercise. The distal end of the limb is moving in OKC exercises so the stress is greater on the knee. Wait until the CKC exercises are performed with ease before prescribing OKC exercises.

The third phase is the functional phase. Identification of the patients' work and/or specific recreational activities is required for this phase. Patients may feel they can return to performing the functions required for work or their sport but if they return too early, they may suffer a reinjury or a new injury. Proprioception and compensatory movement patterns are key to the functional phase. Review the suggested exercises at the end of Chapter 14 for a better understanding of this issue.

Another issue in rehabilitation is cross training to maintain conditioning. If tolerated, alternative activities such as water jogging, swimming, walking, running, or using a stationary exercise bike should be considered while the patient is recovering from the injury or the chronic problem.

Other modalities like heat and electrotherapy may be helpful in decreasing pain and edema, promoting healing, and increasing flexibility. Heating modalities facilitate stretching and strengthening by increasing blood flow to muscle and inducing muscle relaxation. Heat is not used during the acute phase because of increased edema and inflammation. Ultrasound, a deep heating agent, is used to promote heating of the joint and to drive medications into the tissue. Electrical modalities like transcutaneous electrical nerve stimulation (TENS) units are used to modulate the pain response and may help acutely in managing edema.

5. Principle 5

Training errors and the need for orthotics are often overlooked areas in treating MS problems. The patient with medial tibial stress syndrome presented in Chapter 13 is an example of training errors leading to an MS problem. This patient started football practice without conditioning and was wearing an old worn pair of shoes. He was also an unrecognized pronator. His pronation, old shoes, and poor conditioning predisposed him to overstressing his posterior tibial muscles. This stress resulted in a periosteal reaction and the medial tibial stress syndrome. This entity, commonly mistaken for shin splints, will be discussed in more detail in Chapter 13. He responded very well to the use of an orthotic, proper shoe size, exercises, and a more appropriate conditioning program.

Stress fractures are another good example of a training error. Bone responds to overload or additional stress by increasing its rate of turnover and by repairing itself. A balance between bone resorption and bone formation keeps the bone intact. A stress fracture occurs when the repetitive load disrupts the balance, resulting in a spectrum of injury that results in a fracture through the cortex. The balance between normal repair and bone breakdown can be compromised. The majority of the time, excessive training and/or training errors like a change in footwear, training on different surfaces (hard surfaces or the sand on the beach), or failure to modify activities at the onset of symptoms compromises the balance. Stress fractures occur in women or adolescent girls who are less than 75% of the ideal body weight. The primary care clinician is in an excellent position to recognize these training errors and use this knowledge to prevent and treat the associated problems.

6. Principle 6

Older patients with seemingly minor MS complaints may develop significant disability if the problem is not aggressively treated. Aging individuals are likely to have osteoarthritis (OA), past MS injuries, decreased strength secondary to a loss of muscle mass, and less coordination and may be deconditioned because of chronic disease. All of these issues make the elderly individual more susceptible to a minor injury, resulting in major disability.

An example is a 65-year-old woman who is caring for a spouse disabled by a stroke, is mildly depressed, and has type 2 diabetes and OA of her right knee. While lifting her husband she felt a pull in her right thigh. She thought it was a muscle strain and did not seek medical attention initially. Three days after her injury she developed swelling and significant pain in her right knee. She was evaluated by her clinician and treated with an injection of steroids into her knee joint and prescribed NSAIDs. This treatment relieved the knee pain but she began to experience decreased ability to get up from a chair and within 1 week, she was bed-bound. Her blood sugar became more difficult to manage with oral agents and she required injections of insulin. Both she and her husband had to be admitted to a nursing home because they were unable to perform activities of daily living without assistance.

This woman had multiple problems that made her susceptible to what happened. Type 2 diabetes is characterized by decreased glucose delivery to muscle, therefore contributing to the normal muscle weakness associated with aging. The pain of OA of the knee decreases leg extension and leads to weakness of the quadriceps. She then sustained a strain in the quadriceps when lifting her husband. This strain added to the burden of a muscle that was already weak. There was minimal reserve and she quickly lost the ability to use her quadriceps muscle effectively, leading to increased stress on the knee joint and an exacerbation of her OA. Her clinician then treated her OA with NSAIDs and steroids in her joint. Unfortunately, the patient's muscle weakness increased and she became bed-bound and required admission to a nursing home. In the nursing home, she received intensive physical therapy and was able to return to her home and care for herself within 3 weeks. She continues to do her quadriceps-strengthening exercises daily and is now able to take her daily walk because of less arthritic pain in her knee. Increased walking has aided in relieving her depression and increased her diabetes control. If this patient had been instructed in quadriceps strengthening as part of her treatment for OA, it may have prevented her admission to the nursing home. For a more extensive discussion of OA of the knee and knee exercises, see Chapter 12.

7. Principle 7

Exercise is an excellent medication for many chronic diseases. Exercise reduces cardiovascular disease by decreasing low-density lipoprotein (LDL) cholesterol and triglycerides, increasing high-density lipoprotein (HDL) cholesterol, decreasing blood pressure, and improving endothelial function by decreasing the inflammatory mediators of atherosclerosis and improved left ventricular function. It also increases longevity and decreases the risk of the metabolic syndrome and diabetes by decreasing visceral fat. Exercise also prevents and treats disability by decreasing some of the changes attributed to the aging process, reducing the incidence of falls in the elderly and increasing bone mass. It also reduces the incidence of breast and colon cancer and contributes to psychologic health and well-being.

Understanding how to motivate patients and yourself to prescribe exercise is difficult and may require a change in clinician and practice attitude. Patients will not exercise if they do not realize a net benefit. The positives must outweigh the negatives. Patients need to feel comfortable and competent with the exercise prescribed. If these issues are not addressed the exercise prescription will not be followed. Another significant patient barrier is their trust and respect for the clinician. *Patients do not care how much you know until they know how much you care.* Patients respond much better to positive messages than negative ones. Negative messages just increase the feelings of guilt, shame, and depression that accompany obesity, diabetes, and sedentary lifestyle.

Change in patient behavior goes through several stages and patients are at different stages at different times. Different strategies are needed for the different stages. Questions that seek patient partnership are more effective than lectures about exercise. Clinicians who understand the stages of change and have different strategies for each stage are usually more successful in assisting their patients with performing exercises.

The exercise prescription should be individualized and be one that the patient feels is achievable. Write the prescription out on your prescription pad. Give patients an opportunity to disagree or modify the plan. Also, include the little things they can do with their daily activities, like walking up one flight of stairs rather than taking the elevator, parking at a distance rather than close to their work or destination. Chapter 2 provides more discussion on addressing patient and clinician obstacles to exercise.

8. Principle 8

The advice to exercise should always include suggestions that prevent MS problems from developing. Training errors and anatomic issues like pronation increase risk of injury. Training errors are common in individuals who have just begun an exercise program. Exercise has not been a regular part of their lives and they lack knowledge of proper shoe wear, exercise surface, exercise terrain, and stretching and strengthening routines. Even exercises like daily walking requires appropriate preparation. The clinician should be prepared to evaluate current shoe wear by looking at the shoes patients intend to use. Chapter 15 has a good discussion on how to evaluate and purchase shoes. Surface for exercise should be consistent when first starting a program. Switching from one surface to another without acclimatizing to one can create problems. Different terrains create different demands on the lower extremities. Hills stress different muscles when going downhill than when going uphill. Slanted surfaces like those on a beach stress one leg differently than the other. Stretching and strengthening muscle groups, especially the lower leg muscles, aid in the prevention of most common exercise-related MS problems. Chapters 11 to 15 provide good insight into how to stretch and strengthen all muscle groups below the waist.

Anatomic risks if not recognized and treated before an exercise program is started may lead to MS problems. Two good examples are pronation and increased quadriceps (Q) angle in the knee. Pronation is associated with several knee, lower leg, and foot problems like patellar femoral tracking syndrome (PFTS), posterior tibial tendonitis, and plantar fasciitis. These clinical problems may be prevented or minimized with the use of orthotics. Further discussion of the treatment of pronation and use of orthotics is included in Chapter 15. An increased Q angle is more common in women because of their hip anatomy. The increased angle changes the movement of the patella through the femoral groove with knee extension and flexion and increases the risk of PFTS. The size and strength of the lateral quadriceps muscles increase in individuals who start exercise programs. This creates an imbalance between the lateral and medical quadriceps muscles and causes the patella to move more laterally with extension and flexion of the knee. This imbalance can cause the PFTS. The individual with an increased Q angle starts out with an increased risk of PFTS and exercise adds to the risk. The PFTS can be prevented or at least minimized if the patient is taught how to perform quadriceps-strengthening exercises, especially straight leg raising, before the exercise program is started and continues them once the exercise program begins. Chapter 12 further discusses the PFTS. Exercises for PFTS are at the end of Chapter 12.

9. Principle 9

Medications for relief of pain and inflammation are helpful but can also have negative effects, especially in the elderly. Tylenol (acetaminophen) and NSAIDs are the most commonly used medication for pain relief in MS injury.

Tylenol is an analgesic with minimal anti-inflammatory action that is effective in relieving mild to moderate pain. The mechanism of action does not interfere with prostaglandin synthesis, thus giving it a safer gastrointestinal (GI) profile. Its action is mediated through the central nervous system. Acetaminophen is equal to aspirin in analgesic properties and it is unlikely to produce many of the side effects associated with aspirin and aspirin-containing products. Tylenol has to be given in the appropriate doses every 6 to 8 h for it to be effective. When given in doses of 4000 mg a day it works as well as NSAIDs for pain relief. Unfortunately, most patients are not informed of the need to take full doses and lose confidence in Tylenol because of inadequate pain relief. Adult Tylenol comes in a 500- and 650-mg tablets and caplets. If the dose does not exceed 4000 mg a day, the risk of liver toxicity is minimal. Tylenol Arthritis Extended Relief caplets (650 mg) have a two-layer formulation. The first layer dissolves quickly to provide prompt relief while the time-released second layer provides up to 8 h of relief.

NSAIDs are the most frequently prescribed medications for MS problems. They work by blocking the conversion of arachidonic acid to prostaglandin. The side effects include increased incidence of hypertension and heart disease, gastric ulceration, GI bleeding, edema, and renal disease. The incidence of these side effects increases with age, use for greater than 2 weeks, and use with other drugs like alcohol. There are two types of NSAIDs: COX-1 and COX-2 inhibitors. The COX-2 inhibitors are more selective and block only COX-2 enzymes. They have fewer GI side effects but have recently been implicated in increased cardiovascular risk. Some controversy exists about the use of anti-inflammatory drugs with injury. Most view them as helpful by reducing inflammatory response but a few believe that the healing process is blunted by the use of NSAIDs [1].

The evidence for either opinion is limited. The major benefit is pain relief and that is a well-documented effect of NSAIDs. The reader is encouraged to use caution in the use of NSAIDs. Some good rules to follow include limiting use for no longer than 7 to 10 days, not mixing with alcohol or other medications that cause GI distress, and monitoring closely for edema, hypertension, proteinuria, cardiovascular disease, GI distress, and/or bleeding.

10. Principle 10

Physical activity performed at high and low altitudes as well as excessive heat and cold are environments that can lead to problems. The most important role for the primary care clinician is prevention and early recognition of these problems. If the primary care clinician practices in an area where these problems are more likely then recognition and early treatment will be more important to the clinician. All clinicians should be aware of the risks of altitude, heat, and cold and educate their patients about how to prevent problems in these environments. High-altitude illness can be prevented with Diamox taken before ascending to altitudes and limiting the distance climbed to 1000 ft a day. Low altitude or diving illness should not be attempted without proper instruction by qualified teachers. Knowing how to descend and ascend properly will prevent most problems. Heat-related problems could be prevented with proper hydration and common sense. Early recognition of "the need to get out of the heat" is essential. Cold illness prevention is a matter of proper clothing, knowledge of early symptoms, and common sense. Common to all of these environmental problems is the increased risk created by certain medications and age. Chapter 4 covers most of these issues.

11. Principle 11

A URI or infection of any type should not necessarily limit physical activity. How patients feel is the best indicator. If they want to participate, they probably can as long as the activity does not add to their risk. An example might be an adolescent football player who has had diarrhea and/or vomiting for 2 days, is now better, and wants to participate in a game. Because of the outside temperature, and the pads and helmet worn in football, the risk of dehydration is greater. The diarrhea and vomiting have already created fluid loss that makes the individual more at risk for heat illness. Playing in a game will probably cause him to develop heat illness. It would be prudent to advise the parents and/or coach to reacclimatize the athlete to playing slowly. The type of sport will also influence the decision. A game of golf on a cool day would not be as risky. Temperature of greater than 100°F (37.7°C) associated with an infection can be used as a guide to limit activity. Temperature alone is not enough to make the decision. Temperature should be coupled with the other symptoms for a more informed decision.

Infectious MONO is another illness that raises questions about physical activity. There is no evidence that MONO is a contraindication to physical activity. One commonly described worry is splenic rupture in contact sports. If a spleen can be palpated or is enlarged on ultrasound, advice to not participate in contact sports like football is appropriate. That does not mean that the athlete cannot run and stay conditioned or acclimatized to the environment. How persons feel is the key indicator of participation in physical activity. Sometimes, they are fatigued not because of the MONO but because of the depression secondary to not being physically active or participating in their sport.

Reference

1. Gorsline RT, Kaeding CC. The use of NSAIDs and nutritional supplements in athletes with osteoarthritis: prevalence, benefits, and consequences. *Clin Sports Med*. 2005;24:71–82.

2

Exercise as Medication

EDWARD J. SHAHADY

All parts of the body which have a function, if used in moderation, and exercised in labors to which each is accustomed, become healthy and well developed and age slowly; but if unused and left idle, they become liable to disease, defective in growth and age quickly. This is especially so with joints and ligaments if one does not use them.

Hippocrates

Sedentary lifestyle accelerates the aging process, and causes or contributes to many chronic diseases. Exercise is a powerful medication that aids in decelerating the aging process, preventing chronic as well as many other cardiovascular diseases, and provides musculoskeletal benefits. Motivating patients to exercise is a complex challenge. The challenge includes both patient and clinician barriers to implementing an effective exercise plan. Frustration, knowledge deficit, difficulty in motivating and being motivated, and a general lack of enthusiasm for exercise are some of the barriers. This chapter presents information about exercise, its benefits, patient and clinician barriers, and strategies to overcome the barriers.

Good evidence now exists that the observations of Hippocrates were correct. Sedentary lifestyle leads to accelerated aging and the following physiological changes:

- Reduced insulin sensitivity
- Increased visceral fat mass and intramuscular lipid accumulation
- Decreased aerobic capacity, cardiac contractility, stroke volume, and cardiac output
- Increased arterial stiffness and blood pressure (BP)
- Decreased bone mass, strength, and density
- Decreased muscle strength, power, and endurance
- Decreased tissue elasticity, thinning of cartilage, decreased tendon length, and tendon weakness
- Decreased gait stability secondary to impaired proprioception and balance

Some of the changes are age-related and others are secondary to lack of use. There is also overlap between changes related to aging and those related to

13

TABLE 2.1. Benefits of exercise.

1. Reduces the incidence of coronary artery disease
2. Decreases LDL cholesterol and triglycerides
3. Increases HDL cholesterol
4. Decreases blood pressure
5. Improves endothelial function
6. Decreases the inflammatory mediators of atherosclerosis
7. Improves left ventricular function and decreases left ventricular mass
8. Decreases arterial stiffness
9. Decreases visceral fat
10. Prevents or delays the onset of type 2 diabetes
11. Increases longevity and decreases the risk of several common chronic diseases
12. Prevention and treatment of disability
13. Decreases some of the changes attributed to the aging process
14. Reduces falls in the elderly
15. Increases bone mass
16. Reduces the incidence of colon and breast cancer
17. Contributes to psychologic health and well-being

lack of use and/or sedentary lifestyle. Multiple cardiovascular and musculoskeletal diseases and problems result from these changes. Fortunately, many of the changes are modifiable with endurance exercise and strength training. Exercise has several positive benefits as noted in Table 2.1.

1. Cardiovascular Respiratory Response to Exercise

Cardiovascular fitness is attained through physical changes in the heart. The conditioned heart is more efficient if it can deliver more blood to the body with less work. Figure 2.1 is a theoretical description that provides numbers to illustrate the differences in efficiency of the conditioned heart compared with the nonconditioned heart. The conditioned heart is bigger and stronger than the nonconditioned heart and is better able to pump out the blood with every beat. The heart has two phases: diastole and systole. During systole, the heart is squeezing out blood to deliver it to the body. During diastole, the heart is relaxing and filling with blood. The heart can become more efficient if it has more blood available at the end of diastole and squeezes more out by the end of systole. The efficiency is a reflection of the heart becoming larger and stronger and better able to pump out more blood with each beat. Figure 2.1 demonstrates this efficiency. In this theoretical example, the nonconditioned heart has an end-diastolic volume of approximately 120 cc and an end-systolic volume of 50 cc. It has pumped out 70 cc. This is called the stroke volume or cardiac output per beat. The percent of the volume ejected was 58% (70/120 = 58%). This amount is called the ejection fraction. Because the conditioned heart has become more fit with exercise, it has enlarged and increased

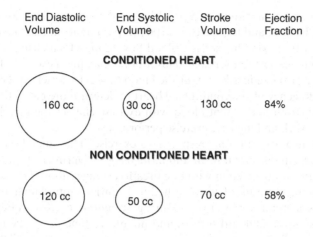

FIGURE 2.1. Differences in the nonconditioned and conditioned hearts.

its ability to contract. The end-diastolic volume has increased to 160 cc and the end-systolic volume has decreased to 30 cc. In the conditioned heart the stroke volume or cardiac output with each beat is 130 cc (160–30) and the ejection fraction is 81% (130/160). The conditioned heart is able to deliver 60 cc more per beat (130–70) to the body than the nonconditioned heart. This efficiency increases the capacity to exercise as well as to conserve cardiac work. Simply stated, the conditioned heart has developed so it can fill up with more blood at the end of diastole and is better able to squeeze that blood out at the end of systole. The conditioned heart delivers more blood per beat than the nonconditioned heart so it can do more work with fewer beats.

In addition to an increased cardiac output, there is a redistribution of the blood flow during exercise, as noted in Table 2.2. This table provides another theoretical example of the redistribution of blood that occurs with exercise. In this example, the cardiac output at rest is 5900 mL per minute and during exercise, it increases to 24,000 mL. The blood flow redistribution with exercise would be as follows: Coronary blood flow at rest is 250 mL per minute whereas at maximum exercise it increases to 1000 cc. Brain flow is 750 mL per minute,

TABLE 2.2. Cardiovascular response to exercise.

	At rest (mL)	During exercise (mL)
Cardiac output	5900	24,000
Coronary flow	250	1000
Brain flow	750	750
Renal, GI tract, liver, and spleen flow	3100	600
Brain flow to muscles	1300	28,850

both at rest and at maximum exercise. Flow to the kidney, the gastrointestinal (GI) tract, the liver, and the spleen is 3100 mL per minute at rest and decreases to 600 mL with maximum exercise. Blood flow to muscles increases from 1300 mL per minute at rest to over 20,000 mL during maximum exercise. Therefore, the majority of the redistribution of the blood flow is to muscle and heart. The increased efficiency of the conditioned heart to deliver more blood to the body and the redistribution of that blood with exercise enables the muscles of the body to do work and increase exercise performance.

There is also a respiratory response to exercise. The lungs become more efficient and can take in more air and more oxygen. During rest, the tidal volume (amount of air taken in with one breath) averages about 500 mL, with a minute volume (amount of air breathed in 1 min) of approximately 6 L/min (12 breaths a minute is average). During strenuous exercise, tidal volume can increase up to 2000 mL/breath and minute volume up to the maximum of 140 L/min. This means a lot more air and oxygen is now available to the body. The increase in tidal volume is attained through taking deeper breaths. As the heart is becoming more efficient with delivering blood to tissue, the lungs are improving their efficiency to deliver more oxygen to that blood. At the tissue level, changes that increase the ability to provide oxygen to muscle are occurring. The size and number of blood vessels increase and there is an increase in capillary density. Mitochondria increase in size and number, enabling muscle cells to extract and use oxygen more efficiently and improve the ability to oxidize fat and carbohydrate. The body is adapting by changing its physiology and anatomy to do more work with less effort.

With exercise and increased activity the body needs to deliver more blood to muscle to enhance the ability to perform that activity. As the body becomes more conditioned the heart increases in size, the lungs take in oxygen more efficiently, and the cells increase their ability to use oxygen and other nutrients.

2. Cardiovascular Disease and Exercise

Disease states such as diabetes, coronary artery disease (CAD), heart failure, peripheral arterial disease, and the metabolic syndrome all change the ability of blood vessels to expand and contract. Less blood flows to the body organs in these disease states. The term used for expansion or dilatation of the blood vessels is vasodilatation. The endothelial lining of the blood vessel is one of the factors involved in vasodilatation. Regular physical activity improves endothelium-dependent vasodilation in patients with all the above diseases. The improved vasodilator function is secondary to endothelial release of nitric oxide (NO). Besides vasomotor tone, exercise also improves the endothelial functions that regulate the clotting factors like fibrinolysis and the inflammatory factors involved in the formation and rupture of arterial plaque.

Inactivity has negative hematological consequences. It causes a lower plasma volume, higher fibrinogen, high hematocrit, elevated blood viscosity, increased platelet aggregation, and diminished fibrinolysis. This hypercoagulable state places the patient at increased risk for thrombophlebitis and pulmonary embolus. Exercise reverses all these negative consequences.

Aging and sedentary lifestyle are associated with increased left ventricular mass, left ventricular diastolic filling abnormalities, impaired endothelial function, increased arterial stiffness, and systemic inflammation. Endothelium-derived NO, a powerful vasodilator, may be the key to many of these abnormalities. A variety of medications commonly used to treat cardiovascular disease, diabetes, and hypertension increase the production of NO. Exercise also increases the production of NO and is an excellent primary or additive medication for cardiovascular disease, diabetes, hyperlipidemia, and hypertension. The positive benefit of exercise is partially explained by its action on NO production. Discussion of this and other physiologic effects of exercise will occur when each disease or problem is presented.

3. Hypertension

Hypertension can be prevented and treated with exercise. The acute response to exercise in a normotensive individual is a rise in systolic pressure to less than 180 mmHg and after a brief rise the diastolic pressure decreases 5 to 10 mmHg. If a patient is hypertensive and exercises, the systolic pressure will rise above 180 mmHg and the diastolic pressure rise will persist. This acute response disappears minutes after exercise stops. With sustained daily exercise or at least five times a week, there is a sustained reduction in both systolic and diastolic pressure. In a meta-analysis of 13 controlled studies of chronic exercise, there was a mean decrease of 11.3 mmHg in systolic pressure and 7.5 mmHg of diastolic pressure. Five to seven days a week of exercise for 30 min a day at 50% to 75% VO_2max was required to sustain the above effect. A simple tool for accessing VO_2max is discussed later. Other studies indicate that chronic exercise in a hypertensive population with left ventricular hypertrophy reduces left ventricular mass.

Hypertension is part of the metabolic syndrome and is associated with diabetes, largely independent of age and obesity. Hypertension is present in 60% of patients who have type 2 diabetes. Diabetes and hypertension are compelling indications for aggressively treating hypertension. There is an estimated doubling of cardiovascular events when hypertension and diabetes coexist although many of these patients will have no cardiovascular symptoms. Intensive BP control is required for reducing cardiovascular events in diabetic patients who have hypertension. Exercise will commonly be coupled with antihypertensive medications to obtain adequate treatment. Exercise is an excellent treatment to not only treat hypertension but delay and prevent hypertension.

4. Type 2 Diabetes, Insulin Resistance, and Exercise

Type 2 diabetes is a genetic disease of insulin resistance that is associated with obesity and sedentary lifestyle. Children whose parents are diabetic have higher fasting insulin levels independent of sedentary lifestyle and obesity. These children have a greater risk of becoming obese and developing a sedentary lifestyle. The insulin resistance initially is manifested by lipid abnormalities and hypertension long before there is an increase in blood sugar. The hyperglycemia will not appear until the pancreas is no longer able to produce the large amount of insulin required to keep the glucose normal. Because of the associated mortality and morbidity, this condition is now called prediabetes or, more appropriately, the metabolic syndrome. The estimated prevalence is 20% in US adults and approaches 50% in older groups. For adults, the risk of progressing from prediabetes to overt diabetes is about 10% over 6 years. There also is a 40% increased risk of mortality, mostly cardiovascular disease, independent of other risk factors in persons with the metabolic syndrome. Type 2 diabetes increases the risk of cardiovascular disease by 200% to 400%. Twenty-five percent of newly diagnosed diabetics have overt cardiovascular disease. All of the above abnormalities can be prevented, reduced, and treated with exercise.

Exercise reduces insulin resistance by 40%. Drugs such as metformin and troglitazone reduce the resistance by 20% to 25%. Insulin resistance decreases the transport of glucose from blood to muscle because of the decreased action of glucose transporters (Glut 4). Exercise training in insulin resistance patients improves glucose transport and enhances the action of insulin in the skeletal muscle. More glucose now reaches muscle where it can be utilized for energy. This movement of glucose to muscle reduces blood sugar acutely and chronically. Exercise training reduces hemoglobin HbA1c. Any type of exercise helps. Motivating diabetics to exercise is difficult as many have physical disabilities. Strategies for helping patients with disabilities are presented in Section 12 (The Exercise Prescription). Exercise also plays a role in the prevention of type 2 diabetes and related metabolic conditions. Men who engage in more than 3 h per week of moderate or vigorous leisure time physical activity are half as likely to develop the metabolic syndrome as sedentary men. Women in the Nurse's Health Study who engaged in light to moderate activity had a decreased risk of developing obesity and the metabolic syndrome. Compared with no treatment, lifestyle changes in the Diabetes Prevention Study reduced the incidence of developing type 2 diabetes by 58% and metformin (glucophage) reduced the incidence by 31%. The lifestyle intervention included 150 min of exercise a week and an average of 7 lb of weight loss.

Heart failure is a frequent consequence of type 2 diabetes, independent of CAD. The most common feature of the diabetic heart is impaired diastolic filling secondary to reduced compliance or prolonged relaxation. Aging and hypertension also contribute to impaired diastolic filling. Exercise improves diastolic filling in diabetes and hypertension. Age-related decline in diastolic filling is less pronounced in older persons who exercise.

The diastolic filling abnormality is secondary to arterial and myocardial stiffening. The stiffening is caused by endothelial dysfunction, decreased NO, and inflammation that accompany insulin resistance, the metabolic syndrome, diabetes, hypertension, and aging. Exercise decreases the stiffening by decreasing endothelial dysfunction and inflammation and increasing NO production.

5. Lipids and Exercise

Serum lipid levels are influenced by exercise especially in the insulin-resistant state. In the normal non-insulin-resistant individual, insulin activates lipoprotein lipase (LPL) lipolysis and causes adipose tissue to store free fatty acids (FFA) for energy. This is most evident following the ingestion of food. Insulin, when its action is not resisted, drives postmeal FFA into adipose tissue and keeps it there until it is needed for energy. In obesity, there is an overflow of FFA secondary to the increased amount of dietary FFA. Insulin-resistant individuals are resistant to LPL activity and are unable to store and/or inhibit the release of a large amount of circulating FFA into the circulation. This increase in serum FFA leads to an atherogenic dyslipidemia (increases in atherogenic small, dense low-density lipoprotein (LDL) and serum triglycerides and decreases in high-density lipoprotein (HDL)). The increased amount of FFA also produces a state of lipotoxicity that contributes to hyperglycemia. Lipotoxicity decreases the ability of the pancreas to secrete insulin, increases hepatic glucose production, and decreases the movement of glucose into muscle.

Exercise reverses all of this by increasing LPL activity. This increase in LPL drives FFA into adipose tissue and helps keep it there until it is needed for energy. This decrease in FFA aids in the decrease of the small, dense LDL particles and triglycerides and increases HDL. Simply stated, exercise produces a reduction in atherogenic dyslipidemia. Exercise also decreases lipotoxicity that in turn reduces hyperglycemia, and helps preserve pancreatic cell function. This provides some explanation for the cardioprotective effect of exercise and the prevention and treatment of diabetes, hypertension, and the metabolic syndrome. All of these effects are additive to all the medications that are used for these problems.

Insulin resistance and sedentary lifestyle also increase the amount of abdominal visceral fat or "pot belly." Visceral fat is an independent predictor of diabetes, hypertension, and cardiovascular disease. Visceral adipose tissue is a major source of proinflammatory cytokines/adipokines. These cytokines contribute to endothelial dysfunction and the increased propensity for the factors that lead to CAD like plaque formation, plaque rupture, and thrombosis. Exercise decreases visceral fat and waist size, sometimes without reducing total body weight. This reduction in visceral fat decreases all the negative factors previously discussed and enhances insulin sensitivity.

6. Inflammation and Exercise

Inflammation is associated with CAD and myocardial infarction. There are now several serum markers for inflammation. Lower concentrations of several inflammatory markers have been reported with exercise. Exercise decreases one of the best surrogate markers for inflammation: highly sensitive C-reactive protein. Patients with chronic heart failure improve exercise tolerance and decrease peripheral inflammatory markers after 12 weeks of moderate-intensity cycling for 30 min, 5 days per week. A reduction in systemic inflammation is an important feature of the training response.

7. Psychological Well-Being and Exercise

Physical activity is associated with a lower prevalence and incidence of depressive symptoms in many adult studies. In these studies of individuals, aged 18 to 91 with clinical depression, aerobic and resistance training produced meaningful improvements in depression with rates from 31% to 88%. Studies of patients with major depression that compared high-intensity aerobic exercise with antidepressant medications found that both approaches produced 60% to 69% recovery.

There was no added benefit of combined exercise and medication. Yoga, resistance training, and aerobic exercise are all equally effective in treating depression. The effects of exercise on depression are most significant in patients with comorbid illness like chronic obstructive pulmonary disease (COPD) and CAD. Exercise also reduces anxiety, distress, and coronary prone behavior and elevates mood, improves self-esteem, and increases intellectual function.

8. Exercise and Cancer

The incidence of colon cancer is decreased in physically active individuals. This is probably secondary to the increased food transit time and less constipation. Exercise also reduces the incidence of breast cancer. Recent studies indicate that physical activity after a breast cancer diagnosis may reduce the risk of death from this disease. The greatest benefit occurred with walking 3 to 5 h per week at an average pace. An average pace would be 2 to 2.9 mph.

9. Musculoskeletal Benefits of Exercise

Muscle mass and strength also change with age. Strength peaks in the third decade of life and begins to decrease after age 40. Muscle mass is 20% less by age 65. Resistance training delays loss of muscle mass, increases flexibility, preserves joint health, and enhances balance. This is of primary importance in the treatment and prevention of osteoarthritis. Immobilization and inactivity lead to muscle shortening. The shortening results in a decrease in the range of motion and a disruption of the shock-absorbing capability. Bed rest or other forms of inactivity are devastating to muscles and joints. One of the most devastating pieces of advice we sometimes give to patients is "take it easy." Some patients interpret this as a command to do nothing, rather than the intended decrease in activity for a while. Remember, "motion is lotion." This is discussed in Section 12 (The Exercise Prescription) (see p.24).

Exercise prevents bone loss, increases bone strength, and decreases the risk of falling by increasing the neuromuscular response that protects the skeleton from injury. Osteoporosis and fracture prevention are two additional benefits of exercise. Inactivity may lead to sarcopenia (decreased muscle mass), followed by muscle weakness and further restriction in activity levels. All of this contributes to the development of osteopenia (less bone), gait abnormalities, and, finally, hip fracture.

Osteoporosis is a disease characterized by low bone mass and deterioration of bone tissue, leading to enhanced bone fragility and an increase in fracture risk. It is most prevalent in postmenopausal white women. Each year, approximately 1.5 million fractures are associated with osteoporosis. Of particular concern is the spine, the most common site of fracture. Weight-bearing physical activity is essential for normal skeletal development during childhood and adolescence and for achieving and maintaining peak bone mass in young adults. Peak bone mass is 95% complete by age 17 in girls and 2 to 3 years later in boys. Bone mass remains relatively stable until about age 50 when progressive loss is detected in men and women. Many factors influence bone mass. Genetics influences up to 70% and the remaining 30% are influenced by habitual physical activity, nutrient intake, and reproductive hormone status.

Bone accommodates to the loads imposed on it by altering its mass and distribution of mass (Wolf's law). When habitual loading increases, bone is gained; when loading decreases, bone is lost. Loading is the sum of all individual daily loading events. An excellent example of the interaction between physical activity and bone mass is the bone loss that follows complete immobilization. Immobilized patients may lose 40% of their original bone mass in 1 year. Studies of bed rest indicate that standing upright for as little as 30 min each day prevents bone loss. Resistance training or mixed endurance/resistance exercise studies show gains in bone mass or a reduction in loss of bone mass in older men and women.

10. Patient Obstacles to Exercise

Patients will not exercise if they do not realize a net benefit. The positives must outweigh the negatives. Some of the negatives include loss of time or competing time demands, negative peer pressure, financial or social costs, and problems with self-identity. Patients need to feel comfortable and competent with the exercise prescribed. It must feel safe and be enjoyable, fit into their daily schedule, and be easy to access on a regular basis. If these issues are not addressed the exercise prescription will not be followed.

Another significant patient barrier is trust and respect for the clinician. *Patients do not care how much you know until they know how much you care.* Patients respond much better to positive messages than to negative ones. Telling them they are going to die if they do not exercise or lose weight or they are lazy is not usually effective. Most patients already know the dangers and feel ashamed that they are unable to start an exercise program. Negative messages just increase the feelings of guilt, shame, and depression. This makes matters worse, not better. Some readers may have a few examples where they think this strategy worked but patients do not return to see the clinician who embarrassed them or increased their guilt. The clinician may of course be aware of this patient in their accounts receivable or through some negative publicity.

Change in behavior is very difficult especially when it comes to physical activity and diet. There are several stages to change and patients are at different stages at different times. The first stage is precontemplation. Most patients are here when you first see them and the stage is reinforced by negative remarks or nonverbal communications of all the clinicians who have seen them in the past. In this stage, only questions are of value. Consider asking them if they have ever tried to exercise in the past. Ask what they think about exercise and its benefits. The challenge here is to get them to the next stage of contemplation, not to get them to exercise. It may take days, weeks, months, or years to reach the next stage but let the patient be in control. Remember they are the ones who have to make the decision. Contemplation is usually reached when they say they want to start an exercise program. Ask them why they want to start. You find out it has nothing to do with you but an incident that happened to them or a family member. The response may be a heart attack in a family member or the onset of chest pain in the patient. The answer will affect your next move. Next is the action stage. It may not follow contemplation as fast as you wish. Questions here should focus on the type of exercise that will most likely be sustainable. Consider all the potential barriers that were mentioned above. The next stage is relapse. This stage is the most important for the patient and clinician. After initial success, patients will relapse to their prior behavior of nonactivity. The patient and clinician need to be ready for the reasons why this happens and have plans ready to address the relapse. The last stage is maintenance. This stage is the last but not the final as patients will relapse periodically and go back and forth between stages. Clinicians who expect this and do not react negatively are more successful in helping patients achieve sustainable exercise programs. Relapse is a normal part of the process and does not mean the clinician or patient are failures.

11. Clinician Obstacles to Exercise

A national survey of exercise counseling found that those who do not exercise are less likely to counsel their patients about exercise. This study identified lack of time and inadequate knowledge/experience as major barriers to counseling. Other obstacles noted were "I don't get reimbursed for it," "I'm frustrated with my lack of success," "I don't think the patient is interested," "I don't feel I have the ability to get people to change," and "it's not my job, it's only common sense."

Clinician frustration with patients is a major barrier to implementing an exercise program. The frustration is based partially on the structure of medical education. Medical education programs are based on the model of acute care rather than chronic care. In the acute care model, patient participation in decision making is minimal to nonexistent. The medical problems in the acute care model will resolve in a short period of time and require minimal follow-up and minimal patient involvement in the treatment. Simply stated, the clinician tells the patient what to do and they do it. Examples are a laceration or a strep throat. The patient is a passive recipient of a wound repair or just takes medication for 7 to 10 days. The patient has very little to change and the clinician's efforts are focused on one or maybe two visits. In chronic diseases like obesity, diabetes, hypertension, osteoporosis, and the metabolic syndrome, the roles of both the patient and the clinician are much different. The clinician now has to rely on an entirely different set of skills that are not taught in the acute care model. The clinician is now a coach, a facilitator, and a salesman. The patient plays the major role of achieving the lifestyle changes.

Clinicians trained in the acute care model feel more in control and are primarily responsible for the outcome. In other words, if failure occurs the clinician is responsible (blame). This feeling of control and blame creates a negative relationship when patients are not successful. There is a tendency to shift the blame to patients and call them noncompliant or "bad" patients because they do not lose weight, take medications, exercise, or follow other instructions. It takes a major shift of thinking and feeling to accept the changed role in chronic disease. The clinician is not in control in the chronic care model as much as the patient is.

Once the control issue is accepted, the possibilities for success multiply quickly. A possible motto that clinicians may find helpful is unconditional positive regard. Simply stated, this means not putting conditions on patients and accepting all of their decisions. This does not mean the clinician is happy with their decisions but accepts them as theirs and does not seek to blame patients or himself/herself. Positive regard for the patient's decision without conditions enhances trust and increases chances of change. The change may not occur today but it may occur tomorrow or next week because of the relationship the clinician has with the patient.

Clinician counseling in the old model usually involves telling patients they need to exercise and giving them a few reasons why and leaves it at that. This method seldom works. Change is difficult and requires clinician and patient understanding of the complexity of change. The stages for change were presented in Section 10 (Patient Obstacles to Exercise). The key is to know what questions to ask and when. Using the following set of questions may enhance success.

1. Have you thought about exercise?
2. What type of physical activity do you now do?
3. What makes it difficult for you to exercise?
4. Do you think exercise is worth the effort?
5. What kind of exercise do you think might be fun?
6. What can I do to help you get started with an exercise program?
7. How do you feel about stretching and using weights to help you?

The major change in this model is the patient telling the clinician rather than the clinician telling the patient. The answers to the questions form the foundation for an exercise prescription that is devised by the patient with the physician's help. The answers to the above questions also help with the discovery of the patient's values, concerns, and obstacles about exercise.

This style makes patients feel their individuality is being considered, gives them control, and increases the chances of a sustainable exercise plan. The prescription is individualized to what is doable at this time given the patient's values, bias, and knowledge. It may not be ideal from the clinician's perspective but it is a start. Perhaps with time and increased confidence on the patient's part the prescription will evolve into one that fits the clinician's ideal.

12. The Exercise Prescription

The exercise prescription should be individualized and be one that the patient feels is achievable. As discussed previously, sustainability is a function of the patient being a partner in the creation of the prescription. Write the prescription out on your prescription pad. Be specific with the prescription, e.g., walk 6 days a week for 30 min in the morning with your spouse at a heartbeat of 110. Give the patient an opportunity to disagree or modify the plan. Also, include the little things they can do with their daily activities, like walking up one flight of stairs rather than taking the elevator, parking at a distance rather than close to their workplace or destination. If the patient cannot walk 30 min in one setting be happy with three to four 10-min sessions a day.

Calculating an acceptable pulse rate is a function of knowing VO_2max. VO_2 is the amount of O_2 per kg/mL/min that is required to do a given amount of work or exercise. VO_2max is also a term used to define the maximum amount of work that the individual can perform at any given moment. The VO_2max serves as a benchmark to determine the amount of exercise that can be safely performed. Precise measurement of VO_2 requires sophisticated instrumentation that is not practical in the usual office setting.

The following is a simple formula for estimating VO_2max. Subtract the patient's age from 220. The resulting number represents VO_2max pulse rate. For example, a 40-year-old patient would reach VO_2max at a pulse rate of 180 and a 60-year-old at a rate of 140. Reaching 100% of VO_2max is not recommended because it can lead to anaerobic exercise and arrhythmias. A percent of VO_2max is used when prescribing exercise. Fifty to seventy-five percent of VO_2max is a reasonable number to use for most patients to obtain conditioning or fitness. Patients who have low initial fitness would start at 50% to 60% and gradually increase their maximal heart rate. For a 40-year-old a pulse rate of 117 to 135 and for a 60-year-old a pulse rate of 104 to 120 would be a safe range to recommend. Very little extra cardiovascular benefit is obtained by increasing the rate beyond 75% for the average patient in the primary care setting.

Include resistance training and stretching in the plan. Emphasize that increasing strength and flexibility help decrease the chances of falls and fractures as well as help in preventing and treating osteoarthritis. Small weights of 5 to 10 lb are all that is needed. A few bricks in an old purse will work. If the patient wants to use increased weights, machines are preferred for safety and ease of use. Handheld weights and barbells can also be used. Figure 2.2 shows common handheld barbells and Figure 2.3 shows ankle weights that

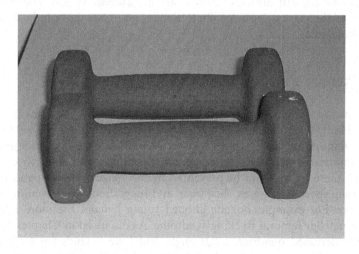

FIGURE 2.2. Bar bells for resistance training.

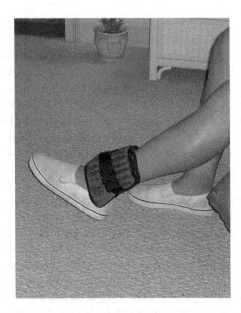

FIGURE 2.3. Leg weights can be used as part of a resistance training program.

can be used for leg exercises. Determining what weight to use can be done by first discovering the maximum weight that can be achieved one time. Then perform 8 to 10 repetitions at 30% to 50% of maximum weight achieved. Rotate to different muscle groups and repeat each set of repetitions three times. Resistance exercise should be done at least twice per week. At a minimum, stretch the major muscles like the quadriceps, hamstrings, the shoulder muscles, and the calf muscles before resistance exercise begins. The chapters on each of these areas have demonstrations of exercises that can be done for all of these areas.

13. Exercise Precautions

The clinician should evaluate risks before prescribing exercise. Nonconditioned individuals are more likely to develop overuse injuries of the knee like patellar femoral tracking, stress fractures, or acute injuries like ankle sprains. These injuries sometimes discourage patients from continuing to exercise. Most of these injuries can be prevented by recognizing at-risk patients and prescribing specific exercises, shoe wear, and suggestions for preventing training errors. For example, nonconditioned young females are more likely to develop patellar femoral tracking syndrome. As discussed in Chapter 12 they have an increased quadriceps (Q) angle and have a tendency to pronate. Exercise will increase the strength of the vastus lateralis and produce a relative weakness of the vastus medialis that will result in patellar femoral tracking. Teaching patients to stretch and strengthen the vastus medialis, use orthotics, and vary their training routine may prevent the injury from occurring.

Most patients with medical problems like diabetes and hypertension can engage in moderate exercise without difficulty. Systolic BP greater than 160 mmHg or diastolic BP greater than 100 mmHg should be controlled before exercise begins because of the increase in BP with exercise. In diabetics, blood sugars less than 60 mg/dL or greater than 400 mg/dL are contraindications to exercise. Patients who use insulin should be instructed to decrease their insulin before they exercise and to not use their extremities as a site for injection before exercise.

References

1. American College of Sports Medicine. Physical activity, physical fitness and hypertension: position stand. *Med Sci Sports Exerc.* 1993;25:1–10.
2. Seals DR, Hagberg JM, Hurley BF, et al. Endurance training in older men and women. I. Cardiovascular responses to training. *J Appl Physiol.* 1984;57: 1024–1029.
3. Ford ES, Giles WH, Dietz WH. Prevalence of the metabolic syndrome among US adults. *JAMA.* 2002;287:356–359.
4. Boyle JP, et al. Projection of diabetes burden through 2050. Impact of changing demographic and disease prevalence in the US. *Diabetes Care.* 2001;24: 1936–1940.
5. Perseghin G, Ghosh S, Gerow K, Shulman GI. Metabolic defects in lean non-diabetic offspring of NIDDM patients: a cross sectional study. *Diabetes.* 1997;46: 1001–1009.
6. Diabetes Prevention Research Group. Reduction in the evidence of type 2 diabetes with life-style intervention or metformin. *N Engl J Med.* 2002;346:393–403.
7. King AC, Taylor CD, Haskell WL, et al. Influence of regular aerobic exercise on psychological health: a randomized clinical trial of healthy, middle aged adults. *Health Psychol.* 1989;8:305–324.
8. Farmer ME, Locke BZ, Moscicki EM, et al. Physical activity and depressive symptoms: the NHANES I epidemiologic follow-up study. *Am J Epidemiol.* 1988; 128:1340–1351.

Suggested Readings

Eden KB, Orleans TC, Mulrow CD, Pender NJ, Teutsch SM. Counseling by clinicians: does it improve physical activity: a summary of the evidence for the U.S. Preventive Services Task Force. *Ann Intern Med.* 2002;137:208–215.

American Geriatrics Society Panel on Exercise and Osteoarthritis. Exercise prescription for older adults with osteoarthritis pain: consensus practice recommendations. A supplement to the AGS Clinical Practice Guidelines on the Management of Chronic Pain in Older Adults. *J Am Geriatr Soc.* 2001;49:808–823.

Huang ES, Meigs JB, Singer DE. The effect of interventions to prevent cardiovascular disease in patients with type 2 diabetes mellitus. *Am J Med.* 2001;111:633–642.

3

Nutrition for Active People

EUGENE TROWERS

1. The Basics

Just as it is important to properly prepare for a particular sport or activity, what you eat or drink before, during, and after can have an important influence on the outcome. Active people require more energy to maintain lean tissue mass, for immune and reproductive function, and for optimum athletic performance. In this chapter we focus on teens and adults. Major issues related to nutrition in sports include weight control, body composition, carbohydrate loading, hydration, eating disorders, and supplementation.

Being well-hydrated before exercise, and consuming adequate liquid during and after performance to balance fluid loss, contributes to better performance and decreased exercise-related injuries. Appropriate selection of foods and fluids, the timing of intake, and supplement choices are important for optimal health and exercise performance. Skipping meals is discouraged. Snacks before and after the activity provide adequate energy to perform and decrease postexercise fatigue. Good choices are high carbohydrate foods such as crackers, fruit, or a bagel with a sports drink. If the individual is overweight the risk of dehydration and heat-related illness is greater. Increased fluids and moderation in snacks are encouraged.

The purpose of the pre-activity meal is to provide the individual with adequate food energy (glucose and glycogen) and fluid to support intense exercise. Foods that are high in fat and protein are discouraged before exercise. These foods are digested slowly and remain in the digestive tract for longer periods of time. The optimal meal before competition is high in complex carbohydrates.

The following contents are recommended for pre-activity meals:

1. **High carbohydrate content.** Carbohydrate should make up 60% to 70% of the total calories of the meal. Athletes should consume at least 200 to 300 g of carbohydrate (800 to 1200 cal) to ensure adequate energy levels for an event. Pasta, rice, and potatoes are good sources of carbohydrates.

2. **Low fat and low protein content.** Fat slows the rate at which food leaves the stomach, thus slowing the digestive process and resulting in the individuals feeling sluggish during the activity.
3. **Low salt content.** High salt levels cause greater water losses from the bloodstream.
4. **Low bulk or low fiber content.** Bulky or high-fiber foods increase intestinal residue, which may lead to cramps or nausea in some individuals. Raw vegetables, although good for the overall diet, should not be eaten at the pre-activity meal.
5. **Adequate fluid content.** Active individuals should drink at least 16 to 32 oz. of water with the pre-activity meals to ensure adequate hydration.

The Internet can be a great source of sports medicine/sports nutrition information. EAT TO COMPETE (www.eattocompete.com) offers the following useful guidelines for refueling the muscles. Concerning pre-activity meal planning tips, remember that there is no single food or "magic potion" that will guarantee success. It is unwise to think that one high-quality pre-activity meal will compensate for a week of poor dietary intake. Likewise, it is unwise to experiment with unfamiliar foods and drinks. Carbohydrates should comprise approximately 60% to 70% of the pre-exercise meal. Keep in mind that when exercising above 65% of your maximum aerobic capacity (see Chapter 2), your body will rely on stored carbohydrate (glycogen) to fuel the body's muscles and brain. Nutrient-dense carbohydrate foods (whole-grain breads, cereals, fruits, and fruit juices) are more readily digested and absorbed than high-protein and high-fat foods such as steak, eggs, burgers, and fries. Low blood sugar, dizziness, and early muscle fatigue during competition can be avoided by consuming a 500-cal meal a few hours prior to competition. In addition, do not neglect to drink fluids (a few cups of water and/or sports drink) along with the pre-activity meal. Naturally, avoid exercising on a full stomach.

Please see Tables 3.1 and 3.2 for sample meal plans. The following guidelines are useful for the timing of the pre-activity meal:

- 3 to 4 h before 500 and 1000 cal
- 2 to 3 h before 300 and 500 cal
- 1 to 2 h before 50 and 300 cal

During exercise that involves multiple events and training lasting longer than 1 h, every 30 min the athlete should consume 80 to 120 cal (20 to 30 g carbs). Possible sources include the following:

- 16 oz. sports drink = 100 cal
- 1 banana = 110 cal.
- 1/2 sports energy bar = 120 cal
- 1 orange = 80 cal.

Every 15 min = at least 8 fluid oz.

TABLE 3.1. High-calorie sample meal plan (approximately 6000 cal).

Breakfast: 3/4 c. orange juice: 1 c. hot cereal with 2 tsp. sugar; 1 egg fried; 1 slice whole wheat toast with tsp. margarine, 1 tsp. jelly; 8 oz. milk (whole)
Total cal. = 620
Snack: 1 peanut butter and jelly sandwich (2 slices bread, 2 Tbsp. peanut butter, 2 tsp. jelly); 1/2 c. raisins; 1 c. apple juice.
Total cal. = 680
Lunch: 1 ham and cheese sandwich (2 slices bread, 1 oz. cheese, 1 oz. ham, 1 Tbsp. mayonnaise); 1 serving french fries; 1 c. tossed green salad with 2 Tbsp. dressing; 10-oz. chocolate milkshake; 4 oatmeal cookies
Total cal. = 1440
Snack: 1 bagel with 2 tsp. margarine and 2 Tbsp. cream cheese; 1 c. sweetened applesauce; 3/4 c. grape juice
Total cal. = 710
Dinner: 2 pieces baked chicken (7 oz. total); 1 c. rice with 1 tsp. margarine; 1 c. collard greens; 1/2 c. candied sweet potatoes; 2 pieces cornbread with 1 Tbsp. margarine; 8 oz. milk (whole); 1 slice apple pie
Total cal. = 1760
Snack: 1 banana; 1/2 c. peanuts; 1 c. chocolate milk (whole)
Total cal. = 720

c., cup; oz., ounce; tsp., teaspoon; cal., calories; Tbsp., tablespoon.

- Water
- Sports drink
- Diluted fruit juices (2:1) water/juice

After/Postexercise—sooner the better

A. 30 to 60 min after exercise
B. 240 to 400 cal. (60–100 g carbs) or 1/2 gram carbo per pound body weight (bagels, yogurt, fruits, juices, carbo load drinks, soft pretzels)
C. Water—a minimum of 1 qt. (32 oz.) of H_2O for each hour of intense exercise or for each pound wt. loss replace w/16 to 24 oz. H_2O.

TABLE 3.2. Sample pre-activity meals (to be eaten 3to 4 h prior to event).

- 3/4 c. orange juice; 1/2 c. cereal with 1 tsp. sugar; 1 slice whole-wheat toast with 1 tsp. margarine and 1 tsp. honey or jelly; 8 oz. skim or low-fat milk; water
- **Total cal. = 450–500**
- 3/4 c. orange juice; 1 to 2 pancakes with: 1 tsp. margarine and 2 Tbsp. syrup: 8 oz. skim or low-fat milk; water
- **Total cal. = 450–500**
- 1 c. vegetable soup; 1 turkey sandwich with 2 slices bread, 2 oz. turkey (white or dark), 1-oz. cheese slice, 2 tsp. mayonnaise; 8 oz. skim or low-fat milk
- **Total cal. = 550–600**
- 1 c. spaghetti with tomato sauce and cheese; 1/2 c. sliced pears (canned) on 1/4 c. cottage cheese; 1 to 2 slices Italian bread with 1 tsp. margarine (avoid garlic); 1/2 c. sherbet; 1 to 2 sugar cookies;4 oz. skim or low-fat milk; water
- **Total cal. = 700**

2. Consequences of Unhealthy Eating

Obesity is defined as a state of excess adipose tissue mass. The most widely used method to gauge obesity is the body mass index (BMI), which is equal to weight/height^2 (in kg/m^2). BMIs for the midpoint of all heights and frames among both men and women range from 19 to 26 kg/m^2 Based on unequivocal data of substantial morbidity, an individual with a BMI greater than 25 is overweight and of 30 is obese in both men and women. Large-scale epidemiologic studies suggest that all-cause, metabolic, cancer, and cardiovascular morbidity begin to rise when BMIs are greater than or equal to 25. There are multiple possible causes for obesity, which include heredity and increased caloric intake versus low energy expenditure. We cannot choose our ancestors but we can control what we eat and how and how much we exercise. A number of pathophysiologic consequences result from obesity including insulin resistance and type 2 diabetes mellitus. Either one of these conditions can result in increased atherosclerotic cardiovascular and peripheral vascular disease, which is the basic etiology of heart attacks and strokes. Just think of it, one could possibly avert or greatly minimize the possible seriously debilitating consequences of top two major health problems in the United States simply by eating a balanced diet and exercising on a regular basis.

Obesity is associated with other disabling reproductive disorders such as hypogonadism in males. In women, obesity may be associated with irregular menses and amenorrhea. Obesity-induced hypertension is associated with increased peripheral resistance and cardiac output, increased sympathetic nervous tone, and increased salt sensitivity. Obesity may be associated with pulmonary abnormalities such as increased work of breathing, decreased total lung capacity, and obstructive sleep apnea. Sleep apnea can greatly impede an active lifestyle. Sleep apnea may preclude patients from driving, operating heavy machinery, or employment that requires constant alertness. Simple tasks such as staying awake during class or everyday conversation or activities may be significantly compromised.

Gallstone disease is associated with obesity. Since gallstone-related surgery is one of the most common surgeries in the United States, a healthy lifestyle might contribute to a reduction of this problem developing. Obesity is also associated with a higher death rate from cancer of the esophagus, pancreas, liver, colon, rectum, and prostate in men. Women who are obese are at greater risk of death from cancer of the breasts, endometrium, cervix, ovaries, gallbladder, and bile ducts.

Bone and joint problems, problems such as osteoarthritis, and gout occur more frequently in obese individuals. Skin abnormalities like acanthosis nigricans (darkening and thickening of the skin) occur more frequently in the obese. Stretch marks and thinning of the skin also occur more often in obese persons.

The approach to helping the obese patient involves a several-pronged attack plan. First, behavior modification is an important first step. Unless patients recognize that a problem exists and are committed to solving the problem, very little can be achieved. Certain techniques that are beyond the scope of this text can be employed to successfully reorient the obese persons' thinking about themselves, dietary habits, and exercise program. Concerning weight reduction and obesity, gradual versus rapid approach is preferred. Monitoring by a qualified health care professional and/or dietician can help enhance compliance and minimize the development of complications seen with a rapid reduction of calories and fluids. Unsafe practices such as enemas, induced vomiting, starvation, laxatives, diuretics, steam rooms, and over-the-counter appetite suppressants should be avoided. Weight loss should occur gradually at approximately 1 to 2 lb per week while the patient consumes well-balanced meals and undergoes a tailored exercise program that has been cleared by the physician.

3. Childhood Obesity

Obesity is an increasing problem in children and adolescents. From 1974 to 2000 the number of obese children increased from 3% to 12%. Obesity in children is defined as 95% of expected BMI for age. Overweight is defined as greater than 85% of expected BMI. BMI tables and graphs for all ages are available at www.cdc.gov. Once in the Web site, place the word "BMI" in the search engine to find excellent information on BMI. Suggested programs for nutrition and physical activity can also be obtained on the Internet. Three such programs and their Web sites are as follows:

1. TAKE 10 (www.take10.net) is a classroom-based physical activity program for kindergarten to fifth-grade students. It contains a curriculum tool for teachers and students, safe and age-appropriate 10-min physical activities, and fun characters that represent organs of the body (The OrganWise Guys).
2. SPARK (www.sparkpe.org) has organized curriculum for teaching children about nutrition and healthy food choices, safety and injury prevention, positive self-talk, goal setting, and balance and moderation in diet and exercise.
3. The National Center for Chronic Disease Prevention and Health Promotion program "Healthy Youth" (http://www.cdc.gov/healthyyouth/index.htm) has sections on healthy eating and physical activity as well as other healthy behaviors in children.

4. Weight Control Issues for Teens

Gymnasts, wrestlers, and endurance athletes, e.g., lightweight rowers, are generally concerned about making their weight classification for competition. Because of increasing pressure to win, these young athletes may engage in various activities to loose weight. Anorexia nervosa, bulimia, starvation diets, fad diets, purging, fluid restriction, laxative ingestion, and improper consumption of stimulants may expose these individuals to possible serious health problems. Proper caloric intake, fluid consumption, nutritional education, and prescribed exercise routines can go a long way in preventing the previously mentioned disorder.

Today's athletes are bigger, stronger, and faster than their predecessors. Some teens may try to gain weight by eating large quantities of fatty and other non-nutritious foods. The main goal of weight gain in the athlete is to increase muscle mass. This is best achieved by an increase in muscle building workout routines and increased caloric intake. Despite the claims of some health food companies there are no special substances that can cause one to magically gain weight. The goal should be to consume a balanced diet and gain approximately 1 to 2 lb per week. This can be accomplished if the average teen consumes an additional 500 to 1000 cal per day. In general, if an athlete gains weight at a faster clip than as mentioned, the increased weight will be in the form of fat as opposed to muscle. See Tables 3.3 and 3.4 for sample meal plans for losing weight and increasing caloric intake via high carbohydrate meals.

TABLE 3.3. Sample meal plan for losing weight.

1800 cal:
Breakfast: 3/4 c. orange juice; 3/4 c. cereal; 8 oz. low-fat milk; 1 slice whole-wheat toast with 1 tsp. margarine
Total cal. = 415
Snack: 1 apple
Total cal. = 80
Lunch: 1 peanut butter and banana sandwich (2 slices bread, 1 Tbsp. peanut butter, 1/2 banana); 5 to 7 carrot sticks; 1 peach; 8 oz. low-fat milk
Total cal. = 485
Snack: 20 grapes; 2 graham crackers
Total cal. = 155
Dinner: 1 hamburger patty (4 oz.) with 1 hamburger bun; 1 c. tossed green salad with 1 Tbsp. dressing; 4 oz. low-fat milk; 1/2 c. ice cream
Total cal. = 715
2400 cal:
Breakfast: 3/4 c. orange juice; 1 slice toast with 1 oz. cheese; 3/4 c. cereal; 4 oz. low-fat milk
Total cal. = 420
Snack: 1 banana
Total cal. = 100
Lunch: 1 slice cheese pizza; 1 cup tossed green salad with 1 Tbsp. dressing; 8 oz. low-fat milk
Total cal. = 425
Snack: 1/2 c. raisin/peanut mix; 1/2 c. apple juice
Total cal. = 360
Dinner: 1 c. macaroni and cheese; 1/2 c. lima beans; 1 c. tomato and cucumber slices with 1 Tbsp. dressing; 1 dinner roll with 1 tsp. margarine; 8 oz. low-fat milk
Total cal. = 895
Snack: 1/2 c. sherbet; 1 granola cookie
Total cal. = 185

TABLE 3.4. High-carbohydrate sample meal plan.

Breakfast: 3/4 c. orange or pineapple juice; 1 egg, fried; 2 slices toast with 2 tsp. margarine and 2 tsp. jelly; 3/4 c. cereal; 8 oz. skim or low-fat milk or hot cocoa

Lunch: 1 or 2 sandwiches, each with 1 oz. meat or 1 oz. cheese or 2 Tbsp. peanut butter; carrot and celery sticks; 1 banana; 8 oz. skim or low-fat milk

Dinner: 5 to 6 oz. baked fish or chicken without skin; 1 baked potato with 1 tsp. margarine; 1/2 c. green beans; 1/2 c. coleslaw; 2 pieces cornbread with 2 tsp. margarine and 2 tsp. honey; 1/2 c. sliced peaches; 8 oz. skim or low-fat milk

Snack: 1 or 2 servings of fruit; 1 or 2 servings of cookies/crackers

Suggested Readings

1. Ray TR, Fowler R. Current issues in sports nutrition in athletes. *South Med J.* 2004;97(9):863–866.
2. Wheeler KB, Cameron AM. Sports nutrition: the pre-event meal. American Rowing pp. 30–32, January/February 1989.

4

Altitude, Heat, and Cold Problems

EDWARD J. SHAHADY

Patients may choose to be physically active in environments that can create illness, like high and low attitudes and the extremes of heat and cold. The primary care clinician needs to be aware of how to prevent and treat problems that are associated with these environments. Age, comorbid disease, and use of certain medications increase risk of environmental illness in some patients. A good working knowledge of the physiological responses to changes in altitude and temperature, clinical symptoms, and principles of treatment and prevention will facilitate effective management of this group of patients. Table 4.1 lists some of the problems that are encountered by the primary care clinician.

1. High-Altitude Sickness

1.1. Acute Mountain Sickness

Thirty-four million people travel yearly to high altitudes for some type of recreational activity. Heights above 5000 ft usually produce some mild symptoms of shortness of breath and mild headache for a few days. Individuals with compromised pulmonary function, the elderly, and those with other chronic diseases may experience more severe symptoms and symptoms at less elevation. Twenty-five percent of those who travel above 8500 ft experience symptoms of high-altitude illness and one in 100 develop serious symptoms. The syndrome of high-altitude illness represents a spectrum of clinical conditions that range in severity from mild acute mountain sickness (AMS) with an unpleasant constellation of symptoms to the life-threatening conditions of high-altitude pulmonary edema (HAPE) and high-altitude cerebral edema (HACE). Acute mountain sickness may also be the early presentation of a process that can progress to life-threatening HAPE or HACE. Although most primary care clinicians practice in areas below 5000 ft they still will encounter altitude sickness. Patients will rely on primary care clinicians for advice on prevention of altitude illness and if they become ill the telephone and the Internet bring patients and clinicians together no matter what the distance.

TABLE 4.1. Classification of environmental problems.

High-altitude illness
- Acute mountain sickness
- High-altitude pulmonary edema
- High-altitude cerebral edema
- Other altitude-related disorders: retinopathy, peripheral edema, venous stasis
- Chronic diseases and altitude

Low-altitude illness
- Barotrauma to ears, sinuses, teeth, skin
- The bends

Heat injury
- Heat cramps
- Heat exhaustion (heat syncope)
- Heatstroke

Cold injury
- Hypothermia—mild, moderate, severe
- Frostbite
- Chilblains

The symptoms of mild AMS are similar to a viral syndrome, a hangover, or physical exhaustion. These vague symptoms have led to misdiagnosis in some cases. In a setting of high-altitude exposure, these vague symptoms should be considered AMS until proven otherwise.

The diagnosis of AMS can be made when a patient has had a recent exposure to increase in altitude for several hours and complains of a headache plus at least one of the following symptoms: nausea, vomiting, loss of appetite, fatigue, dizziness, light-headedness, and difficulty in sleeping. The headache may be mild but is usually bitemporal and throbbing in nature. The other symptoms described may range in severity from mild to incapacitating.

Acute mountain sickness symptoms usually develop within a few hours after arrival at high altitude and reach maximum intensity in 24 to 48 h. Most individuals become symptom-free by the third or fourth day. The onset of symptoms may be delayed in some individuals for up to 4 days and a few may have symptoms that may be prolonged for up to 1 month. Most people tolerate or treat their symptoms by remaining at the same altitude until the illness resolves.

Acute mountain sickness is rare below 8000 ft and is more common with rapid ascent to altitudes greater than 10,000 ft. Difficulty with breathing on exertion is common at high altitudes but if the difficulty is present at rest, HAPE may be present. Similarly, any alteration in mentation or signs of ataxia suggests the presence of HACE. Any hint of HAPE or HACE should be taken seriously.

1.1.1. Treatment

The mild forms of AMS may not require specific treatment. It usually resolves spontaneously if further ascent and exercise are avoided. Halting ascent or activity to allow further acclimatization may reverse the symptoms; however, continuing the ascent exacerbates the underlying pathologic processes and may lead to disastrous results. Further treatment is indicated if the symptoms become severe enough to interfere with the individual's activities.

Acetazolamide (Diamox) speeds the process of acclimatization and, if given early in the illness, leads to a more rapid resolution of symptoms. A dose of 250 mg of acetazolamide given at the onset of symptoms and repeated twice daily is effective therapy. If AMS does not respond to maintenance of altitude, rest, and pharmacologic intervention within 24 h, the patient should descend to a lower altitude. A descent of 1500 to 3000 ft effectively reverses high-altitude illness in most cases. Oxygen, if available, addresses the primary insult of high-altitude exposure, corrects hypoxemia, and relieves the headache. For persistent difficulty in sleeping, it can be given in small amounts (1 to 2 L/min) during sleep. Insomnia generally results from periodic breathing, which is experienced by most visitors to altitude. This is best treated with the respiratory stimulant acetazolamide. Doses of acetazolamide as low as 62.5 mg at bedtime may be adequate to prevent periodic breathing and eradicate insomnia. Avoid the use of benzodiazepines and other sedative hypnotics because of their tendency to decrease ventilation during sleep.

Dexamethasone is an effective treatment for AMS. It is usually used for patients who cannot tolerate acetazolamide, or in more advanced cases of AMS. Trials have used 8 mg initially, followed by 4 mg every 6 h.

1.1.2. Prevention

The symptoms of AMS can be unpleasant enough to interfere or interrupt travel, business, or vacation plans. The majority of individuals with AMS report a decrease in activity. Allowing adequate time for acclimatization by slow ascent is the best method of prevention. This may not be possible for a short vacation period. The altitude where the individual sleeps is the key altitude. The ideal first-night altitude is no higher than 8000 ft, with a subsequent increase of not more than 2000 ft each night. If the journey begins at 10,000 ft, then three nights should be spent acclimatizing. Daytime excursions to higher altitudes with a return to a lower sleeping altitude are acceptable. Mild to moderate exercise aids acclimatization but overexertion may contribute to AMS. Intake of a high-carbohydrate diet and maintenance of adequate hydration are helpful.

Acetazolamide (Diamox) is very effective in preventing AMS. Lower dosages provide similar prophylaxis with fewer adverse reactions than higher dosages. The current recommended dosage is 125 mg twice daily starting 24 h before ascent and continuing for the first 2 days at high altitude. The dosage for children is 2.5 mg/kg/dose up to 125 mg total, given twice daily. Acetazolamide is a carbonic anhydrase inhibitor that induces a mild diuresis and stimulates respiration. This respiratory stimulation is particularly important during sleep, when the hypoxemia caused by periodic breathing is eradicated by acetazolamide. The diuretic effects reduce fluid retention in AMS. This drug also lowers cerebrospinal fluid (CSF) volume and pressure, which may play an additional role in prevention and treatment of cerebral edema.

The most common adverse reactions to acetazolamide include paresthesias and polyuria. Less common reactions include nausea, drowsiness, tinnitus, and transient myopia. The flavor of carbonated beverages such as soft drinks or beer may change. Acetazolamide is a sulfa drug, so patients allergic to sulfa drugs may have a reaction. Dexamethasone can prevent AMS but should be reserved for individuals who cannot tolerate acetazolamide. The lowest effective dosage is 4 mg every 12 h.

Other issues that aid with prevention include carbohydrate ingestion and avoiding alcohol and smoking. Some but not all studies suggest carbohydrates as the most efficient form of fuel for digestion. This fuel consumes less oxygen and may leave more oxygen available for other bodily activities. Avoidance of alcohol and smoking optimizes acclimatization. Alcohol depresses respiration and produces dehydration. Smoking cigarettes decreases oxygen-carrying capacity.

1.2. High-Altitude Pulmonary Edema

HAPE is the most common fatal manifestation of severe high-altitude illness. It is uncommon below 10,000 ft but can occur at 8000 ft related to heavy exercise. At higher altitudes, it may also occur at rest or with light activity. The symptoms may start a few hours after reaching the higher altitude but usually begin slowly 2 to 4 days after arrival at high altitude. Dyspnea on exertion, fatigue with minimal to moderate effort, and dry cough are early manifestations of the disease. These symptoms may be subtle but noticeable when comparing the victim with others in the group. The symptoms of AMS are also usually present. As HAPE progresses the dyspnea intensifies with effort and is unrelieved by rest. The cough becomes productive of copious amounts of clear watery sputum, and with time, hemoptysis. This may be followed by ataxia and altered mentation secondary to hypoxemia and/or cerebral edema. Examination reveals an increased respiratory and heart rate, with audible rhonchi and gurgles.

1.2.1. Treatment

Descent to a lower altitude, bed rest, and supplemental oxygen are the most effective methods of therapy. Descents of 1500 to 3000 ft should be adequate to allow for a rapid recovery. After recovery, the victim may be able to reascend in 2 or 3 days. Mild cases may be treated without descent and 1 or 2 days of bed rest. The rate of improvement is increased with oxygen. At ski resorts, victims of mild HAPE are given oxygen in their hotel rooms and are able to recover, avoid descent, and continue their ski holidays. Any treatment plan that does not include descent mandates serial examinations of the patient by clinicians with experience in managing high-altitude illness. For a discussion of treatment for more severe pulmonary edema, consult the readings suggested at the end of this chapter.

1.2.2. Prevention

Nifedipine, 20 mg three times daily, taken before ascent and continued at altitude for 3 days is effective in preventing a recurrence of HAPE. Acetazolamide may be useful in the prevention in susceptible individuals because of respiratory stimulation caused by acetazolamide. Avoiding extreme exertion during the first 2 days at altitude also helps in individuals with a prior history of HAPE. Gradual ascent that allows time to acclimatize and immediate cessation of further ascent at the onset of symptoms are the most effective means of prevention.

1.3. High-Altitude Cerebral Edema

HACE is not as common as HAPE but is a most severe form of high-altitude illness. Most cases occur above 12,000 ft. The usual time course is 1 to 3 days for the development of severe symptoms. HACE has developed in as little as 12 h or as long as 5 to 9 days following AMS. The symptoms of HACE usually include those of AMS and HAPE. Headaches, fatigue, vomiting, cough, and dyspnea are present along with the symptoms of HACE, which include ataxia, slurred speech, and altered mentation. The mental changes can range from mild emotional lability or confusion to hallucinations, and decreased levels of consciousness. Ataxia is the most sensitive early indicator of cerebral edema because of the sensitivity of the cerebellum to decreased oxygen. The appearance of ataxia alone is an indication for immediate descent. Early recognition and initiation of descent are the keys to successful therapy of HACE. Long-term neurologic deficits, such as ataxia and cognitive impairment, are possible after recovery from an episode of HACE. For a complete discussion of treating HACE, consult the readings suggested at the end of this chapter. Prevention is the same as that discussed with HAPE and AMS.

1.4. Other Altitude-Related Disorders

High-altitude retinal hemorrhage can occur with high altitude and high-altitude illness. These hemorrhages usually occur at altitudes over 17,500 ft. They also occur at lower levels when strenuous activity is involved or the patient has suffered from HAPE or HACE. The hemorrhages are usually asymptomatic, only discovered with retinal examination, and resolve without treatment in 2 to 3 weeks. Occasionally, the macular region is involved and central scotomata may be noticed. The scotomata gradually resolve in a few months but a few cases of permanent visual defects are reported.

Peripheral edema is associated with high altitudes. It is usually benign and resolves with descent to lower altitudes. Venous stasis and thrombophlebitis are increased with high altitudes. Patients with increased risk of thrombophlebitis at lower altitudes may require prophylactic anticoagulation when they go to higher altitudes.

1.5. Chronic Diseases

Chronic disease may be aggravated by hypoxic atmosphere at high altitude and have a higher predisposition for the development of high-altitude illness. Chronic obstructive pulmonary disease (COPD) is a risk factor for the development of AMS. Oxygen saturation remains more than 90% in healthy individuals until an altitude of 8000 ft but patients with COPD may desaturate below 90% at lower altitudes. Patients with COPD may need oxygen supplementation when traveling to higher altitudes. Patients with asthma usually have fewer problems with increases in altitude, probably secondary to decreased allergies and pollutants.

No studies indicate risk to individuals with cardiovascular disease. Because of decreased oxygen availability, these individuals should be attentive to any increase in symptoms but there is no absolute contraindication to travel to higher altitudes. All travelers to high altitude experience increased sympathetic activity in the first 3 days. This results in increased heart rate, blood pressure (BP), cardiac work, and increased need for oxygen.

Recommendations for travelers with stable coronary artery disease should include gradual ascent, limitation of activity, and continuation of medications. Caution individuals who have more severe, symptomatic coronary disease or those in a high-risk group who are about to travel to high altitudes. An exercise stress test would be an effective means of accessing ability to ascend to higher elevations. Improved cardiovascular fitness as discussed in Chapter 2 will increase the heart and lungs' ability to bring more oxygen to the body.

Patients with hypertension require BP monitoring because high-altitude travel produces a mild increase in BP secondary to increased catecholamine activity. The increase begins in the first few days and reaches maximum in 2 to 3 weeks. The BP returns to baseline values at high altitude or with return to prior altitude. Monitor BP periodically to ensure adequate control of BP with current medication.

Patients with sickle cell (SC) disease are affected by hypoxemia at 5000 to 6500 ft. Those with the SC trait may not experience symptoms until they reach higher altitudes. Some individuals may not know they have SC trait until they suffer a vaso-occlusive crisis at higher altitudes. See the discussion of SC trait in Chapter 4.

2. Low-Altitude Illness

2.1. Barotrauma

Recreational diving continues to attract more participants every year. Approximately 100 people per year die in the United States because of diving, and many others suffer barotrauma and decompression sickness. On a yearly basis, Florida leads the nation in the incidence of these injuries. Many patients may not develop symptoms for 24 to 48 h after their dive experience and others may suffer symptoms that they may not associate with the dive experience. Primary care clinicians, no matter their location, will need to know the principles of prevention and recognition of the symptoms associated with low-altitude illness.

2.1.1. Gas Principles

At sea level, the body has an ambient air pressure of 14.7 lb/in.^{2} exerted on it [1]. This is also known as 1 atm of pressure. Increasing altitude decreases atmospheric pressure and decreasing altitude increases atmospheric pressure. At an altitude of 18,000 ft, the atmospheric pressure is decreased 50%. Pressure exerted on the body increases by 1 atm for each 33 ft of depth. For instance, at a depth of 33 ft, ambient pressure is 2 atm. The effects of pressure under water involve Boyle's law and Henry's law. Boyle's law states that the volume a gas occupies is inversely related to the pressure that is unique to that environment. As pressure increases, the volume that the gas will occupy decreases. As the body goes to more depth the volume of gas decreases because of the increased pressures at these depths. When the body rises, the gases will occupy more volume [1]. Think of the impact this will have on the areas of the body with gas-filled spaces like the ears, sinuses, teeth, and lungs.

Henry's law states that gas enters a given volume of liquid in proportion to the partial pressure of the gas. Nitrogen, like other gases during descent, becomes increasingly soluble in blood and tissue. During ascent, the same gases become less soluble and form bubbles. Unlike oxygen, nitrogen is not metabolized and so is free to accumulate and coalesce into larger bubbles if the ascent takes place too quickly. This helps understand decompression illness (DCS) (i.e., the bends).

2.1.2. Ear Barotrauma

Middle ear barotrauma, also known as barotitis or "ear squeeze," is the most common complaint of scuba divers. Thirty percent of novice divers and 10% of experienced divers develop this problem. As the diver descends, each foot of water exerts an additional 23 mmHg pressure against the intact tympanic membrane (TM). Normally the diver performs maneuvers to force passage of additional air into the middle ear through the eustachian tubes, maintaining an equal pressure on the TM. Ear squeeze occurs when a negative differential pressure is created within the middle ear. As the TM stretches, sharp pain is experienced. Further pressure increases can cause the TM to rupture. If the TM ruptures the middle ear is exposed to cold water, inducing a caloric-induced nystagmus and vertigo. Persistent discomfort with a hyperemic TM may lead the inexperienced clinician to diagnose a bacterial or virus-induced otitis media. External ear barotrauma is less common and results from the outward bulging of the TM during descent. The external auditory canal is usually filled with water during descent. If air becomes trapped in the external canal because of obstruction from cerumen, stenosis, earplugs, or a tight-fitting wet suit hood, a relative negative pressure develops in the external canal. As the TM bulges outward against the negative pressure, pain develops. Inner ear barotrauma results in damage to the cochleovestibular apparatus. The mechanism of injury is similar to middle ear barotrauma where negative pressure develops in the middle ear because the diver is unable to equalize pressure during descent. Sudden equilibration of pressure in the middle ear or a vigorous Valsalva maneuver may rupture the round window or cause hemorrhage into the inner ear. Symptoms and signs include hearing loss, vertigo, nausea, vomiting, tinnitus, nystagmus, positional vertigo, ataxia, and fullness in the affected ear. Evaluation by an ear, nose, and throat (ENT) physician is indicated.

2.1.3. Sinus Barotrauma

The air-filled maxillary, frontal, and ethmoidal sinuses are all susceptible to the effects of volume–pressure changes. If the nasal passages are obstructed by mucosal thickening, polyps, pus, or a deviated septum, equilibration of pressure within the paranasal sinuses may not occur. Obstruction predisposes to sinus barotrauma. The diver will complain of pain over these sinuses with descent and ascent. Treatment is for the problem that caused the obstruction.

2.1.4. Facial Barotrauma

Facial barotrauma results from negative pressure generation in the airspace created by a dive mask over the eyes and nose. As water pressure increases during descent, a negative pressure develops within the mask. Forced exhalation through the nose will equalize the pressure. If not adequately performed the negative pressure produces facial and conjunctival edema, diffuse petechial hemorrhages on the face, and subconjunctival hemorrhages of the sclera. Rarely, optic nerve damage can result from severe facial barotrauma. Physical examination should include a careful ophthalmologic examination, including determination of visual acuity. If no eye problems are noted, the treatment is symptom relief.

2.2. Decompression Sickness (DCS)

The clinical manifestations of DCS are divided into type I and type II. Type I DCS affects the musculoskeletal system, skin, and lymphatic vessels.

Type II DCS involves any other organ system. Type II DCS is more commonly reported and more serious than type I.

Type I DCS is also called "the bends." The symptoms are periarticular pain in the arms and legs. The elbow and shoulder joints are most commonly affected. The diagnosis may be confirmed by pain relief with inflation of a BP cuff to 150 to 200 mmHg over the affected joint [2].

Skin manifestations of DCS type I may include pruritus, erythema, and marbling. Skin marbling, known as cutis marmorata, is a true form of DCS and results from venous stasis. It may begin as severe pruritus and progress into an erythematous rash and then to skin mottling. Cutis marmorata commonly involves the trunk and torso. Type II DCS symptoms can also involve the central nervous system (CNS), the inner ear, and the lungs. The spinal cord, especially the upper lumbar area, is more often involved than the cerebral tissue. Symptoms include limb weakness or paralysis, paresthesias, numbness, and low back and abdominal pain. Limb symptoms often begin as a distal prickly sensation that advances proximally, followed by progressive sensory or motor loss. Decompression illness should be managed in a decompression chamber.

2.2.1. Prevention

The potential for development of DCS increases with the length and depth of a dive. Other risk factors include fatigue, heavy exertion, obesity, dehydration, fever, tobacco, and alcohol, cold ambient temperature after diving, diving at high altitude, and flying after diving. The US Navy has constructed a series of dive tables that calculate the amount of nitrogen that will accumulate during a dive at a particular depth and duration [3]. The tables calculate amount of time a diver may spend at a maximum depth and return to the surface without sufficiently exceeding the solubility of nitrogen at sea level to produce DCS. The diver still must ascend in a slow, controlled manner to allow the gradual release of nitrogen. Off-gassing continues after the diver has surfaced; it takes up to 12 h at the surface for nitrogen stores to return to normal sea level values. Repeat dives within several hours result in accumulation of tissue nitrogen and shorter dive limits. Submersible dive computers are being used increasingly by sport scuba divers to calculate maximum dive times.

3. Heat Illness

There is an increase in the number of individuals adversely affected by heat because of the trend toward more hot and humid summers. Each year, 175 to 200 people on average die from heat-related illnesses [4]. Heat illness presents a spectrum of disease ranging from mild heat exhaustion to severe heatstroke. Body temperature increases about 36°C in the early morning to 37.5°C in the late afternoon. This range reflects the balance between heat production and heat dissipation. Heat is produced by all metabolic processes and when external temperatures exceed the body temperature. Body temperature increases when the rate of heat production exceeds the rate of heat dissipation.

In response to this rising temperature, the thermal center in the hypothalamus activates the autonomic nervous system to produce vasodilation and increase the rate of sweating. Vasodilation dissipates heat by convection, and sweat dissipates heat by evaporation.

Increased body temperature occurs when heat regulatory mechanisms are overwhelmed by excessive metabolic production of heat, excessive environmental heat, or impaired ability to dissipate heat. Age, certain disease states, medications, and types of clothing all can decrease the body's ability to respond to heat production.

3.1. Heat Cramps

These cramps are very painful muscle spasms in the calves, hamstring, or quadriceps muscles and occasionally in the arms and back. They usually occur after strenuous exercise or heavy labor. Heat cramps were previously thought to be purely secondary to dehydration associated with significant electrolyte loss but recent research has proven this is not accurate. These cramps can occur in a cool environment. They are probably due to a combination of excessive work, dehydration, and lack of conditioning. Muscle fatigue in susceptible individuals is the underlying problem. Hydration, cardiovascular fitness, and adequate stretching before and after exercise should prevent most heat cramps. Treatment consists of stretching and fluid replacement with cool isotonic solutions. A common mistake is to rely on thirst to indicate dehydration.

3.2. Heat Exhaustion (Heat Syncope)

Fatigue, flu-like symptoms, orthostasis, dehydration, nausea, vomiting, headache, and collapse may all occur. Heat exhaustion results from dehydration and heat retention that is not severe enough to cause heatstroke. Mental status is normal and body temperature is normal or mildly elevated. Rehydration, rest, and supportive care in a cool environment are usually all that is required to treat heat exhaustion. The symptoms will range from mild to more severe. If the patient collapses, they may have significant dehydration and require intravenous (IV) therapy. Do not rely on thirst alone to determine the amount of fluid that is needed. As much as 1000 cc or 33 oz. of fluid can be lost in 1 h with activity in the heat [5]. This is equal to four to five tall glasses of fluid. Cold water and sports drinks like Gatorade® and Powerade® are excellent drinks to use before, during and after exercise. Heat cramps may also be present and should be treated with stretching. Place the patient in an environment that is out of the heat Remove all extra clothing and pour cool water over them. Rapid cooling is not usually required, but patients should be observed for progression to heatstroke, as heat exhaustion and heatstroke are a continuum of one disease process.

3.3. Heatstroke

Heatstroke is a true state of thermoregulatory failure that results from overwhelmed normal heat dissipation mechanisms and elevated core body temperature. Two forms of heatstroke exist: nonexertional and exertional. Nonexertional heatstroke occurs during summer heat waves in the elderly, poor, and others with impaired mobility. Dehydration, lack of air conditioning, obesity, chronic disease, impaired mentation, and medications that interfere with heat dissipation like phenothiazines, diuretics, anticholinergics, anti-depressants, and cold medications predispose this population to heatstroke. Exertional heatstroke results from strenuous physical activity. It is more common in poorly acclimatized, unconditioned athletes; military recruits; and individuals who perform heavy physical labor in hot, humid conditions.

The exact degree of hyperthermia necessary to produce heatstroke in humans is unknown but ranges of 40° to 45° are considered sufficient. The pathophysiology of heat stroke is similar to the acute inflammatory response seen in sepsis. Hypoperfusion results in alterations of immunologic functions. This leads to an inflammatory response and coagulation abnormalities. The result is multiorgan dysfunction, including disseminated intravascular coagulation.

In a setting of exposure to heat the symptoms and signs of heat stroke may include all the symptoms of heat exhaustion, hypotension, hyperventilation, and tachycardia; rectal temperature greater than 40°C; ataxia; altered mental status; disorientation; stupor; or coma. Lack of sweating is a late sign of heatstroke and is not a reliable diagnostic sign. Consider the diagnosis of heatstroke in patients exposed to heat who have mental status changes even if they are sweating. Primary care clinicians should be expert in recognition and prevention of heat stroke and other heat-related illness.

Rapid cooling is necessary to prevent further damage and reverse heat stress. Remove clothing, pour cold water over the patient, and arrange for emergency transport to the nearest hospital. Patients with heatstroke require hospitalization because of multiple organ dysfunctions and the need for close monitoring.

4. Cold Injury

Our knowledge of cold injuries comes from the military experience with this problem. Throughout history, armies have suffered extensive injuries from cold, wet conditions. Interest in prevention with new clothing and footwear has increased in the nonmilitary population as more individuals become active in outdoor activities in the snow and wet environments like rafting.

Unlike cold-adapted animals, peripheral cold injuries are unique to humans. As the external environment cools, human physiology gives priority to maintaining the body's core temperature. Vasoconstriction and shunting of blood away from the extremities occur in order to keep the core temperature elevated. Blood flow to the skin averages about 200 to 250 mL/min in normal temperatures [5].

If the outside temperature is increased, vasodilatation increases skin blood flow up to 7000 mL/min to aid heat loss. When the outside temperature decreases, vasoconstriction reduces blood flow to keep body temperature up. The blood flow may decrease 10-fold to less than 50 mL/min. This results in decreased heat distribution to the extremities and cold injury.

The fingers, toes, ears, nose, and penis are most susceptible to cold injury. The injury results in both freezing and nonfreezing syndromes. Frostbite is the most common freezing injury. Exposure to wet cold causes trench foot and immersion foot, which are nonfreezing injuries. Dry cold causes a nonfreezing injury called chilblains (pernio).

The symptoms of cold injury reflect the severity of the exposure. Numbness produced by vasoconstriction, the most common early symptom, is present in 75% of patients. Patients state they feel clumsy or their feet feel like a piece of dead wood. "Frostnip" is a superficial cold insult manifested by transient numbness and tingling that resolves after rewarming. No tissue destruction occurs.

Pain is usually with reperfusion. The dull continuous ache evolves into a throbbing sensation in 48 to 72 h. This often persists until tissue demarcation several weeks to months later.

Chilblains (pernio) is a mild form of dry cold injury that follows repetitive exposure. Symptoms may include itching, redness, swelling, plaques, blue nodules, and ulcerations. The sores appear in the first 24 h after exposure and usually affect facial areas, dorsa of the hands and feet, and the pretibial areas. Patients with Raynaud's phenomenon are at risk. Management of the chilblain syndrome is usually supportive. Nifedipine (20 to 60 mg daily) may be an effective treatment for refractory symptoms.

Trench foot (immersion foot) is produced by prolonged exposure to wet cold at temperatures above freezing. It usually develops slowly over several days and results in neurovascular damage. Immersion foot commonly develops while a person is wearing sweat-dampened socks or vapor-barrier boots. Symptoms include cool pale numb feet that later appear cyanotic and edematous. Leg cramping is often present. The skin remains erythematous, dry, and very painful to touch, after rewarming. Bullae commonly develop. Protracted symptoms of pain during weight bearing, cold sensitivity, and hyperhidrosis often last for years. Prevention of trench foot often just requires continual wearing of dry socks.

Frostbite can be classified into degrees. Lack of feeling and redness are characteristic of first-degree frostbite. Superficial vesiculation surrounded by swelling and redness is considered second degree. Third-degree frostbite produces deeper blood-filled vesicles. Fourth-degree injuries extend below the skin into muscle and bone. The initial presentation of frostbite is deceptive. Most patients do not arrive with frozen tissue that has no feeling. The tissue appears mottled or violaceous-white, waxy, or pale yellow. After thawing, partial return of sensation should be expected until blebs form. Favorable initial symptoms include normal sensation, warmth, and color. A residual violaceous hue after rewarming is ominous. Early formation of clear large blebs that extend to the tips of the digits are more favorable than delayed appearance of small hemorrhagic blebs. These dark vesicles are produced by damage to the subdermal vascular plexuses. Vesicles and large bullae eventually form in 6 to 24 h. Lack of edema formation suggests significant tissue damage. Post-thaw edema usually develops in less than 3 h. In severe cases, frostbitten skin forms an early black, dry eschar until mummification and apparent demarcation.

The incidence and severity of cold injury correlates with the predisposing factors like chronic diseases and medications that effect vascular response. Most cases of cold injury result from inadequate protection during exposure to cold. Minimal to no cold injury occurs in individuals who have adequate protection for anticipated and unanticipated climatic changes.

The major role of the primary care clinician in cold injury is prevention and early recognition. Educating patients about their risk for cold injury and injury prevention will eliminate most cases of cold injury. Recognizing those patients who need more than simple rewarming and either providing or obtaining the needed treatment for them is also an important role. For a more extensive discussion of treatment of cold injury, consult the suggested reading provided at the end of the chapter.

References

1. Kuo DC, Jerrard DA. Environmental insults: smoke inhalation, submersion, diving, and high altitude. *Emerg Med Clin N Am.* 2003;21:475–497.
2. Beckman T. A review of decompression sickness and arterial gas embolism. *Arch Fam Med.* 1997;6:491–494.
3. Commander, Naval Sea Systems Command. *US Navy Diving Manual.* Vol. 1, revision 3. Flagstaff, AZ: Best Publishing; 1993:8–45.
4. Coris EE, Ramirez AM, Van Durme DJ. Heat illness in athletes: the dangerous combination of heat, humidity and exercise. *Sports Med.* 2004;34(1):9–16.
5. Ulrich AS, Rathlev NK. Hypothermia and localized cold injuries. *Emerg Med Clin N Am.* 2004;22:281–298.

Suggested Readings

Biem J, Koehncke N, Classen D, Dosman J. Out of the cold: management of hypothermia and frostbite. *CMAJ.* 2003;168(3).

Gallagher SA, Hackett PH. High altitude illness. *Emerg Med Clin N Am.* 2004;22: 329–355.

Kuo DC, Jerrard DA. Environmental insults: smoke inhalation, submersion, diving, and high altitude. *Emerg Med Clin N Am.* 2003;21:475–497.

Part II

Upper Extremity

5

Shoulder Problems

Edward J. Shahady, Jason Buseman, and Aaron Nordgren

The shoulder is second only to the knee as a common site for musculoskeletal problems encountered by the primary care practitioner. The problems range from rotator cuff disease in the middle-aged and older population to adhesive capsulitis (AC) joint separation and shoulder dislocations in younger patients. A good working knowledge of the epidemiology, anatomy, associated symptoms, and examination reduces confusion and enhances the diagnostic and therapeutic process.

Caring for problems is easier if a few simple organizational steps are followed:

1. Step 1 is to realize that 95% of patients seen in the office with shoulder complaints can be classified into the categories of problems noted in Table 5.1.
2. Step 2 is to obtain a focused history that segments the categories into acute trauma, overuse trauma, medical disease, and pediatric problems. This process reduces the list to a manageable number for initiating further evaluation.
3. Step 3 is to perform an examination that is directed by the focused history and epidemiology. With a focused history and examination you now most likely have a diagnosis. Your knowledge of the usual history and examination associated with the most common problems has facilitated this process.
4. Step 4 is ordering confirmatory studies if needed (many times they are not).
5. Step 5 is to start treatment. (This may include appropriate consultation.) Five percent of the time the diagnosis will not be so obvious. But not being one of the 95% is usually obvious. That is when additional confirmatory studies and/or a consultation will be required.

Rare or not so frequent problems are usually the ones we hear about because they are missed in the primary care setting. Having a good working knowledge of common problems provides an excellent background for recognizing uncommon problems. Always look for the common problems first. As soon as it is clear the problem is not a common one the hunt for the rare should begin.

TABLE 5.1. Classification of shoulder problems.

Acute trauma
Clavicle fractures
Shoulder (acromioclavicular AC) separation
Proximal humerus fracture
Shoulder (glenohumeral) dislocation
Rotator cuff tears
Labrum injury

Overuse trauma
Shoulder instability
Rotator cuff impingement syndrome
Adhesive capsulitis

Medical problems
Osteoarthritis
Rheumatoid arthritis
AC joint arthritis

Pediatric problems
Little leaguer's shoulder

Caring for shoulder problems is impossible without an understanding of basic shoulder anatomy (Figure 5.1). The shoulder is a unique joint because it allows for significant motion in all directions. Unlike the hip, there is no bony acetabulum to restrict motion. It is the most mobile joint in the human body and allows the upper extremity to rotate up to 180° in three different planes, enabling the arm to perform a versatile range of activities. The downside is the decrease in stability that accompanies the increase in flexibility. The flexibility of the shoulder and the elbow are critical to activities of daily living. Loss of motion in one or both of these joints seriously hampers the

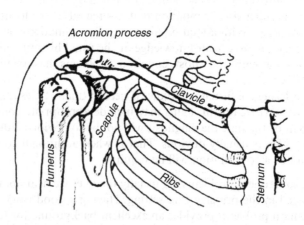

FIGURE 5.1. Anatomy of the shoulder. (Reproduced from Shahady E, Petrizzi M, eds. *Sports Medicine for Coaches and Trainers.* Chapel Hill, NC: University of North Carolina Press; 1991:51, with permission.)

ability to independently eat and dress. Shoulder stability and function is dependent on soft tissues like the glenoid labrum, capsular ligaments, and the rotator cuff muscles.

The shoulder includes the proximal humerus, the clavicle and the scapula, and the ligaments, tendons, and cartilage that connect them to each other (Figure 5.1 and Table 5.2). Joints included are the glenohumeral, acromio-clavicular, sternoclavicular, and scapulothoracic articulation. The gleno-humeral joint capsule consists of a fibrous capsule, ligaments, and the glenoid labrum. Its lack of bony stability makes it the most commonly dislocated major joint in the body. The rotator cuff is composed of four muscles: the supraspinatus, infraspinatus, teres minor, and subscapularis (Figure 5.2). The rotator cuff muscles depress the humeral head against the glenoid. Torn or weak cuff muscles lead to the humeral head migrating upward within the joint because of unopposed action of the deltoid.

1. Focused History

Establish whether the problem is acute (recent onset) or chronic (present for 3 to 6 months) and if other chronic diseases like osteoarthritis or diabetes are present. This will get you started down the right path. The mechanism of injury will many times pinpoint the anatomy involved in the injury. A fall on an outstretched arm places the rotator cuff in tension and may cause it to rupture. Falling on the outstretched hand places more stress on the femoral neck in the elderly and produces a femoral neck fracture. In patients under 40, a fall on the outstretched hand is more likely to produce wrist or elbow fractures. The clinician should be alert for fractures in both areas. A direct

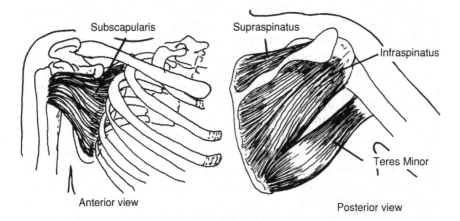

FIGURE 5.2. Diagram of rotator cuff muscles. (Reproduced from Shahady E, Petrizzi M, eds. *Sports Medicine for Coaches and Trainers.* Chapel Hill, NC: University of North Carolina Press; 1991:51, with permission.)

TABLE 5.2. Anatomy and function of the various ligaments, muscles, and other structures that provide stability and movement for the shoulder.

Structure	Anatomy	Function
Glenoid labrum	A fibrocartilaginous rim around the glenoid fossa, covers 1/3 of humeral head	Stability and cushioning
Glenohumeral ligaments	Three ligaments: the superior, medial, and inferior	Stability in all directions
Subscapularis	Originates on the anterior scapula and inserts on the lesser tuberosity of the humeral head	Internal rotation
Infraspinatus and teres minor	Originates on the posterior scapula and inserts on the greater tuberosity of the humeral head	External rotation
Subacromial bursa	Located over the supraspinatus and under the deltoid and acromion	A closed sac in an area subject to friction
Supraspinatus	Originates on the superior scapula and inserts on the greater tuberosity of the humeral head	Abduction
Anterior deltoid	Originates on the clavicle, acromion, and scapula and attaches to midshaft of the humerus	Forward flexion
Medial deltoid	Originates on the clavicle, acromion, and scapula and attaches to midshaft of the humerus	Abduction
Posterior deltoid	Originates on the clavicle, acromion, and scapula and attaches to midshaft of the humerus	Backward extension

blow to the superior aspect of the shoulder may rupture the AC ligament and produce an AC joint separation. The movements that recreate the pain help pinpoint the anatomic structures involved in the injury. Abducting the arm to 90° impinges the supraspinatus muscle under the corocoacromial ligament. In addition, pain produced with this movement indicates the presence of the rotator cuff impingement syndrome. Occupation and sporting activities are associated with specific shoulder problems. Painters and auto mechanics whose work requires recurrent overhead activity are susceptible to rotator cuff injury and the impingement syndrome. Throwing sports like baseball in little league athletes are associated with growth plate injury in the proximal humerus. Adolescent swimmers can develop laxity and subluxations.

Past injuries may predispose to specific types of shoulder problems. Prior stingers or brachial plexus injuries lead to rotator cuff muscle weakness and recurrent subluxations. A prior dislocation in adolescents is usually followed by recurrent subluxations.

Do not forget to ask about other medical problems. Diabetics have a greater incidence of shoulder problems especially impingement syndrome and adhesive capsulitis (AC). Primary osteoarthritis is unusual in the shoulder. Rheumatoid arthritis and polymyalgia rheumatic can cause shoulder pain but it is usually bilateral. Other parts of the history will usually be positive if these diseases are present. Intrabdominal pathology like a ruptured spleen or abdominal tumor can refer pain to the shoulder. It would be unusual for shoulder pain to be the only symptom of intrabdominal pathology.

2. Focused Physical

2.1. Inspection

The patient should have all clothes removed from the upper body to inspect for atrophy and deformity. It is okay to allow female patients to keep on their bra for the start of the examination but they may need to remove it for a complete evaluation. Patients in pain are more concerned about symptom relief than modesty. Adequate explanation of the reasons for exposing all the shoulder structures and a chaperone (if needed) is usually sufficient to reduce patient and clinician discomfort. Observe the posterior scapula for atrophy. Atrophy in this area indicates a rotator cuff tear with weakness of the infraspinatus and teres minor muscles. Pathology of the subscapularis muscle is unusual compared with that of other muscles and tendons of the rotator cuff. The shoulder becomes square with shoulder dislocation rather than its usual rounded appearance. Rotator cuff disease causes relative imbalance of the cuff muscles. This imbalance causes the humeral head to move forward and be easily palpable. Clavicle fractures and AC joint separations will have obvious deformities.

2.2. Palpation

The AC joint will be tender in AC joint separation and AC arthritis (Figure 5.1). Clavicle fractures will acutely be tender and later have a palpable callus (Figure 5.1). Many times, rotator cuff disease will be associated with tenderness over the anterior shoulder.

2.3. Range of motion (ROM)

Compare one side to the other noting any difference.

- Abduction (Figure 5.3) is normal up to 180°.
- Forward flexion (Figure 5.4) is normal up to 180°.
- Backward extension (Figure 5.5) is normal up to 80°.
- Internal rotation (Figure 5.6) is normal is up to 80°.
- External rotation (Figure 5.7) is normal up to 45°.

Evaluate internal and external rotation with the arm at the side rather than abducting the arm. If impingement syndrome is present, abduction creates impingement (pain) and the patient does not want to move the shoulder.

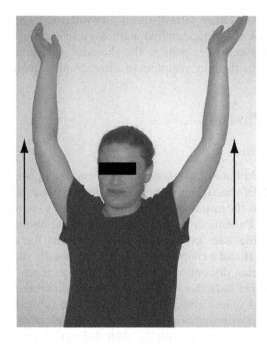

FIGURE 5.3. Abduction of the shoulders.

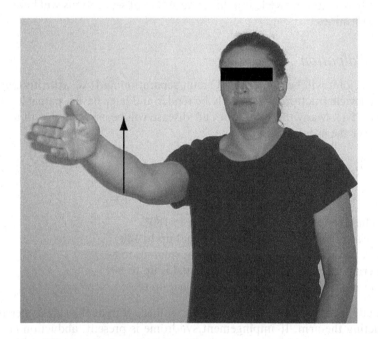

FIGURE 5.4. Forward flexion of the shoulder.

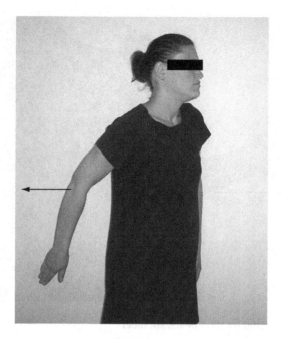

FIGURE 5.5. Backward extension of the shoulder.

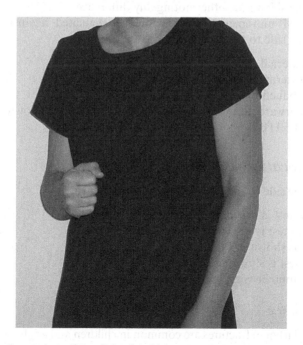

FIGURE 5.6. Internal rotation of the shoulder.

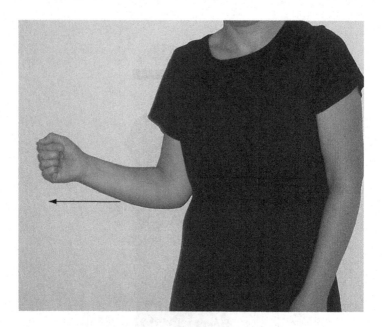

FIGURE 5.7. External rotation of the shoulder.

2.4. Resistance testing

Compare one side to the other noting any difference.
All the ROM movements should now be evaluated against resistance.
Compare one side to the other and note the difference.

- Resisted internal rotation is shown in Figure 5.8.
- Resisted external rotation is shown in Figure 5.9.
- Resisted abduction is shown in Figure 5.10.
- Resisted forward flexion and backward extension are shown in Figures 5.11A and 5.11B.

2.5. Provocative tests

Compare one side to the other noting any difference.

- Crossover test is shown in Figure 5.12.
- Empty can test is shown in Figure 5.13.
- Neer test is shown in Figure 5.14.
- Hawkins test is shown in Figure 5.15.
- Anterior apprehension test is shown in Figure 5.16.

Fractured clavicle

Clavicle (collarbone) fractures are common in children and adults. The fracture is caused by some type of direct trauma such as a fall or a direct blow to the

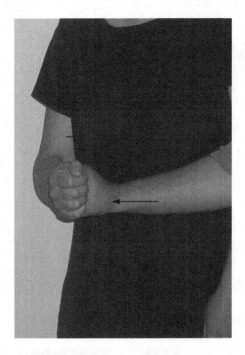

FIGURE 5.8. Resisted internal rotation of the shoulder.

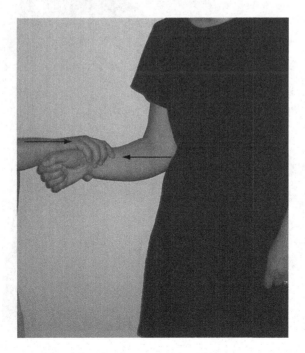

FIGURE 5.9. Resisted external rotation of the shoulder.

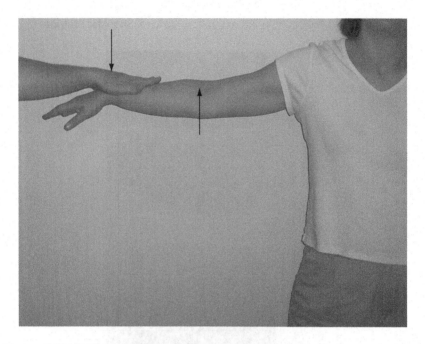

FIGURE 5.10. Resisted abduction of the shoulder.

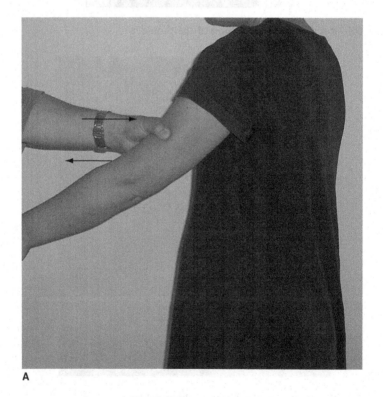

A

FIGURE 5.11. (A) Resisted forward flexion.

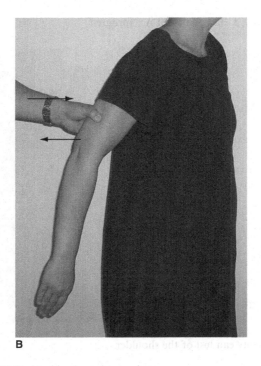

FIGURE 5.11. (B) Resisted backward extension.

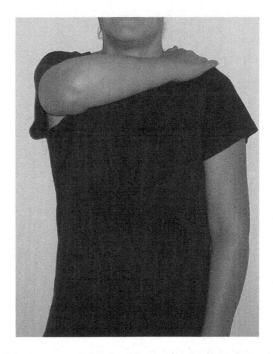

FIGURE 5.12. Crossover test of the shoulder.

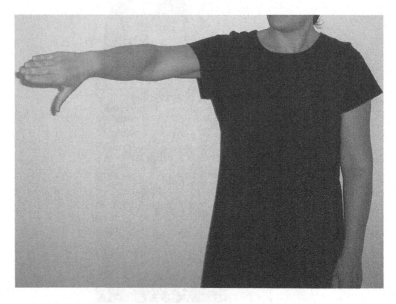

FIGURE 5.13. Empty can test of the shoulder.

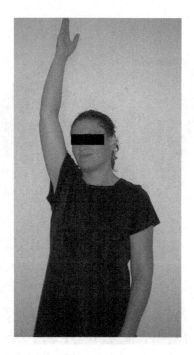

FIGURE 5.14. Neer test of the shoulder.

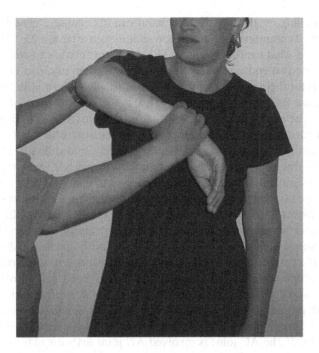

FIGURE 5.15. Hawkins test of the shoulder.

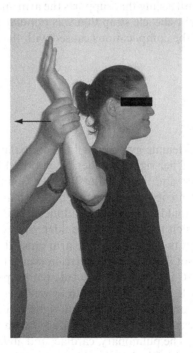

FIGURE 5.16. Anterior apprehension test of the shoulder.

shoulder. Falling on the outstretched hand can also cause a clavicle fracture. They are most common in males and are seldom seen after age 25. They usually heal no matter what treatment is used. The statement "clavicle fractures will heal as long as the two ends are in the same room" is often made to indicate how unusual it is for them not to heal. The break is usually at the middle third of the clavicle where the curvature changes. This is the weakest part of the bone. The racture interrupts weight transmission from the arm to the axial skeleton. The resulting deformity is produced by the weight of the arm, which pulls on the lateral fragment through the coricoclavicular ligament and draws it downwards. The medial fragment, as a rule, is minimally displaced. Once the swelling decreases, a significant lump may be present for 3 to 6 months. The lump is secondary to the original bony displacement and the healing callus formation.

In all patients with a clavicle fracture, your examination should include a neurovascular assessment of the involved extremity. The fracture will decrease muscle power but no sensory loss should be present. Also observe for signs of obstruction to the flow in the subclavain vein and artery. These are rare complications but if found indicate the need for more extensive evaluation and consultation. Other indications for consultation include any fractures that break the skin and distal clavicle fractures. Fractures of the distal 1/3 of the clavicle are not as stable and may require a special brace to provide stability. If the AC joint is involved AC joint arthritis may occur in the future. The vast majority of clavicle fractures are located in the midshaft. They heal very well with a sling that supports the arm and adequate pain control. The figure of eight-clavicle strap that was popular in the past is seldom used now because of the complications caused with the strap.

3. Case

3.1. History

A healthy 17-year-old female gymnast fell from a balance beam directly on the anterior portion of her right shoulder. She noticed immediate pain over the anterior shoulder and pain with shoulder abduction on the right. Examination revealed no obvious deformity but she had discomfort when she abducted the right shoulder to 90° and adducted the shoulder across her body so she could touch the opposite shoulder. She was able to withstand downward pressure on the elbow with the arm crossed over but the maneuver produced significant discomfort (positive crossover test, Figure 5.12). She was tender over the AC joint on the right side but no pain or deformity was present over the clavicle. There was no pain or weakness with right shoulder internal and external rotation. The additional right shoulder provocative tests were difficult to do because of the pain produced with abduction, but none seemed to be positive. The pulmonary, cardiac, and abdominal examinations were within normal limits. The left shoulder examination was normal.

3.2. Thinking Process

A direct blow to the anterior shoulder can cause fractures of the clavicle, AC joint separations, and rotator cuff tears, as well as contusions. The lack of pain over the clavicle and no obvious deformity palpated over the clavicle shaft rule out clavicle fracture. It is highly unlikely that a clavicle fracture would be present without significant clavicular tenderness and palpation of a deformity. Limitation of abduction is suggestive of either rotator cuff tear or AC joint separation. Pinpoint tenderness and a positive crossover test are highly suggestive of AC joint separation. Once you have positive findings suggestive of another diagnosis a contusion is ruled out as the only diagnosis. An imaging study like a plain X-ray is usually not needed unless a fracture is suspected.

This patient was diagnosed with a right shoulder first-degree AC joint separation. She was treated with a sling and nonsteroidal anti-inflammatory drug (NSAIDs) for 7 days. A rehabilitation program was started while she was in the sling. Within 2 weeks she was able to return to her activities as a gymnast.

4. Joint Acromioclavicular Separation (AC joint separation)

AC joint separation can occur under many different circumstances. Yet, in almost all cases it can be attributed to a specific incident or traumatic event. Patients that play football, rugby, or any other high-impact activities are at an increased risk of having this type of injury. AC joint separation can occur in nonathletes as well, for example, by falling on an outstretched hand. Do not overlook the patient that may show signs of AC separation, but may not necessarily be the most athletic. Active individuals who work in construction, roofing, or even simple yard work are susceptible to falls and AC separation.

4.1. Mechanism of Injury and Anatomy

AC joint separation occurs when enough force is applied to the joint to disrupt the joint proper or the surrounding ligaments that hold the joint in its anatomical position. The AC joint lies between the acromial end of the clavicle and the acromion. Both the clavicle and the acromion are covered by fibrocartilage. This cartilage is damaged during acute injury, and with time, this damage leads to cartilage loss and osteoarthritis. The joint capsule is formed by several ligaments, which are named based on their origins and insertions, the acromioclavicular, coricoclavicular, and corocoacromial ligaments (Figure 5.17). The joint has a capsule surrounding its articular margin and a ligament (acromioclavicular) located between the clavicle and acromion.

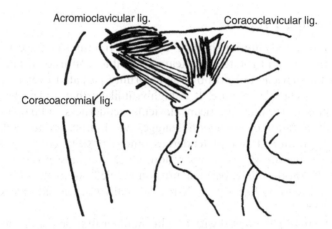

Acromioclavicular lig.   Coracoclavicular lig.

Coracoacromial lig.

FIGURE 5.17. Drawing of acromioclavicular, coricoclavicular, and corocoacromial ligaments. (Reproduced from Shahady E, Petrizzi M, eds. *Sports Medicine for Coaches and Trainers*. Chapel Hill, NC: University of North Carolina Press; 1991:52, with permission.)

AC separation can be graded by the amount of trauma that occurs to the joint and the acromioclavicular and coricoclavicular ligaments. There are five grades of injury but in the primary care office setting only three grades of injury are usually seen. In the emergency room setting a grade 5 injury will be seen with more severe trauma.

- Grade 1—Injuries consists of only a slight sprain to the acromioclavicular ligament (Figure 5.18). There is no deformity noted.
- Grade 2—Injuries consists of a ruptured or torn acromioclavicular ligament as well as a sprain or partial tear of the coricoclavicular ligament. A deformity occurs with the torn AC ligament because the acromion drops below the clavicle and the clavicle rides higher with the decrease in ligamentous stability (Figure 5.19).
- Grade 3—Injuries consists of complete rupture of the acromioclavicular and coricoclavicular ligament, a more serious injury. A deformity occurs for similar reasons as grade 2 (Figure 5.20).

4.2. Presenting History and Examination

The usual patient will present with pain in the anterior shoulder over the AC joint following an episode of trauma. The pain is worse with abduction and crossing over of the injured shoulder. On examination, what seems to be a lump to the patient is the deformity created by the loss of integrity of the AC

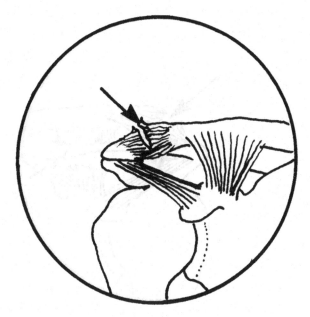

FIGURE 5.18. Grade 1 AC tear. (Reproduced from Shahady E, Petrizzi M, eds. *Sports Medicine for Coaches and Trainers*. Chapel Hill, NC: University of North Carolina Press; 1991:52, with permission.)

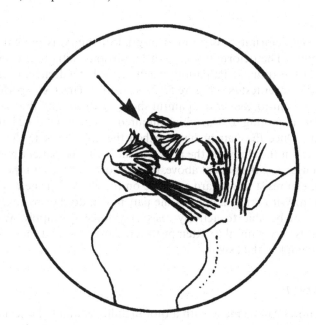

FIGURE 5.19. Grade 2 AC tear. (Reproduced from Shahady E, Petrizzi M, eds. *Sports Medicine for Coaches and Trainers*. Chapel Hill, NC: University of North Carolina Press; 1991:52, with permission.)

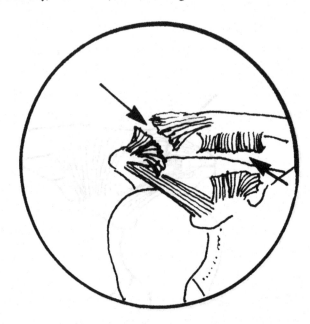

FIGURE 5.20. Grade 3 tear. (Reproduced from Shahady E, Petrizzi M, eds. *Sports Medicine for Coaches and Trainers*. Chapel Hill, NC: University of North Carolina Press; 1991:52, with permission.)

ligament. The deformity, not present in grade 1 injury, is present in grade 2 and 3 injury. The deformity may not be obvious initially because of the edema from the trauma. Palpation usually reveals tenderness over the AC joint. The crossover test (see Figure 5.12) is positive. This test is performed by asking the patient to abduct the painful shoulder to 90° and then adduct the shoulder by attempting to touch his uninjured shoulder with the hand of the injured side. Once the patient has touched the opposite side the examiner pushes down on the elbow of the affected side while the patient resists. With grade 1 injuries, like the patient above, the crossover maneuver is possible and the patient can resist downward pressure on the elbow but there will be significant pain. With grade 2 injuries the patient can do the crossover maneuver but is not be able to actively resist any force you apply. With grade 3 injuries it is very painful to attempt the crossover test and they usually are unable to complete the task.

4.3. Imaging

Most diagnoses can be made with a thorough history and physical examination. If a fracture is suspected plain film X-rays of the shoulder are usually sufficient to make the diagnosis. Magnetic resonance imaging (MRI) would not be indicated unless other injuries are suspected.

4.4. Treatment

For grade 1 to 3 AC injuries, ice and NSAIDs are the mainstay of initial treatment. Most AC separations will heal without surgical intervention. A sling is recommended until the pain subsides. The pain lasts for 1 to 6 weeks depending on the grade of separation. Within a few days, initiate a rehabilitation program in order to restore a full ROM. The patient is asked to remove the arm from the sling and slowly begin to make circular motions. The circle of the motion is gradually increased as tolerated. The time needed for complete healing varies from 1 week to up to 12 weeks depending on the grade of the tear. Resume full activity when the patient has a full ROM and there is no tenderness in the AC joint region on palpation. Treatment by a physical therapist may be needed in grade 2 and 3 injuries.

It is important to tell the patient that the deformity or lump will not go away but it does not lead to a decrease in ROM or function. For some patients the cosmetic result is not acceptable and they wish to have surgery. Surgery for grade 3 injuries may also be indicated for elite athletes or laborers who are dependent on a more speedy recovery and a more stable AC joint that can endure significant stress earlier in the recovery process. Consultation with an orthopedic surgeon will help with this decision.

5. Acromioclavicular Joint Arthritis

In some patients who sustained a grade 1 injury at a younger age the symptoms of AC joint discomfort may return. The usual time period is 15 to 20 years after the initial injury. The patient usually has forgotten about the initial injury and complains of the gradual onset of anterior superior shoulder pain that is made worse with abduction and adduction of the shoulder. The patient may have been treated unsuccessfully for other diagnosis before this one is considered. The examination will be negative for rotator cuff disease. Tenderness is present over the AC joint and the crossover test is positive similar to a grade 1 injury. Over 50% of these patients respond to an injection of lidocaine and a steroid into the joint and the shoulder strengthening exercises described at the end of the chapter. If there is no response to injections, consultation with an orthopedic surgeon for possible surgery should be considered.

6. Fractured Proximal Humeral Head

Humeral head fractures can occur in patients over 55 who fall on their outstretched arm. Falling on the outstretched arm is a mechanism of injury for several fractures and/or soft tissue injuries. Injuries more common in younger patients include rotator cuff tear, AC joint separation, and fractures of the scaphoid, radius, and ulna. Fractured radial head in the elbow and fractured humeral head in the shoulder are more common in older patients. Be alert for the possibility of more than one injury occurring with this type of fall. The primary care clinician can treat many of the proximal humerus fractures.

Once the diagnosis of fracture of the proximal humerus is suspected, a neurologic and vascular evaluation of the upper extremity should be conducted. Injuries to the axillary nerve and brachial plexus as well as the axillary and brachial artery are rare but possible. A good radial pulse and no sensory or motor loss of the deltoid region and the lower arm will rule out these possibilities.

X-rays help not only with the diagnoses but also with decisions about treatment. Because of the insertion of the rotator cuff tendons, the proximal head of the humerus generally fractures along four predictable cleavage lines. Regardless of the number of fragments, proximal humerus fractures are classified by the displacement and degree of angulation. Neer 1 fractures have no more than 1-cm displacement of any fragment and no more than 45° of angulation. More than 85% of proximal humerus fractures are nondisplaced Neer 1 and can be treated nonoperatively. The radiologist should help with diagnosing the degree of displacement and angulation. Any fracture that is open or associated with neurological or vascular deficit requires referral.

Treatment of Neer 1-part fractures includes a sling for comfort and early ROM exercises (about 5 to 10 days after the injury). Patients should begin with pendulum exercises with the injured arm out of the sling. They perform this movement by bending at the waist, allowing the arm to fall toward the floor, and rotating it in a circle. With time, the size of the circle is increased and the sling removed during the exercise (see Fig. 5.30).

Early movement is important to reduce residual stiffness and deformities. Two weeks following the injury start the following:

1. Abduct the shoulder by progressively walking the fingers up the wall.
2. Internally rotate by placing the hand of the fractured shoulder behind the back and progressively move up the back.
3. Increase elbow ROM by flexing and extending the elbow when it is out of the sling.

Discontinue the sling gradually after 4 to 6 weeks. Physical therapy referral may be helpful if the patient is having difficulty with achieving the exercises. This is especially true in the elderly.

7. Case

7.1. History

A 16-year-old male football player presents to your office directly from football practice complaining of left shoulder pain that began after attempting a tackle with the left arm. His past health is excellent and he has no past shoulder problems or a family history of shoulder problems. Upon examination, he is in acute distress with shoulder pain. He is holding his left arm close to his abdomen to protect it from movement. He thinks he heard his shoulder pop when he was making the tackle and has been in extreme pain since that time. On observation of the left shoulder, with his shirt removed, the lateral shoulder looks square compared with the roundness of the right shoulder. A bulge is present below the distal clavicle. There is no deformity or tenderness over the AC joint or the clavicle. The bulge is tender and there is an empty space under the acromion laterally. He resists any attempt to move the arm away from the abdomen, and attempts to externally rotate or abduct the shoulder are very painful. There is no sensory loss over the deltoid region or any part of the shoulder and arm. He has good pulses and no loss of color in the extremity.

7.2. Thinking Process

Think of how the injury occurred. Preparing for a tackle the patient internally rotated both shoulders in order to grab the runner. The runner overpowered his internal rotation grasp and forced the shoulder into external rotation. The most likely injury given the mixture of forces would be an anterior dislocation or subluxation of the humeral head outside the glenoid fossae. Other injuries still need to be considered. This is not the usual mechanism of injury for AC joint separation and clavicle fracture but palpation of those areas is important to rule out these possibilities. As noted previously, there was no deformity or tenderness over the AC joint or the clavicle so these diagnosis are not likely. Subluxation is probably ruled out by the lack of history of a prior shoulder injury. The physical examination will be the same for both a subluxation and a dislocation. The remaining parts of the examination are classical for a dislocation. Refusing to move the arm, a square shoulder, a tender bulge, and emptiness where the humeral head should be are all characteristic of both dislocation and subluxation. As there is no history of recurrent subluxation the diagnosis of dislocation is most likely in the presence of this type of trauma. The diagnosis or dislocation was made and the shoulder was reduced using an active countertraction force as noted in Figure 5.21. After the reduction, an X-ray of the shoulder was performed and it revealed no evidence of fracture. A 6-week rehabilitation program was prescribed and the patient was able to return to his usual activities following the rehabilitation.

8. Glenohumeral Joint Dislocations

The glenohumeral joint lies between the glenoid fossa and the humeral head. The flat surface of the glenoid provides no bony stability like that provided by the acetabulum of the hip for the head of the femur. The stability of the joint is dependent upon soft tissue structures like the glenoid labrum, glenohumeral ligaments, and rotator cuff muscles. Injury to any of these soft tissue structures makes the joint susceptible to dislocation, instability, and/or subluxation. The relative lack of stability makes the joint one of the most

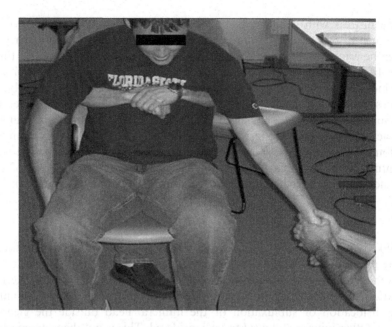

FIGURE 5.21. Relocating a shoulder dislocation by countertraction in a chair.

commonly dislocated joints. Ninety percent of shoulder dislocations are anterior, with the rest being posterior. Inferior dislocations are rare. In younger patients, most shoulder dislocations are caused by sports injuries whereas falls are the usual cause in the elderly. For anterior dislocations, the mechanism of injury is an excessive external rotation or abduction force, while posterior dislocations usually occur when the humeral head is driven posteriorly.

The usual symptoms are immediate pain and an unwillingness to move the affected arm. The patient tends to cradle the affected arm with the other arm. Inspection reveals a square shoulder, a bulge where the humeral head now rests, and emptiness beneath the acromion. Before considering reduction, a neurovascular evaluation should be done. After comparing the radial pulses assess for axillary nerve deficit. Axillary nerve deficit is the most common neurologic deficit associated with shoulder dislocation. Contraction of the deltoid is not possible when an axillary nerve deficit is present. To test for deltoid function, place a hand on the patient's elbow while the arm is at the patient's side. Ask him or her to gently abduct the shoulder while you resist the attempt to do so. If there is no nerve injury, you will feel the deltoid contract.

8.1. Imaging

Order standard three-view X-rays to rule out humeral fractures. Obtain the X-rays after the reduction unless there is an open fracture or a neurologic deficit. Delaying reduction makes relocation more difficult.

8.2. Treatment

Muscle spasm sets in shortly after dislocation, making reduction more difficult. The quicker the reduction is performed the easier it is for the patient and the clinician. Early reduction also requires less force and provides dramatic relief from pain. Numerous reduction techniques can be used, for example, the self-reduction technique (Figure 5.22) in which the patient interlaces his or her fingers and places them around the flexed knee on the same side of the dislocation. The patient then leans backward, and the reduction occurs. This technique works well for recurrent subluxations. In the gravity method, the patient is placed prone with the affected shoulder supported and the arm hanging over the examination table, bench, or training room table with a weight attached to the hand. A weight of 5 lb usually is sufficient (Figure 5.23). Gravity stretches the muscle spasm and reduction occurs. The traction–countertraction method has the patient sitting on a chair or a bench and leaning forward as an assistant places his arms around the patient's torso to provide countertraction (see Figure 5.21). Gentle but steady pressure is then applied to the affected arm as the countertraction is increased. The pull is gradually increased until the shoulder relocates. There is an older method known as the hippocratic method. In this technique, the clinician places a foot in the axilla to apply countertraction while providing traction on the

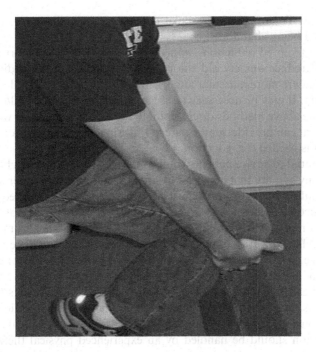

FIGURE 5.22. Self-reduction of a dislocation of the shoulder.

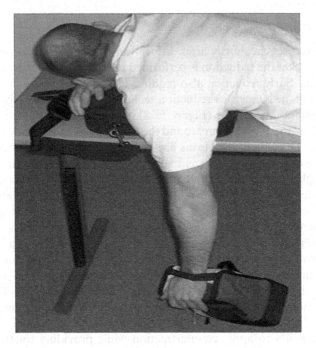

FIGURE 5.23. Gravity reduction of the shoulder.

affected arm. Potential neurovascular damage to the axillary area has led to this method being abandoned.

For all attempted reductions, applying ice to reduce discomfort and reassurance to reduce anxiety aid the process. Reduction is more difficult for patients that are more muscular and when the reduction is delayed for greater than 20 min. It may be necessary to use an injectable narcotic and/or an anxiolytic if the above methods do not initially work. This of course will require a setting that can provide appropriate monitoring. On rare occasions, general anesthesia is needed for reduction.

It is essential to advice patients younger than 20 to wait 6 weeks before they return to any activity that may lead to stressful combined shoulder abduction and external rotation. Contact sports as well as some work-related activities may produce this type of stress. These patients may feel capable of resuming participation after 2 to 3 weeks, and they may seek clearance from their primary care clinician. It is important that the 6-week rule be adhered to in this younger age group to decrease the incidence of repeated dislocations. In older patients, the time required for recovery is less. A rule of thumb is 5 weeks for 20- to 30-year-olds, 4 weeks for 30- to 40-year-olds, and 3 weeks for 40- to 50-year-olds. For patients older than 50 years, the shoulder should be mobilized as soon as symptoms permit (similar to the fractured proximal humerus). Rehabilitation should be handled by an experienced physical therapist that will help motivate the patient to adhere to their exercises. The primary care clinician also needs to help with this motivation. Surgery can be an option initially but the majority opinion is to attempt nonsurgical treatment first and reserve surgery for the patient who fails conservative management because of recurrent dislocations. If the patient experiences recurrent dislocations, imaging studies should be done to access for indications that the subluxations have damaged parts of the glenoid or the humerus. Defects in the anterior inferior aspect of the glenoid rim are referred to as Bankart lesions and those in the posterior lateral aspect of the humeral head are known as Hill–Sachs lesions. Both plain films and MRI demonstrate these lesions.

9. Rotator Cuff Tears

Rotator cuff disease represents a spectrum of conditions that begins with inflammation of the cuff tendons that may progress to impingement of the cuff and a tear. Tears can also occur acutely with trauma. Rotator cuff tears are classified as acute, chronic, and chronic with an acute extension. They are then divided further into full- or partial-thickness tears. Full-thickness tears are more common in younger patients under age 35 and are usually the result of a traumatic event like a fall. Partial tears are more characteristic of chronic tears. The incidence of tears increases with age and many of the chronic tears are not symptomatic.

Knowledge of the anatomy of the rotator cuff provides an understanding of cuff function and pathology. The cuff surrounds the anterior, posterior, and superior portions of the glenohumeral joint. The cuff consists of the tendons from the subscapularis, supraspinatus, infraspinatus, and teres minor muscles. The subscapularis attaches to the lesser tuberosity of the humerus and the other three attach to the greater tuberosity. The primary function of the cuff is to provide a compressive force that keeps the humeral head centered in the glenoid. The subacromial bursa lies between the coracromial arch and the rotator cuff. The bursa provides a frictionless surface for movement and limits contact between the cuff and the acromion. Instability occurs when cuff muscles are weak. Unopposed movement of the deltoid muscle now causes the humeral head to move away from the center of the glenoid, leading to the cascade of inflammation, impingement, subluxation, and in some cases a tear (impingement cascade).

The patient with a chronic rotator cuff tear may have a history of recreational or work-related overhead motion activities. Overhead activities predispose to rotator cuff injury by creating repeated microtrauma. The microtrauma leads to the impingement cascade and eventually to microtears. The other parts of the history and physical are the same as those listed in the impingement syndrome that will be discussed in Section 9.1. Some specific parts of the examination that are more indicative of rotator cuff tear include atrophy in the infraspinatus and supraspinatus fossae, lift-off test shown in

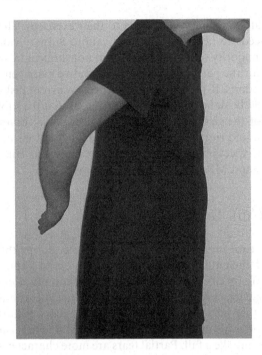

FIGURE 5.24. Lift-off test for subscapularis weakness of the shoulder.

Figure 5.24 (inability to lift the internally rotated arm off the back) for sub-scapularis tear, and the drop arm test (Figure 5.25). During the drop arm test the patient is asked to abduct the arm to 180° and then gradually lower it to the side. At 90° the arm will quickly drop to the side. No matter how many times the motion is tried once 90° is reached the arm drop cannot be controlled. This indicates a rotator cuff tear.

Injecting the subacromial space with 5 to 10 cc of lidocaine helps differentiate rotator cuff tears from other forms of rotator cuff disease. Patients without tears experience dramatic improvement in all provocative tests for impingement and the above tests for tears. If there is no improvement after the injection in these tests a tear is more likely.

9.1. Treatment

Patients with acute rupture following trauma usually have full-thickness tears. These patients are younger and have no prior history of shoulder problems. They may benefit from surgery and should be evaluated by an orthopedic surgeon but do not be surprised if the treatment chosen is non-surgical.

Chronic tears whether they be full or partial thickness may be asymptomatic or associated with all the symptoms characteristic of the impingement

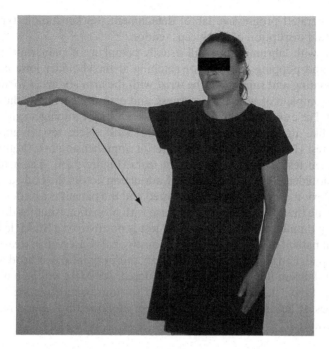

FIGURE 5.25. Drop arm test of the shoulder is positive when the patient is unable to keep the arm abducted to 90° and the arm drops to the patient's side.

syndrome. The treatment is nonsurgical and consists of the rehabilitation program of shoulder exercises described at the end of this chapter.

10. Labrum Tears

As previously discussed, the glenoid labrum is a fibrocartilaginous rim around the glenoid fossa. It functions to increase the area and depth of the glenoid cavity and contributes to the stability of the glenohumeral joint. Before the use of shoulder arthroscopy and MRI, glenoid labrum lesions were unusual except in association with anterior shoulder subluxation and dislocation. In the mid 1980s, labrum lesions that involved the long head of the biceps (LHB) were being noted in throwing athletes who had shoulder problems. Because the LHB is contiguous with the superior labrum, both the labrum and the LHB pulled off the glenoid in these throwing athletes. This led to the definition of labral injuries as superior labrum anterior posterior (SLAP) lesions. SLAP lesions were categorized into four types. Type I has minimal degenerative changes with no avulsion of the biceps tendon and the labrum edges are firmly attached to the glenoid rim. Types II through

IV demonstrated progressive labral detachment, bucket handle type tears, and eventual disruption of the biceps tendon.

Patients with labrum injury will usually complain of pain with overhead activities and popping, clicking, or catching at the shoulder joint especially when pronating and supinating the wrist with the arm abducted to 90°. They may also complain of weakness, stiffness, and pain while lying on the affected extremity. The examination will reveal positive tests for impingement and subluxation like the empty can test (Figure 5.13), Neer test (Figure 5.14), Hawkins test (Figure 5.15), and the anterior apprehension test (Figure 5.16). The O'Brien test is helpful for labrum tears (Figure 5.26). The arm of the painful shoulder is brought into 90° of adduction across the body and 90° of forward flexion. Forward flexion is resisted and the patient is asked to pronate and supinate the wrist. If the pain is worse with pronation (thumbs down) and relieved by thumbs up (supination), the test is positive for a SLAP lesion.

When a patient is not responding to nonsurgical conservative treatment for shoulder pain and a history of subluxation and/or painful overhead activities is present, labrum injury should be considered. An MRI will help make this diagnosis. Type 1 lesions usually respond to nonsurgical treatment but the other types of lesions usually require surgery followed by a good rehabilitation program.

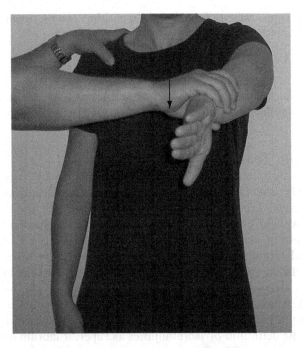

FIGURE 5.26. O'Brien test for labrum tears. Forward-flex the arm to 90° and place downward pressure on the arm. Ask the patient to resist. Thumbs down causes pain and thumbs up reduces pain in labrum tears.

11. Case

11.1. History

A 48-year-old man presents to your office with a 1-year history of intermittent right shoulder pain that has become worse over the past 6 weeks. The pain now awakens him at night and he cannot sleep on his right shoulder. He works as an auto mechanic, is an avid tennis player, and is right hand dominant. The pain is worse when he raises his arm above his shoulder, making it difficult to work, play tennis, and comb his hair. He has not worked the past week. He has no history of shoulder trauma and does not experience clicking or catching of the shoulder with any movements. The pain is dull, achy, and not burning in character. The pain is located over the anterior deltoid area, does not radiate, and neck movements do not intensify the pain.

The left arm is abducted first when removing his shirt and the right arm is not abducted as he removes his shirt. When observing the shoulders anteriorly and laterally the humeral head of the right shoulder is more forward than the left. Observing the shoulders from the rear reveals obvious atrophy over the right scapula in the area of the supraspinatus and infraspinatus fossa. Active motion comparing right with left reveals limited abduction to 90° on the right compared with 180° on the left (Figure 5.3), external rotation is limited to 15° on the right compared with 45° on the left (Figure 5.7). Internal rotation is 80° on both sides (Figure 5.6). Both the Neer and Hawkins tests are positive for impingement (Figures 5.14 and 5.15). Resisted external rotation (Figure 5.9), resisted abduction (Figure 5.10), and the empty can test (Figure 5.13) reveal normal 4/4 strength on the left and decreased strength of 2/4 on the right. The apprehension test (Figure 5.16) is positive for significant discomfort. The O'Brien test for a labrum tear is negative.

The crossover test is negative (Figure 5.12). The Spurling maneuver (see Figure 9.6) with head compression does not reproduce the pain. Sensory evaluation of cervical nerves C4 through C8 reveals no sensory loss. Motor function is difficult to evaluate because of the pain-limiting muscle movement.

11.2. Thinking Process

This is obviously a chronic problem with a long history and no prior trauma. Acute rotator cuff tear is unlikely but a chronic tear may be a possibility. Cervical nerve root compression is unlikely given the lack of radiating or burning pain, negative Spurling maneuver, and lack of sensory nerve loss. The most obvious issue with this patient is the difficulty with raising the arm above his head (shoulder abduction). His pain is aggravated by all work and recreational activities as well as activities of daily living that involve abduction. Pain with abduction suggests impingement syndrome. The tests for impingement (Neer and Hawkins) are both positive so impingement is present. However, this patient has more than impingement.

The observation of the humeral head being more forward on the right suggests weakness of the external rotators. This weakness is confirmed by the atrophy noted over the infraspinatus fossa of the posterior scapula, the location of the external rotators (infraspinatus and teres minor), the limitation of active external rotation to only 15°, and the strength of external rotation reduced to 2/4. Atrophy of the supraspinous fossa and the reduced strength of the empty can test (2/4) confirm weakness of the supraspinatus muscle, the rotator cuff abductor. The other significant positive test is the anterior apprehension test. This indicates subluxation of the humeral head on the glenohumeral joint.

The most likely diagnosis given the history and examination is inflammation and impingement of the supraspinatus muscle and tendon accompanied by atrophy of the external rotators of the cuff and subluxation. Partial-thickness tears may also be present. Recurrent subluxation can lead to tears of the labrum as well as defects in the glenoid rim (Bankart lesions) and the humeral head (Hill–Sachs lesions). The O'Brien test is negative so a SLAP lesion or labrum tear is not likely. Both plain films and MRI should be performed to demonstrate the presence of defects in the glenoid rim, humeral head, and labrum tears.

The plain film was negative and his MRI revealed areas in the supraspinatus consistent with microtears. He was treated with NSAIDs for 10 days and referred to a physical therapist for extensive rehabilitation. He responded very well to the rehabilitation and after 6 months has regained most of his strength, is back to full-time work, is playing tennis, and is able to raise his arm above his head without difficulty.

12. Rotator Cuff Disease

Rotator cuff pathology is the most common cause of shoulder pain. Most of the time, a spectrum of pathology is present. Early on in the process, one diagnosis may be appropriate but as the process continues, multiple diagnoses are appropriate. Because the treatment is similar for the majority of the diagnoses, searching for only one diagnosis is nonproductive. However, understanding the spectrum of pathology helps the clinician perform a focused history and physical examination and then put the pieces of the puzzle together.

12.1. History and Physical

The most common scenario for the shoulder pain of rotator cuff pathology is a middle-aged patient with chronic shoulder pain who has the impingement syndrome. This syndrome involves impingement of the supraspinatus tendon and the subacromial bursa against the corocoacromial arch when the arm is abducted. The impingement leads to inflammation, edema, small tears, and formation of scar tissue. These pathological changes lead to decreased movement and eventual atrophy of the rotator cuff muscles, especially the supraspinatus, infraspinatus, and teres minor. The weak rotator cuff muscles decrease the stability of the humeral head and it moves off the glenoid fossae (subluxation) with abduction and external rotation. Subluxation increases the chances of injury to the labrum, glenoid fossa, and the humeral head.

The early symptoms may only be periodic achy shoulder pain that is worse at night. This is the first sign of inflammation caused by the impingement syndrome. As the process progresses, it becomes more painful to abduct and rotate the shoulder. Patients will now complain about discomfort with combing their hair, fastening their bra from the back, and performing occupational or recreational activities that require placing the arm above the shoulder. Examination at this time will demonstrate positive impingement tests (Neer and Hawkins, Figures 5.14 and 5.15) and pain and weakness with the empty can test (Figure 5.13). The rotator cuff tendon is now more edematous and microtears may be present. Weakness of the cuff muscles now begins to play a part in the symptoms. The humeral head is not held as tightly in the glenoid fossae and the patient notices clicking and catching of the shoulder. The shoulder may come "out of place" and "pop back" in place with or without additional effort by the patient (subluxation). Each patient may express the symptoms of subluxation differently. Some may say it just feels limp and they cannot use it for a few seconds while others may only say it feels "funny." The examination now has additional positive signs that include weakness of abduction and internal and external rotation (Figures 5.8 to 5.10). The apprehension test for subluxation (Figure 5.16) may also become positive. The problem in some patients may progress to a complete tear of the cuff. If it is an acute tear in a chronically inflamed cuff there may be noticeable increase in symptoms and a positive drop arm test (Figure 5.25). If the cuff tear is gradual, there will not be an abrupt change in symptoms and the only additional physical signs are the atrophy noted over the infraspinatus fossae and supraspinatus fossa of the posterior scapula. There, of course, would be marked weakness of the external rotation and abduction accompanying this atrophy. Some patients, especially older women with type 2 diabetes, may progress to a frozen shoulder. This will be discussed in Section 13 (Adhesive Capsulitis, see p. 83).

The above scenario described the usual story for a patient over the age of 45. If the patient is younger, the process is a little different. Teenagers and young adults usually start out with subluxation and then proceed on to impingement. These patients will first complain of the dead or limp arm and then progress to the symptoms of impingement. So the apprehension tests may be the first positive examination signs followed by the more traditional signs of inflammation and impingement. As noted in Section 10 (Labrum Tears) patients can acutely tear the cuff with a fall. Labrum tears are also possible with recurrent subluxation. Attempt to elicit a history of pain with wrist pronation/supination while the arm is abducted and adducted 90° and perform the O'Brien SLAP test to access for labrum tears (see Fig. 5.26).

12.2. Imaging

If a fracture, Bankart, or Hill–Sacks lesion is suspected, obtain X-rays. Magnetic resonance imaging is expensive and is used only in those circumstances where rotator cuff tears are possible. An orthopedic consultation is more cost-effective than an MRI. The history and physical is usually sensitive and specific enough to make a preliminary diagnosis of rotator cuff tear. Do not rely on the MRI to make a diagnosis. It only confirms the diagnosis. The goal of treatment is to reduce discomfort and return the patient to adequate use of the shoulder to perform activities of daily living. Waiting for the MRI to make the diagnosis delays treatment and prolongs disability. It also gives the patient the feeling that the diagnosis cannot be made without the image.

12.3. Treatment

The mainstay of treatment is effective shoulder exercises as outlined at the end of this chapter. If properly taught and properly performed, the vast majority of the time patients will respond very well to strengthening and stretching exercises. However, both patients and clinicians have difficulty understanding the importance of performing these exercises correctly and continuously. Most patients will do them for a few days, not see dramatic improvement, and quit. Most clinicians do not emphasize the need to do them correctly and continuously. The ideal is for the clinician to provide a verbal and written explanation of the exercises, teach the patient how to do them, and then have the patient demonstrate the exercises to the clinician. At each follow-up visit, the patient should again demonstrate the exercises to the clinician. Most patients do not do them correctly initially and need three to four reminders. Referral to a physical therapist also helps assure that the exercises are done correctly and continuously. It is still important to ask the patient to demonstrate what the physical therapist has taught them and reinforce the importance of continuing to do the exercises. Most patients with shoulder problems will prevent recurrence if they continue some of their shoulder exercises for life. The exercises at the end of the chapter are excellent for rotator cuff problems. Make copies and give them to your patients.

The patient can also take NSAIDs for 4 to 7 days and use heat before exercise and ice massage after exercise. Chapter 1 discusses proper use of NSAIDs, ice, and heat. Injections with lidocaine and steroids into the subacromial bursa or the glenohumeral joint may also be of benefit especially if it is difficult for the patient to do the exercises because of pain with rotation and abduction. These injections are discussed in Section 13 (Adhesive Capsulitis).

13. Adhesive Capsulitis

Adhesive capsulitis or frozen shoulder in pathological terms is a contracted, thickened joint capsule around the humeral head. There is absence of synovial fluid in the capsule and chronic inflammatory changes within the subsynovial layer of the capsule. In clinical terms, there is an initial loss of internal rotation followed by loss of forward flexion, external rotation, and abduction. The patient has 50% loss of internal and external rotation and shoulder abduction is limited to 70° to 80° at best.

Several conditions have been associated with AC, including diabetes mellitus (up to five times more), cervical disk disease, hyperthyroidism, intrathoracic neoplasms, post stroke and trauma. It is most common in women over age 50, and almost all patients experienced a period of immobility preceding the onset of AC. There are two types of AC: primary and secondary.

Primary AC is divided into three phases. Phase I is characterized by a gradual onset of diffuse shoulder pain over a period of weeks. The pain usually is worse at night and is increased by lying on the affected side. The patient uses the arm less and stiffness ensues. During Phase II the patient seeks pain relief by restricting movement. Sometimes, unfortunately, the clinician advises this decreased movement. The stiffness phase usually lasts 4 to 10 months. Patients now describe significant restriction of internal rotation like inability to reach their wallets in the case of men and fastening brassieres in the case of women. As the stiffness progresses a dull ache is present most of the time but especially at night. The patient will also experience sharp pain at the limits of their ROM. This leads to decreased desire to reach these limits and a continuous decrease in the limit of their ROM. The old adage "if you don't use it you lose it" is certainly true here. Phase III is the "thawing" phase. This phase lasts for weeks or months, and as motion increases, pain diminishes. Without treatment (other than benign neglect), motion return is gradual in most but may never return to normal. Patients may say they feel near normal because of their adjustment to living with limited ROM. Treatment still has value at this stage.

Secondary AC is different only because of the presence of an acute precipitating event. The event can be an acute injury like a fall. The patient will usually not move the shoulder after the trauma (as sometimes suggested by the clinician). The three phases of a classic frozen shoulder may not all be present and may not follow the previously described chronology. The stiffness phase (II) sets in quickly and the time frame may differ depending on the degree of intervention.

13.1. Examination

The examination will differ depending on the phase of AC. Initially the patient may be holding the involved arm to the side and have great difficulty with any movement. The key movements that are very difficult are shoulder abduction and internal and external rotation. Two movements, the Apley scratch tests, help discover the degree of disability. The posterior Apley scratch (Figure 5.27) is performed by placing the arm behind the back as far up on the back as possible. One side is compared with the other by measuring how far up the back the hand can reach to scratch the back. There usually is a little difference with the dominating arm lagging behind the other arm. This tests the limit of internal rotation and in a patient with a frozen shoulder, the arm usually cannot go back any further than the iliac crest without significant discomfort. Perform the anterior Apley scratch (Figure 5.28) by elevating the arm above the head and attempting to scratch the back on the opposite side. Compare the symptomatic side with the asymptomatic side. The patient with AC is usually unable to elevate the arm above the shoulder (90° of abduction) and cannot reach the back on the opposite side. Injecting the shoulder joint with 3 cc of lidocaine helps determine how much of the limitation is secondary to pain versus actual adhesive capsulitis. The patient with AC will not achieve much improvement with the lidocaine injection.

13.2. Treatment

Treatment for primary and secondary AC is the same. It is mainly conservative using intra-articular injections, heat, gentle stretching, NSAIDs, and

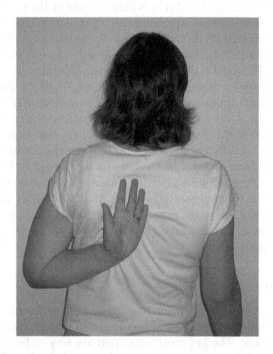

FIGURE 5.27. Posterior Apley scratch.

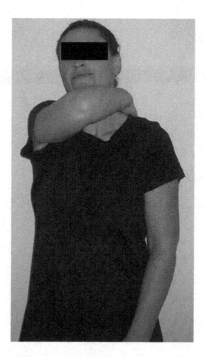

FIGURE 5.28. Anterior Apley scratch.

physical therapy modalities. Adhesive capsulitis is usually self-limited. Once the pain has subsided, it is not that disabling. A thorough explanation of how much time it will take for the condition to improve is mandatory. I usually say it may take 1 year but find that it is more like 4 to 6 months if they do their exercises faithfully. Closed manipulation and surgery may be needed in patients who do not respond to conservative measures. Avoiding excessive immobilization is the key to prevention of AC.

Injection of lidocaine and steroids into the glenohumeral joint may be of help. There are no randomized studies that demonstrate that these injections influence outcome. Many clinicians, including this author, feel positive about their experience with these injections. The injections do help decrease discomfort for a period of 2 to 3 weeks and in some cases increase the chances that the patient will be able to be successful with exercises. Some authors report success with distention of the glenohumeral joint using up to 50 cc of fluid. The fluid is a mixture of 3 cc of lidocaine and the rest is normal saline. Injecting the bursa or the joint can be accomplished through an anterior or posterior approach. In most patients with shoulder pathology, the humeral head is moved forward making a posterior approach easier. Landmarks, as noted in Figure 5.29, help identify the site of the injection. About 1 cm below the acromion, posteriorly, the humeral head boundaries are identified. Internal and external rotation of the shoulder with the elbow at the side helps

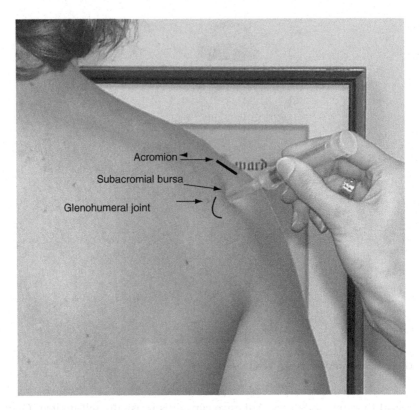

FIGURE 5.29. Shoulder injection with landmarks.

with this identification. There is an obvious sulcus or indentation at the medial border of the humeral head. As noted in Figure 5.29, the subacromial bursa is about 1 cm below the acromion and the glenohumeral joint about 3 cm below the acromion. Careful insertion of the needle just barely avoiding the medial border of the humeral head places it in the correct location. The depth of the insertion is usually about half the depth of a 1.5-in. 22-gauge needle. Patient bulk also influences the depth of insertion. With AC, the injection into the glenohumeral joint will be met with resistance because of the contracted, thickened joint capsule. If large amounts of fluid are injected after the first 5 cc the resistance will decrease. Injections can be repeated more than once. A good rule of thumb is no more than two injections in a month or three injections a year. This is an anecdotal rule and no good evidence exists to support it. Also, remember that many of these patients are diabetic or have the metabolic syndrome and can become diabetic with stress. Steroids can elevate the blood sugar and patients should be warned so they can adjust their medications accordingly. This does not mean steroids cannot be used in diabetics.

14. Arthritis of the Shoulder

The most common inflammatory arthritis of the shoulder joint is rheumatoid arthritis. Other systemic disorders like lupus erythematosus, psoriatic arthritis, ankylosing spondylitis, Reiter's syndrome, gout, pseudogout, and scleroderma may cause glenohumeral degeneration but are rare causes. It is unlikely that shoulder pain would be the presenting symptom for one of these diseases.

Any patient with known inflammatory arthritis who has shoulder pain should be evaluated for inflammatory arthritis in that joint. These patients are still more likely to have the more common shoulder problems but deserve evaluation to access for signs of the inflammatory arthritis. Treatment is initially conservative and directed toward controlling pain, inducing a systemic remission, and maintaining joint motion by physical therapy. The use of intra-articular steroids may help. Patients with progressive loss of motion or radiographic destruction should be referred for possible surgical treatment.

Osteoarthritis of the glenohumeral joint is less common because it is a non-weight-bearing joint. If a patient has prior trauma like a dislocation or fracture, osteoarthritis should be considered. Osteoarthritis may also be present in patients who have engaged in activities like boxing, heavy construction, or chronic use of a pneumatic hammer. Pain is the usual presentation, but it is generally not as acute or associated with the spasm seen in inflammatory conditions. Plain radiographs show narrowing of the glenohumeral joint, osteophyte formation, sclerosis, and some cyst formation. Patients with osteoarthritis of the glenohumeral joint do well with conservative therapy.

15. Little Leaguer's Shoulder

A stress fracture of the growth plate or physis of the proximal humerus is commonly known as little leaguer's shoulder. It occurs in high-performance pitchers between 11 and 13 years of age. In addition to shoulder pain, the common finding is radiographic evidence of widening of the proximal humeral physeal plate. Repeated rotational and compressive stress from throwing produces the stress on the physis. Treatment is usually nonoperative. Like in the case of little leaguer's elbow, rest for the remainder of the season is the key. Encouraging coaches and athletes to develop good pitching skills can prevent shoulder problems in the skeletally immature athlete. Speed should be the last skill developed and only after proper technique and control are established. Many physical therapists and trainers are adept at teaching these techniques. The primary care clinician's role is early recognition and prevention. You will be called on to provide advice. Just prescribing cessation of activity is not enough. Helping coaches and parents understand how to prevent and rehabilitate is an important additional role. Pitching technique and number of pitches are associated with injury. Recommendations are to avoid throwing breaking pitches between the ages of 9 and 14 years. Pitchers should focus on fastball and change-up pitches, avoiding a split-finger change-up. Many authors agree with the *USA Baseball News* recommendations for limiting of pitches per game to the following: limits of 52±15 pitches per game for 8- to 10-year-olds, 68±18 for 11- to 12-year-olds, and 76±16 for 13- to 14-year-olds.

16. Shoulder Exercises

Repeat each of the following exercises two times a day. Rotate from one exercise to the other. Do one set of exercises and then rotate to another exercise and do a set. Do not exercise past the point of pain. Pain means stop.

A. **Pendulum exercises (Figure 5.30)**: Usually the first shoulder exercise done once pain has diminished. Bend over and let injured arm hang loose at your side. Begin to make small circles and gradually increase the circle size. Pain is the only limiting factor.

B. **External and internal rotation 1 (Figure 5.31)**: Place a hand weight or a can of soup in your hand and lie on your back in bed. With the elbow flexed to 90° and tucked tightly to or at your side rotate your arm out and then back

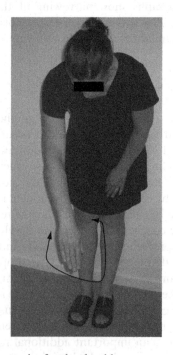

FIGURE 5.30. Pendulum exercise for the shoulder.

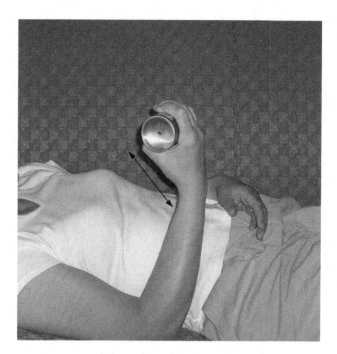

FIGURE 5.31. External and internal rotation 1 exercises.

to your stomach. Remember to keep the elbow tucked to your side at 90°
of flexion. Hold the outer and inner movements for 10 seconds each at
their peak. Repeat 10 to 15 times for one set. Do three sets.

C. **External and Internal rotation 2 (Figure 5.32)**: Place a hand weight or a can
of soup in your hand and lay on the uninjured side in your bed. With the
elbow flexed to 90° and tucked tightly to or at your side rotate your arm
out and then back to your stomach. Remember to keep the elbow tucked
to your side at 90° of flexion. Hold the outer and inner movements for 10 s
each at their peak. Repeat 10 to 15 times for one set. Do three sets.

D. **Supraspinatus strengthening (Figure 5.33)**: Standing with the shoulder
abducted to 90°, elbow straight, arm crossed over about 20°, and thumbs
down, begin to move the arm up and down. Initially use no weight but
within 1 week or so add a small hand weight or a can of soup. Hold each
up and down movement for 5 s and repeat 10 to 15 times. Do three sets.

E. **Forward flexion (Figure 5.34)**: Stand with the injured arm at your side,
elbow straight and a small weight or can of soup in the hand. Forward-
flex the shoulder as high as you can without pain. You may want to start
without a weight and add one as your strength increases. Hold each up
and down movement for 5 s and repeat 10 to 15 times. Do three sets.

F. **Backward extension (Figure 5.35)**: Stand with the injured arm at your
side, elbow straight and a small weight or can of soup in the hand.

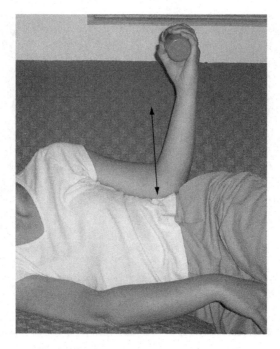

FIGURE 5.32.   External and internal rotation 2 exercises.

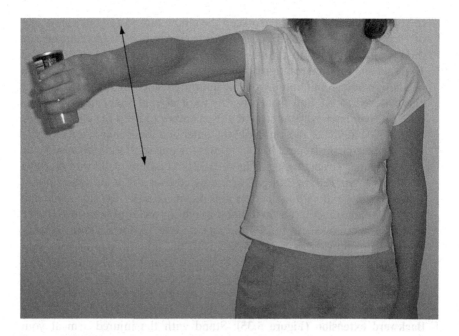

FIGURE 5.33.   Supraspinatus strengthening exercise.

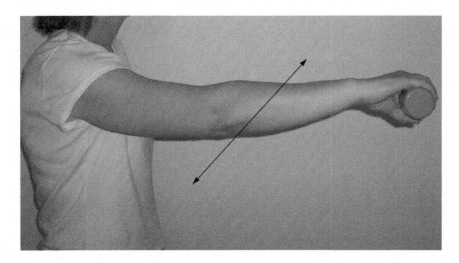

FIGURE 5.34.   Forward flexion exercise.

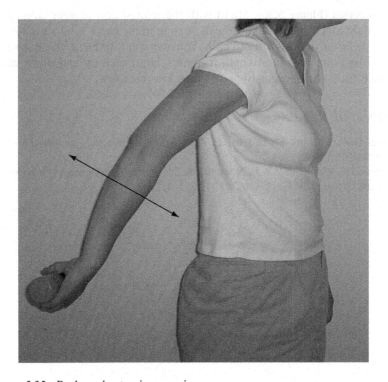

FIGURE 5.35.   Backward extension exercise.

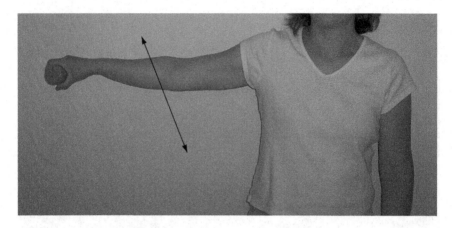

FIGURE 5.36. Abduction exercise.

Backward-extend the shoulder as far back as you can without pain. You may want to start without a weight and add one as your strength increases. Hold each up and down movement for 5 s and repeat 10 to 15 times. Do three sets.

G. **Abduction (Figure 5.36)**: Stand with the injured arm at your side, elbow straight and a small weight or can of soup in the hand. Abduct the shoulder as far as you can without pain. You may want to start without a weight and add one as your strength increases. Hold each up and down movement for 5 s and repeat 10 to 15 times. Do three sets.

Suggested Readings

Quillen DM, Wuchner M, Hatch RL. Acute shoulder injuries. *Am Fam Physician.* 2004;70(10):1947–1954.

Mantone JK, Burkhead WZ Jr, Noonan J Jr. Nonoperative treatment of rotator cuff tears. *Orthop Clin North Am.* 2000;31:295–311.

6

Elbow Problems

EDWARD J. SHAHADY

Elbow movement facilitates rotation and positioning of the hands. Inability to position or rotate the hands correctly impedes ability to perform activities of daily living (ADL) such as eating and dressing as well as participating in throwing sports and certain occupations. Activities of daily living are adequately performed in the range of 30° to 130° of flexion and 50° of pronation and supination. If the range of motion (ROM) is less than these numbers, ADL become more difficult to perform and disability becomes a problem. These numbers should always be kept in mind when evaluating and treating elbow problems.

The most common elbow problem seen in primary health care is lateral epicondylitis, i.e., tennis elbow. It is fairly easy to diagnose but satisfactory treatment results are difficult to obtain. Other elbow problems are more of a challenge to evaluate but a thorough knowledge of the anatomy, epidemiology, and mechanism of injury helps sort out the diagnostic and therapeutic challenges.

Caring for elbow problems becomes possible with a few simple organizational steps. Table 6.1 divides elbow problems into three major categories: acute trauma, overuse trauma, and medical disease. Further differentiation is now possible based on several factors. Knowledge of the patient's age helps, as certain problems are more common in the pediatric adolescent age group, e.g., little leaguer's elbow and osteochondritis dissecans (OCD). Pain location also helps in making the correct diagnosis. Lateral elbow pain is present in tennis elbow, whereas golfer's elbow is associated with medial elbow pain. Knowing the mechanism of injury also helps. Falling on the outstretched hand transmits a force that can cause a radial head fracture and if an occupation requires repeated shaking of hands, lateral epicondylitis, politicians' elbow, may be the diagnosis. Your knowledge of the usual history and examination associated with these problems facilitates the diagnostic process. Confirmatory studies like plain X-rays are of help in many cases but not always needed.

Conducting a focused history and physical and ordering needed confirmatory studies will provide the diagnosis in 95% of the patients. Five percent of

TABLE 6.1. Classification of elbow problems.

Acute trauma
- Fractures
- Dislocations
- Nursemaids' elbow

Overuse trauma
- Lateral epicondylitis
- Medial epicondylitis
- Olecrenon bursitis
- Throwing-related injury
  1. Medial epicondyle traction apophysitis (little leaguer's elbow)
  2. Ulnar collateral ligament injury
  3. Ulnar nerve injury (cubital tunnel syndrome)
  4. Panner's disease
  5. Osteocondritis dissecans

Medical problems
- Arthritis associated with other diseases like rheumatoid, posttraumatic gout, and pseudogout

the time the diagnosis will not be so obvious. That is when additional studies and/or a consultation will be required.

Rare or not so frequent problems are usually the ones we hear about because they are missed in the primary care setting. Having a good working knowledge of the characteristics of common problems provides an excellent background to help recognize the uncommon.

1. Focused History

The first question is usually related to the acuteness of the problem. Did it just start or has it been present for a long period of time? The next question would depend on the answer to the first. If the onset is acute, then ask about a fall especially one that involved breaking the fall with the outstretched hand. Chronic overuse problems can also be made worse by acute trauma so inquiring about prior discomfort is helpful. If the onset is not acute ask about occupations, hobbies, or sports that involve repeated flexion and extension of the wrist or throwing. Pain can be referred to the elbow from shoulder and wrist problems, so inquiring about pain or problems in the wrist or shoulder is appropriate. As a general rule of thumb, it is appropriate to inquire about the joints below and above the problem area. Recent changes in occupation and intensity or style of activity are important. A pitcher may have just started to throw curve balls or the length of time spent throwing or working on the computer may have increased over the past few weeks. Joint swelling or nodules around the elbow may be indicative of rheumatoid or psoriatic arthritis.

2. Focused Physical Examination

First observe the carrying angle of the elbow. Ask patients to fully extend the arm and place it at their side with the hand in the anatomic position (palm side up), as demonstrated in Figure 6.1. The angle in a female is usually 10° to 15° as noted in the patient as compared with 5° in a male. Compare one side with the other. Differences in the angle may indicate a problem. Next have the patient flex and extend the arm. Normal extension (Figure 6.2) is 0° and occasionally to −10°. Normal unassisted flexion (Figure 6.3) is 145°. Use a goniometer (Figure 6.3) to assess the exact degree of flexion and extension. Trauma and synovitis is associated with limitation of elbow flexion and extension. Exact measurements provide an accurate means of comparing one arm with the other and judging effectiveness of therapy. Observe and palpate the elbow. Stand behind the patient to view the posterior elbow. Ask the patient to extend the shoulder and flex the elbow 20° to view all the posterior landmarks. Observe for any fluid over the olecrenon process and palpate the medial and lateral epicondyles for tenderness and crepitus (Figure 6.4). Nodules may be present over the extensor surface (back) of the upper arm and lymph nodes are palpable medially. For the anterior elbow stand in front of the patient and observe the cubital fossa for swelling. Ask the patient to pronate (palm facing down) and supinate hands (palm facing up) (Figure 6.5)

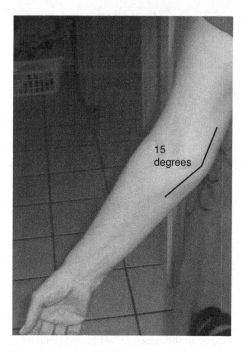

FIGURE 6.1. Elbow carrying angle of 15° in a female subject.

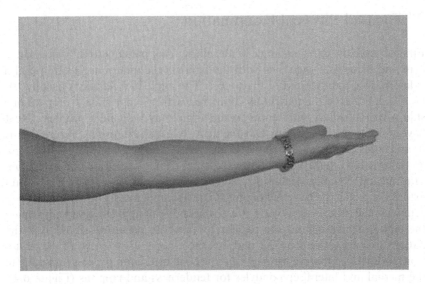

FIGURE 6.2. Elbow extension.

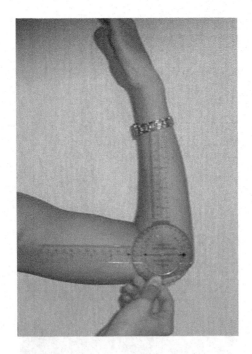

FIGURE 6.3. Elbow flexion to 90° measured with a goniometer.

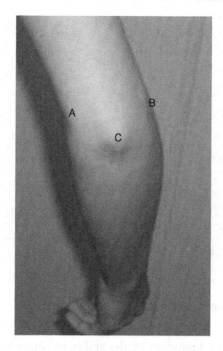

FIGURE 6.4. Posterior elbow. (A) Medical epicondyle; (B) lateral epicondyle; (C) olecrenon.

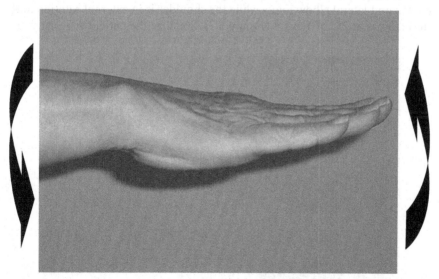

Pronation   Supination

FIGURE 6.5. Supination and pronation.

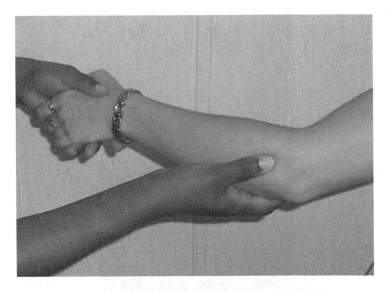

FIGURE 6.6. Radial head palpation.

to see if there is any limitation of the ability to rotate 80° to 85° in either direction. Palpate the radial head (Figure 6.6) for tenderness and while palpating pronate and supinate the hand to see if the pain is increased. Test the collateral ligaments for stability. Apply a valgus and then a varus force to the medial and lateral elbow joints while the shoulder is in external rotation and the elbow is at 25° of flexion (Figure 6.7). Stabilize the patient's arm at your

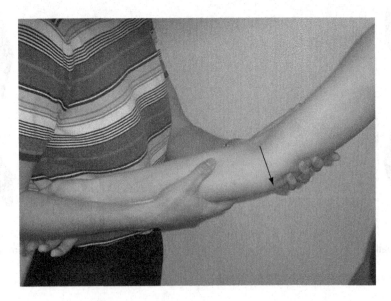

FIGURE 6.7. Valgus stress for medial (ulnar) collateral ligament stability.

side. Place one hand on the lateral side of the lower arm and grasp the posterior elbow with the palm of your hand along the lateral joint line and exert a valgus force on the lateral elbow to evaluate the degree of medial instability. Apply a varus force to the medial joint to test lateral stability.

3. Case

3.1. History

A 68-year-old woman comes to your office with pain in her right elbow. She reports that she fell on her outstretched hand last evening. She was unable to sleep very well because of the pain. Examination reveals she is holding her elbow in 90° of flexion with her left hand. Any attempt to flex or extend her elbow is resisted and she is tender over the radial head (see Figure 6.6). Pronation and supination are also difficult for her to perform (see Figure 6.5). She has no pain or limitation of movement of her shoulder and wrist. There is no gross deformity. There is no numbness, tinkling, or loss of neurological function. No vascular deficit is noted. X-rays of the elbow reveals a possible fat pad sign on the lateral film.

3.2. Thinking Process

At age 68, osteopenia (thin bones) is more likely, especially in a woman. Osteopenia increases the risk of a fracture. Falling on the outstretched hand is associated with fractures because of significant force transferred to the scaphoid bone in the wrist, the radial head in the elbow, and the humeral head in the shoulder. Falling on the outstretched hand may transmit 90% of body weight across the radial head when the hand is pronated. Elbow dislocations can also occur after falling on the outstretched hand but a deformity is usually present and the pain is usually so extreme the patient seeks immediate medical attention.

Age may determine location of fractures. The neck of the humerus is more susceptible to fracture in the older age group. The radial head can fracture in all ages except the very young and scaphoid fracture is more common in patients between age 20 and 50. A fracture in more than one of these areas at the same time is also possible. Adequate examination of all three anatomic areas is important. Elbow fractures can be associated with neurovascular compromise secondary to the swelling or a displaced facture. As noted previously, there is no loss of motor or sensory function and the radial pulses are bounding and equal bilaterally.

Humeral neck fracture is associated with the pain in the upper shoulder and difficulty in abducting the shoulder. The patient has no tenderness in the shoulder and can abduct (see Figure 5.3) with no shoulder pain. She has no pain with ulnar deviation of the wrist and no pain in her anatomic snuffbox (see Figure 7.10). The pain over the radial head accompanied by pain with supination and pronation is indicative of radial head pathology. The most likely diagnosis is a fractured elbow, with the radial head being the most likely bone involved.

Plain film X-rays, anteroposterior (AP) and lateral, are indicated. Radial head fractures are common and occur in 17% to 19% of all elbow trauma and account for 33% of all elbow fractures. The fractures are divided into four types:

- Type I: undisplaced
- Type II: displaced (marginal or neck fracture)
- Type III: comminuted
- Type IV: radial head fracture with associated dislocation

Type I undisplaced fractures are difficult to see on plain film X-ray but intra-articular bleeding or effusion may displace the fat pad posteriorly, producing a radiolucent area behind the lower humerus on the lateral X-ray. This is the fat pad sign. In the pediatric age group the fat pad sign usually means supracondylar fracture. In adults, it usually is associated with radial head fractures. No additional studies like magnetic resonance imaging (MRI) or computerized tomography (CT) are usually required when assessing elbow fractures in the primary care setting.

3.3. Treatment

Type I undisplaced fractures (which this patient probably has) are best treated with 5 to 7 days of splinting with a sling and encouraging early motion. The first few days use ice to reduce swelling and Tylenol or nonsteroidal anti-inflammatory drug (NSAIDs) to reduce discomfort. After the first week, gradually remove the arm from the sling and begin flexion and extension exercises (see suggested elbow exercises at the end of this chapter). Many of these patients end up with difficulty completely extending, so encourage extension. Consulting a physical therapist to help the rehabilitation program is beneficial. This patient was treated with a sling for 7 days. She gradually was able to keep the arm out of the sling in an additional week. After 3 weeks she was pain-free and able to perform all her ADL. She did have a 15° limitation of extension at that time. She was treated by a physical therapist for an additional 3 weeks and now has a normal ROM of her elbow.

Type II, III, and IV radial head fractures should be referred to the orthopedist. Some of these fractures may require operative therapy and/or manipulation. Supracondylar fractures are not as common as radial head fractures in adults but are more common in children and adolescents. Supracondylar fracture may be associated with neurovascular compromise. The orthopedic surgeon should evaluate these types of fractures.

4. Dislocations of the Elbow

Dislocation of the elbow is the most common type of dislocation in children and secondmost common in adults, second only to shoulder dislocation. Sports activities account for the majority of the dislocations. The majority of the dislocations are posterior. The usual history is extreme pain, swelling, and inability to bend the arm after a fall on the outstretched hand. Neurovascular injury is common, so evaluation of the radial pulse and tests for sensation in the palmar and dorsal surfaces of the hand and fingers should be performed in all elbow dislocations. Motor evaluation is more difficult because extreme pain limits the patient's ability to flex and extend the lower arm.

The elbow should be reduced as soon as possible. Infusing lidocaine into the hematoma facilitates the reduction. Once adequate anesthesia is obtained, have an assistant hold the patient's upper arm to provide counter-traction. Grab the patient's hand and forearm and apply steady firm traction. Both you and the patient usually feel the reduction. After the reduction have the patient pronate and supinate the hand and gently extend and flex the elbow to determine the ability to move in all directions. Next, obtain a postre-duction X-ray to access for adequacy of reduction, intra-articular loose bodies, and fractures (radial head fractures occur in 10% of dislocations). Obtain an orthopedic consultation if there is X-ray evidence of any of these three.

Once complete reduction is obtained, apply a posterior splint extending from the wrist to just below the axilla for 10 days. No elbow splint should remain on for more than 3 weeks as prolonged immobilization produces elbow contracture. Once the splint is removed the patient should begin ROM exercises. A physical therapist can help with decreasing the chances of loosing the ability to extend and flex the elbow.

5. Nursemaids' Elbow (Subluxation of the Annular Ligament)

This common problem usually occurs in children 2 to 3 years of age. But it has been reported between the ages of 9 months and 7 years. Some young children have more lax joints so they are more susceptible to this occurring. The typical history is that of a parent, babysitter, or older sibling pulling or swinging the child with the hand pronated and the elbow fully extended. This longitudinal traction on the upper extremity causes the radial head to move distally and the annular ligament of the elbow slides over the radial head and becomes partially entrapped in the radiohumeral joint. The child will no longer move that arm and the arm is held in a flexed position with the hand pronated (palm facing the floor). The child refuses to move the hand.

The child will cry and resist any examination. If the history is classical, the child is holding the arm and hand in the classical position and no reasons exist to suspect any other type of problem. Tell parents the diagnosis and explain your treatment plan. The best treatment is to forgo the examination and have the parent hold the child while you rotate the hand and forearm to a supinated position with pressure over the radial head and flex the elbow. This usually reduces the annular ligament and restores normal use of the extremity but not for a few minutes. Inform the parents the child will cry after the manipulation and will be afraid to move the arm. The examiner can leave the room for a few minutes. By the time you return, the child will be using the arm normally and you are now a hero. Occasionally, if the injury is more than a few hours old it may take more than one try to relocate the ligament. Radiographs are not necessary before or after the reduction unless some other type of injury is suspected. Occasionally, the child may be sent to have an X-ray before reduction and the technologist will reduce it by placing the hand in supination. Being familiar with the usual presentation of nurse-maids' elbow eliminates the need for the X-ray.

6. Case

6.1. History

A 43-year-old right-handed male painter presents to your office with a 4-month history of right lateral elbow pain. He has no history of acute trauma. The pain is increasing in intensity and is limiting his ability to work. When he awakens, the pain is less but as the day goes on it is worse. It is a dull aching pain over the lateral elbow that occasionally radiates up to the middle of the arm and down to the wrist. He notes increasing difficulty in grasping the paintbrush and in shaking hands. His grasp is weaker and grasping of any type causes pain especially toward the end of his workday. Physical examination reveals no gross observed deformities. Palpation produces pain over the vicinity of the lateral epicondyle where the wrist extensor muscles attach (Figure 6.8). Resisted wrist extension produced significant pain with the elbow fully extended (Figure 6.9). Less pain was produced when the elbow was flexed 90°.

6.2. Thinking Process

The lack of a history of trauma and the 4-month history of symptoms that are worse as the workday progresses suggest an occupational overuse syndrome. The lateral elbow location of the symptoms makes lateral epicondylitis likely. This diagnosis is confirmed by an increase in the pain with resisted wrist extension with the elbow in full extension and/or partial flexion. Early on in the disease process the pain is only present in full elbow extension. As the disease progresses the pain is present in flexion although usually not as severe. Equally severe pain in both flexion and extension indicates a more

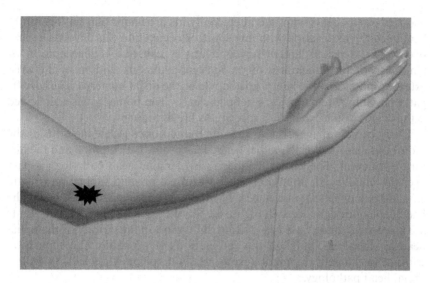

FIGURE 6.8. Point of maximal tenderness in lateral epicondylitis.

significant problem that will require more extensive measures to treat. A test that will confirm the diagnosis has been called the chair test. Ask the patient to try to lift a chair with the elbow extended, hand pronated, and the shoulder adducted. Significant pain and inability to lift the chair is diagnostic of lateral epicondylitis.

Lateral epicondylitis, or tennis elbow, is the most common elbow problem seen in primary care. The term tennis elbow is a misleading term as only

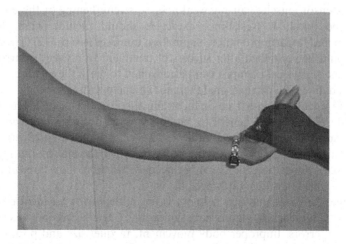

FIGURE 6.9. Resisted wrist extension for lateral epicondylitis.

about 5% of patients with lateral epicondylitis are tennis players. The problem is seen in association with any sport or occupation that involves repetitive wrist extension. Lateral epicondylitis is caused by degeneration or tendinosis of the attachment of the musculotendinous tendons of the wrist extensor muscles to the lateral epicondyle of the distal humerus. The specific pathophysiology remains to be defined clearly. The primary muscle involved is the origin of the extensor carpi radialis brevis muscle.

The only other diagnosis that should be entertained is osteoarthritis of the radiocapitellar joint or the radial head. This is not that common and the history is different. The key to the diagnosis of radial head pathology is pain over the radial head, limitation of elbow pronation, and supination (Figure 6.5) and pain with that movement. The radial head is palpated just below the lateral epicondyle, as noted in Figure 6.6. As the extensor muscle attachments are in close proximity, it is easy to find discomfort in the vicinity of the radial head in lateral epicondylitis. But the motions of pronation and supination will not be limited or produce pain in lateral epicondylitis as they will in radial head pathology.

The vast majority of the time no additional studies are needed to make the diagnosis of lateral epicondylitis. If you suspect radiocapitellar osteoarthritis because of difficulty with elbow pronation and supination, plain film imaging will be needed. Magnetic resonance imaging is rarely indicated.

6.3. Treatment

The initial treatment goals are to decrease pain and inflammation. Therapy begins with activity modification, ice massage, and NSAIDs. Limit any recreational or occupational activity that requires repeated wrist extension. An exercise program should also begin with the initial visit. Start with passive and active ROM exercises of the wrist and elbow. Pain decreases firing of the extensor muscles causing weakness, so strengthening of these muscles should be initiated. Resistance exercises should include wrist flexion–extension and forearm pronation–supination exercises (see p. 112). These exercises should be continued after successful treatment to prevent recurrence of symptoms. A physical therapist can be consulted to teach the exercises and use other modalities. An occupational therapist can help with job-specific exercises.

Steroid injections with 1 cc of local anesthetic and 1 cc of a long-acting corticosteroid can be of benefit to patients who do not respond to conservative measures. Use a sterile technique and a 3-cc syringe with a 25-gauge needle. Identify the area of maximum tenderness for the site of the injection (Figure 6.8). Repeat injections may be needed. No more than three injections should be given in a 12-month period.

A trainer or coach may also help in treating athletes who are involved in racquet sports. Some tennis players have symptoms of lateral epicondylitis because of training errors. Improper body movement, racquet size and position, and one-hand backhand strokes increase stress on the extensor muscles. Measuring for racquet size and learning proper body movement and types of strokes will reduce and eliminate lateral elbow pain in many recreational athletes.

Counterforce bracing can also be used. The brace is applied just distal to the elbow over the extensor muscles origin. The brace provides a constraint over the extensor musculature and distributes forces to nondiseased portions of the extensors.

Indication for surgical intervention is a failure to improve after completing a well-controlled nonoperative treatment program. About 5% of patients with lateral epicondylitis will require surgery. A minimum of 6 to 12 months of nonoperative treatment is recommended before considering surgery. Both open and arthroscopic options can be considered. Good results are expected in the hands of an experienced surgeon.

7. Medial Epicondylitis

Medial epicondylitis, also known as medial tennis elbow or golfer's elbow, is less common than lateral epicondylitis. It is caused by overuse of the flexor and pronator muscles that attach to the medial epicondyle. Overuse occurs with any activity that produces a valgus stress on the medial joint line (see Figure 6.12). Racquet sports, golf, and throwing sports are examples of activities that are associated with medial epicondylitis. The history is usually one of a dull ache over the medial elbow and an occupation or sport that requires repeated elbow pronation–supination or flexion–extension. Examination will reveal tenderness over the medial epicondyle and medial elbow pain with resisted wrist flexion (Figure 6.10). This is in contrast to lateral epicondylitis where the pain is located on the lateral side and is increased with resisted wrist extension (Figure 6.9). Care should be taken to evaluate the ulnar collateral ligament (UCL) and the ulnar nerve. This will be discussed further in Section 10 (Ulnar collateral ligament injury) and Section 11 (Ulnar Nerve Injury (Cubital Tunnel Syndrome)).

Radiographs are usually not needed unless fractures are suspected. Treatment is similar to lateral epicondylitis and includes activity modification, ice massage, NSAIDs, resistance exercises, and corticosteroid injections. Mechanical analysis of sport or occupation technique may provide diagnostic and therapeutic information.

8. Olecrenon Bursitis

The position of the olecrenon (see Figure 6.4) and its overlying bursa makes it susceptible to injury. Bursitis in this area has also been called student's elbow and miner's elbow. These occupations are noted for a large amount of time spent leaning on the elbows. The bursitis can be either acute or chronic.

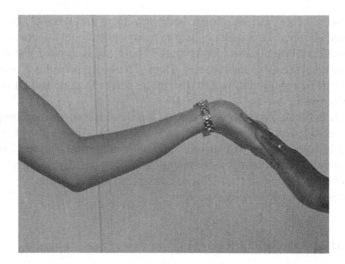

FIGURE 6.10. Resisted wrist flexion for medial epicondylitis.

Acute bursitis can be caused by prolonged pressure or repeated trauma. The fluid can either be clear or hemorrhagic. Initial therapy includes ice, NSAIDs, a compression ace wrap, and elimination of the causative factors. If the bursa is tense and painful it can be aspirated. Elbow pads should be used in any occupation that requires prolonged pressure or repeated trauma to the olecrenon area of the elbow.

Chronic bursitis is characterized by thickening of the bursal walls. Repeated trauma leads to the formation of granulation tissue that grows into the bursal sac. Examination will reveal a firm rubbery mass that may or may not be fluid filled. The history is usually one of repeated trauma like falling on the elbow. There may have been an acute traumatic episode superimposed on chronic bursal disease. Treatment is similar to acute bursitis except the occasional patient that might need surgical excision of the bursa.

Suppurative or septic bursitis is not as common as acute and chronic bursitis. Bacteria can be introduced into the bursa from a puncture wound or a laceration. Erythema, warmth, bursal distention, significant pain, and limitation of motion may be present. Aspiration and identification of the organism, most often staphylococcus, followed by antibiotics is appropriate treatment. Suppurative bursitis, on some occasions, has resulted from an aspiration for acute traumatic bursitis. The blood-filled bursa is an ideal culture medium for bacteria introduced by the aspiration.

Both acute bursitis and suppurative bursitis can cause warmth but the fluid is usually bloody or clear in acute bursitis and cloudy in suppurative. Gout and pseudogout can also present with fluid in the olecrenon bursa. So an analysis of the fluid for crystals, white blood cell (WBC) type, and bacteria is appropriate when you are suspicious of one of these entities.

Aspiration of the bursa should be done under sterile conditions. There should be adequate cleansing of the area and gloves and sterile instruments should be used. Also use an 18-gauge needle because the fluid may be too thick for aspiration with a smaller gauge needle.

9. Case

9.1. History

A 13-year-old right-handed boy presents to your office with elbow pain. He is a pitcher on the baseball team and has noted increased pain as the season has progressed. Initially the pain was vague and only occurred after a game that he pitched. The pain now appears after he pitches two to three innings and he is not able to finish the game. The pain is now localized in the medial aspect of his right elbow. He also complains of pain with twisting motions and flexion of the right elbow. Examination reveals a 10° limitation of elbow extension and an ability to flex only to 100°. Tenderness is noted over the medial epicondyle and the cubital tunnel (area between the olecrenon and the medial epicondyle). Tapping over the cubital tunnel produces some tingling, radiating down to the fifth digit. No other neurological deficit is noted. Valgus stress (see Figure 6.7) of the elbow in 25° of flexion reveals some laxity compared with the left elbow.

9.2. Thinking Process

The first thing that comes to mind in this case is little leaguer's elbow. Little leaguer's elbow unfortunately has become a term that includes any elbow problem that occurs in a young throwing athlete. This wastebasket diagnosis does not help properly diagnose and treat this boy. Three entities—Panner's disease, OCD, and medial epicondyle traction apophysitis (META)—need to be considered in a young athlete with elbow pain. The age of the patient and the location of the pain help start the process of differentiating the three entities. Panner's disease and OCD are problems that result in lateral elbow pain whereas the epicondyle traction apophysitis results in medial pain. Panner's disease is a problem of young children between 7 and 10 years of age and OCD occurs most commonly in 13- to 16-year-olds (see p. 111). The age of occurrence of META is dependent on the skeletal maturation of the athlete and occurs between 11 and 16 years of age. Once the medial epicondyle fuses the ligamentous structures are more susceptible to injury, and medial (ulnar) collateral ligament injury is more likely. With the location of the pain on the medial side and the age of the patient, META is more likely. Osteochondritis dissecans is still possible and an X-ray will help rule out OCD. The laxity on valgus stress probably indicates some separation of the medial epicondyle from the rest of the humerus. The tingling noted when the cubital tunnel is

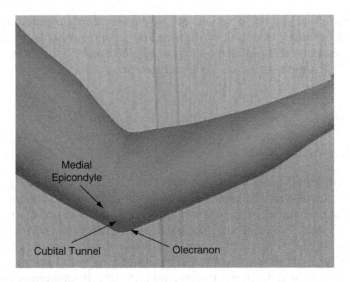

FIGURE 6.11. Medial elbow with landmarks.

tapped (Figure 6.11) is associated with pressure on the ulnar nerve. The nerve is located just below the medial epicondyle under the medial collateral ligament. Swelling in the area places pressure on the nerve and causes ulnar nerve symptoms.

The stresses placed on the elbow joint by throwing sports provide an explanation for the above-mentioned clinical problems. Throwing motion is not simple flexion and extension. The elbow goes through significant medial and lateral stress that can stretch or tear the ulnar (medial) collateral ligament and radial (lateral) collateral ligament and fracture the distal portions of the humerus and the proximal portions of the radius and ulna. When the growth plates are not closed, portions of bone can be separated (avulsed) from the distal humerus. These stresses can be appreciated by taking your own arm or a patient's through the throwing motion while palpating the medial and lateral joints. Figure 6.12 demonstrates the locations of the medial and lateral joints and their collateral ligaments as well as the capitellum and trochlea of the humerus and the radial head and ulna. As the arm is brought into the cocked position the articulation between the capitellum and the radial head is impacted together (Panner's disease and OCD) and the medial side UCL or the medial epicondyle is pulled (META). As the arm is now accelerated, the object released, and deceleration begins, the lateral side radial collateral ligament is now stretched and the bony articulation between the ulna and the humeral trochlea is impacted together. During this phase the radial head impacts with the capitellum because of pronation. This is especially true when attempting to throw a curve ball. It is easy then to see how collateral ligament injury as well as micro- and macrobone fractures can occur.

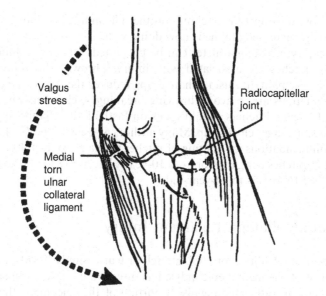

FIGURE 6.12. Mechanism of injury in throwing sports. (Reproduced from Richmond J, Shahady E, eds. *Sports Medicine for Primary Care.* Cambridge, MA: Blackwell Science; 1996:354, with permission.)

Understanding the mechanism helps explain the why and also offers thoughts on prevention and treatment.

Plain films are a necessity with these types of problems. Avulsion or fragmentation of the medial epicondyle will be noted in META. Always request a film of the opposite side to compare for differences as well as normal variants in the skeletal immature athlete. Multiple views are recommended to rule out the presence of loose bodies. Bone scan, CT scans, and MRI may be helpful. These more expensive entities should be reserved for those patients who do not respond to conservative treatment or have more extensive disease on plain films.

9.3. Treatment

Medial epicondyle traction apophysitis can usually be treated with conservative measures depending on the amount of separation observed on the X-ray. If the avulsion is 5 mm or greater, surgery may be indicated. The above patient had minimal separation and was treated with 3 weeks of no throwing, ice, and NSAIDs. Steroid injections are never indicated. He was allowed to be a pinch hitter during the 3 weeks and encouraged to maintain general conditioning so that he remained fit. After the 3 weeks he was gradually allowed to return to activity. Range of motion and resistance exercises to strengthen the flexors are indicated. He was first allowed to play outfield and then after

4 weeks allowed to start his pitching routine. The number of innings pitched was gradually increased and he is now doing well.

Elbow injury in young athletes can be prevented. Pitching technique and number of pitches are associated with injury. Throwing breaking pitches increases elbow pain and using change-ups reduces the rate of elbow pain. Recommendations are to avoid throwing breaking pitches between the ages of 9 and 14 years. Pitchers should focus on fastball and change-up pitches, avoiding a split-finger change-up. Many authors agree with the *USA Baseball News* recommendations for limiting of pitches per game to the following: limits of 52 ± 15 pitches per game for 8- to 10-year-olds, 68 ± 18 for 11- to 12-year-olds, and 76 ± 16 for 13- to 14-year-olds.

10. Ulnar Collateral Ligament Injury

The mechanism of injury for UCL stretch or tear is similar to META. If the growth plate of the medial epicondyle has fused, valgus stress will stretch or tear the ligament rather than avulse a portion of the epicondyle that occurs in META. These patients are older, usually young adults, who are engaged in throwing sports. Symptoms and examination are similar to META. If UCL rupture occurs the patient may report a sudden event and loss of function. The hallmark of UCL rupture is valgus instability. Stability of the ligament can be accessed by applying a valgus force to the medial joint while the shoulder is in external rotation and the elbow is at 25° of flexion (see Figure 6.7). The arm is stabilized by placing the patient's hand in your armpit, one hand on the lateral side to exert the valgus force and the other on the medial joint line to assess the degree of instability. Treatment depends on the expectations for returning to competitive competition. Surgical management is indicated if the patient wishes to return to competitive overhead throwing. Conservative treatment with ice, NSAIDs, and splinting followed by stretching and strengthening exercises is usually sufficient for treatment if return to competition is not contemplated. It also can be attempted for recreational throwing athletes for a 3- to 6-month period.

11. Ulnar Nerve Injury (Cubital Tunnel Syndrome)

The ulnar nerve is susceptible to injury with trauma to the medial side of the elbow. The ulnar nerve enters the cubital tunnel behind the medial epicondyle. The tunnel is made up of the UCL and other lateral ligamentous structures. The nerve is vulnerable to injury from traction, compression, and direct trauma that accompanies any problem that involves the medial complex. This includes META, UCL rupture, and medial epicondylitis. Common symptoms are medial elbow pain that is increased with flexion, numbness and tingling of the fourth and fifth digits, and a positive Tinel's sign (tingling induced by tapping over the cubital tunnel, Figure 6.11). Treatment is symptomatic and aimed at the primary condition that has produced the compression or edema. If this treatment is not successful or ulnar motor nerve weakness is present surgical correction may be needed.

12. Panner's Disease

Children of age 7 to 10 are affected and complain of lateral elbow pain with throwing. The repetitive force of throwing compresses the radial head into the capitellum. The disorder affects the ossification center. Initially there is necrosis or degeneration of the ossification center followed by regeneration and recalcification. Physical examination will reveal pain over the lateral joint between the capitellum and radial head (Figure 6.12). Range of motion is usually not limited. The diagnosis is made by X-ray. The capitellar ossification center is fragmented and the epiphysis is irregular and smaller compared with the opposite elbow. This is usually a self-limited problem. Discontinuation of throwing, ice, and NSAIDs will produce relief of symptoms. Follow-up X-rays are needed to document healing. The capitellar epiphysis usually remodels and returns to a normal appearance. The child can usually return to throwing within a 6- to 8-week period.

13. Osteochondritis Dissecans

Osteochondritis dissecans (OD) is a more serious problem than Panner's disease that affects young adolescents between 13 and 16 years of age. The cause is thought to be a combination of repetitive stress to the radiocapitellar joint and an interruption of the vascular flow to the capitellum. Both throwing athletes and gymnasts are susceptible to OD. The story is one of gradual onset of lateral elbow pain, clicking, locking, and decreased ROM. The pain increases with throwing or in a gymnast with routines that rely on the arms to bear all the weight of the body like hanging from a bar by the hands. Examination will reveal lateral joint line tenderness and limitation of flexion and extension. With the elbow in full extension, pain may be elicited with attempts to pronate and supinate because of radial head involvement. Plain X-rays commonly show the characteristic radiolucent focal defect in the capitellum. If this is noted a loose body may be present. If the defect is present without a loose body noted, a CT scan with contrast should be obtained to search for the loose body. Magnetic resonance imaging can help with early identification of OD. Because of the poorer prognosis with OD a consultation with an orthopedic surgeon is recommended if you suspect OD.

14. Medical Problems

14.1. Rheumatoid Arthritis

Elbow involvement occurs in at least half the patients with rheumatoid arthritis. Soft tissue abnormalities such as joint swelling, olecrenon bursitis and rheumatoid nodules along the extensor surfaces, warmth, and tenderness are the earliest findings. Another early finding, often unnoticed by the patient, is a loss of full extension. Symptoms isolated only to the elbow are a rare occurrence. The majority of the time, rheumatoid symptoms are also present in the shoulders, hands, and wrist as well as the elbow. Early recognition is critical to limiting deformity. Early referral to a physician who can administer disease-modifying drugs is indicated.

14.2. Osteoarthritis

Osteoarthritis is not common in the elbow as it is not a weight-bearing joint. If present it is caused by post-traumatic overuse. Loss of motion rather than pain is what prompts the patient to seek medical attention. Osteophytes and loose bodies will be noted on plain film radiographs. Treatment is symptomatic. Surgical decompression is sometimes required to restore functional motion.

14.3. Other Medical Problems

Gout and pseudogout need to be considered when there is a joint effusion. Gout or pseudogout should be suspected if the effusion is acute and other joints like the big toe (gout) or the shoulder (pseudogout) are involved. Examination of aspirated fluid for crystals should be included if either disease is suspected.

15. Elbow Exercises

Tell patients to perform these exercises two times a day. Rotate from one exercise to the other. Do one set of one exercises and then rotate to another exercise and do a set. Do not exercise past the point of pain. Pain means stop.

1. **Wrist range of motion (Figure 6.13A and 6.13B)**: Bend your wrist forward and backward as far as you can. Hold each movement for 5 seconds (s) and repeat 10 times.
2. **Wrist flexion stretch (Figure 6.14)**: With the injured hand in 30° of flexion begin to flex the wrist against the resistance of the other hand. Resist the movement for 15 s and repeat five times.
3. **Wrist extension stretch (Figure 6.15)**: With the injured hand in 30° of extension, begin to flex the wrist against the resistance of the other hand. Resist the movement for 15 s and repeat five times.

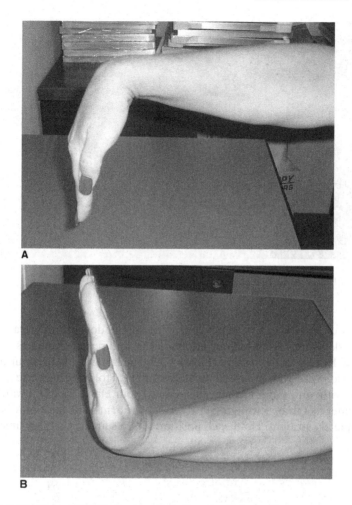

FIGURE 6.13. (A and B) Wrist range of motion.

4. **Wrist flexion exercise (Figure 6.16)**: Hold a weight like a can of soup with your palm facing up. Flex the wrist (bend it upward), hold wrist in maximum flexion for 15 s, and return to the starting position slowly. Repeat five times.

5. **Wrist extension exercise (Figure 6.17)**: Hold weight like a can of soup with your palm facing down. Extend the wrist (bend up) and hold in maximum extension for 15 s. Return to the starting position slowly and repeat five times.

6. **Wrist radial and ulnar deviation strengthening (Figure 6.18A and 6.18B)**: Hold a weight like a can of soup in your hand with your thumb facing up

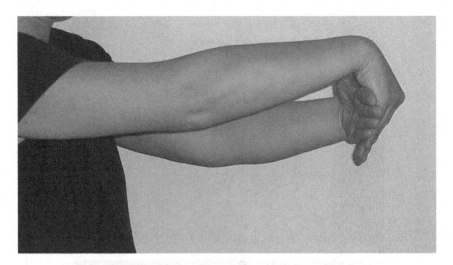

FIGURE 6.14. Wrist flexion stretch.

and your wrist sideways. Move your wrist up and down through radial and ulnar deviation. Hold each position for 15 s and repeat five times.

7. **Elbow flexion and extension (Figure 6.19A and 6.19B)**: Place your arm at your side with your elbow completely straight. Hold a weight like a can of soup with your palm face up. Flex (bend) your elbow slowly toward your shoulder as far as it will go. Slowly lower the arm until the elbow is again completely straight. Hold each position for 15 s and repeat five times.

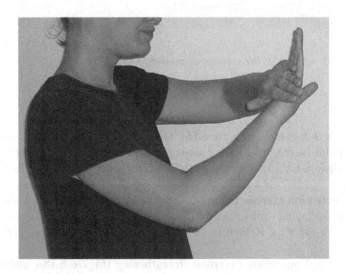

FIGURE 6.15. Wrist extension stretch.

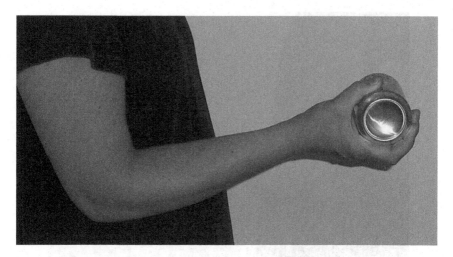

FIGURE 6.16. Wrist flexion exercise.

8. **Pronation and supination of the forearm (Figure 6.20A and 6.20B)**: Place
   your elbow at your side and bend the elbow 90°. Rotate the hand from a
   palm-upward to palm-downward position. Hold each position for 15 s and
   repeat five times. Add a weight like a soup can once the movements can be
   performed easily without a weight.

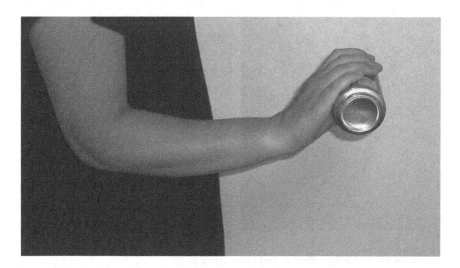

FIGURE 6.17. Wrist extension exercise.

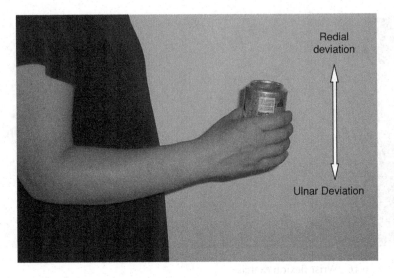

FIGURE 6.18. Wrist radial and ulnar deviation strengthening.

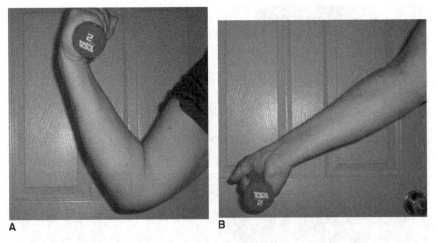

FIGURE 6.19. (A) Elbow flexion and (B) extension.

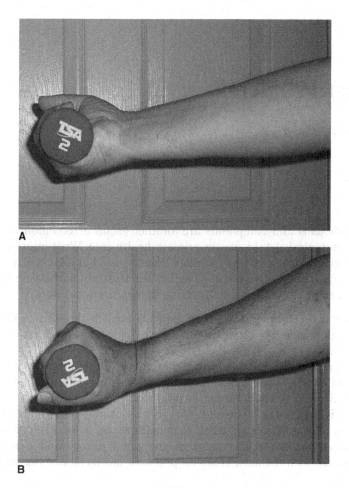

FIGURE 6.20. (A) Pronation and (B) supination of the forearm.

Suggested Readings

1. Lyman S, Fleisig G, Andrews J, Osinski E. Effect of pitch type, pitch count, and pitching mechanics on risk of elbow and shoulder pain in youth baseball pitchers. *Am J Sports Med.* 2002;30(4):463–468.
2. Andrews J, Fleisig G. How many pitches should I allow my child to throw? *USA Baseball News.* 1996;4:5.

7

Wrist Problems

Edward J. Shahady

Wrist problems and complaints are another group of common and frustrating musculoskeletal issues in primary health care. Wrist injuries can be intimidating because of the complex anatomy and concern for potential long-term disability. Overcoming the fear and frustration of caring for wrist injury becomes possible with a few simple organizational steps:

1. Step 1 is to realize that 95% of patients seen in the office with wrist-complaints can be classified into three categories and six to seven problems.
2. Step 2 is to take a focused history that segments the categories into acute trauma, overuse trauma, and medical disease. You now have a manageable list (Table 7.1) to begin further investigation.
3. Step 3 is to perform a focused thorough wrist examination. With a focused history and a thorough wrist examination you most likely now have the diagnosis. Your knowledge of the usual history and examination associated with the most common problems has facilitated the diagnostic process.
4. Step 4 is ordering confirmatory studies if needed (many times they are not).
5. Step 5 is to start treatment. (This may include appropriate consultation.) Five percent of the time the diagnosis will not be so obvious. However, not being one of the 95% is usually obvious. That is when additional studies and/or a consultation becomes necessary.

Rare or not so frequent problems are usually the ones that receive the most press. How often do you hear the words "I got burned once" mentioned about a rare problem that was missed in the primary care setting. Having a good working knowledge of the characteristics of common problems provides an excellent background to help recognize the uncommon. The uncommon is easy to recognize once you know the common. Be driven by the search for the common rather than the expensive intimidating search for the rare birds.

TABLE 7.1. Classification of common wrist problems.

Overuse trauma
- Carpal tunnel syndrome
- De Quervain's tenosynovitis
- Other tendonitis

Acute trauma
- Fractured scaphoid bone of the wrist
- Scapholunate ligament rupture
- Wrist sprain

Medical problems
- Arthritis associated with other diseases like rheumatoid arthritis

1. Focused History

The first question is whether the onset of the problem was acute. Did it just start or has it been present for a prolonged period of time? The next question would depend on the answer to the first. If the onset is acute, then ask about a fall, especially one that involved breaking the fall with the outstretched hand (a common mechanism in wrist injury). If the onset is not acute, ask about occupations, hobbies, or sports that involve repeated wrist movement like computer use, painting, and throwing sports. A recent change in occupation or intensity of activity is also important. Ask about any chronic disease. Wrist pain can accompany collagen vascular diseases like rheumatoid arthritis.

2. Focused Physical Examination

Begin by asking the patient to go through four motions without your help. This examination establishes a marker for severity of the injury and a baseline to assess degree of recovery. The four wrist motions are ulnar deviation (Figure 7.1); radial deviation (Figure 7.2); wrist extension (Figure 7.3); and wrist flexion (Figure 7.4).

It is important to start every examination by defining range of motion (ROM) and noting any difference between one wrist and another. Use a goniometer to precisely assess degrees of motion. The remaining examination will be dictated by the focused history.

3. Case

3.1. History

A 33-year-old female secretary presents to your office with right wrist pain for the past 6 months. It was relieved by taking a few ibuprofen tablets but now the pain is persistent and makes it difficult for her to type. She also notes

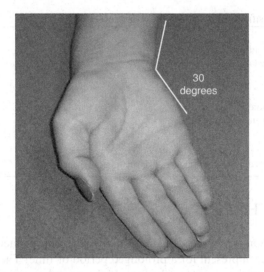

FIGURE 7.1. Ulnar deviation; 30° is normal.

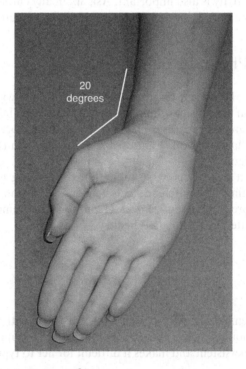

FIGURE 7.2. Radial deviation; 20° is normal.

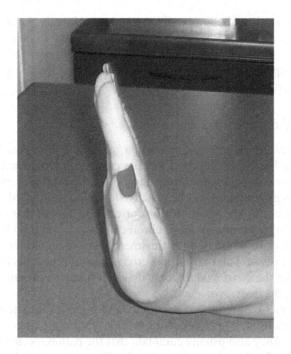

FIGURE 7.3. Wrist extension; normal is up to 80°.

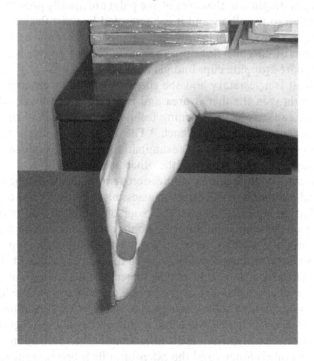

FIGURE 7.4. Wrist flexion; normal is up to 80°.

some weakness when she grasps objects and occasionally she drops her coffee cup. She is frustrated by her inability to open jars or twist off lids. She feels like she is an old woman before her time. She reports no falls and she has no other complaints. Her general health is excellent. She is a power walker and takes no medications.

3.2. Thinking Process

The lack of a fall or other acute trauma makes the diagnosis listed under acute trauma less likely. Still perform the examination maneuvers to assess for trauma as some patients forget the fall that occurred some time ago. Probably this examination will be negative for acute trauma. Medical causes are also unlikely, as she has no history of chronic disease that suggests this. If this is the first sign of a systemic chronic disease, it will soon become obvious by a lack of response to your treatment and appearance of other symptoms of that disease. This makes an overuse syndrome most likely. Additional questions and the wrist examination that will focus on overuse syndromes should make the diagnosis.

Carpal tunnel syndrome is a possibility and it has a characteristic history. These patients usually have occupations that require prolonged or repeated wrist flexion. They also usually complain that the pain is located on the palm of the hand in the thenar area (thumb side). The pain may radiate the elbow. Numbness and tingling in that area of the palm are usually present. The pain may radiate up to the elbow and it is aggravated by wrist flexion and extension. These patients may also awaken at night with pain and numbness because the wrist falls into flexion with sleep. Grasping objects is painful and they may report dropping cups and glasses.

This patient is a secretary and she spends 6 h a day with computer data entry. Her pain is in the thenar area and is accompanied by numbness and tingling. She awakens in the morning feeling like she needs to rub or shake her hand to "get the circulation back." The diagnosis of carpal tunnel syndrome is most likely. The physical examination should be preformed to confirm this diagnosis and to rule out the other possibilities.

Carpal tunnel syndrome is a compression neuropathy of the median nerve. The physical examination will focus on assessing the sensory and motor functions of that nerve. First observe the palm of the hand and compare the thenar area of the injured hand to the noninjured hand to look for atrophy. Next, tap over the median nerve at the wrist (Figure 7.5). A positive test (Tinel's sign) is the production of tingling on the palmer surface of the thumb, index finger, and a portion of the middle finger. Test the strength of the thenar muscles by assessing the ability of the thumb to move toward the little finger against resistance (Figure 7.6). Placing the wrists together in maximum flexion (Phalen's test) for 45 s or less will cause numbness or aching. (Figure 7.7).

De Quervain's tenosynovitis is an inflammation of the tendon sheaths of the abductor pollicis longus and the extensor pollicis brevis at the first dorsal

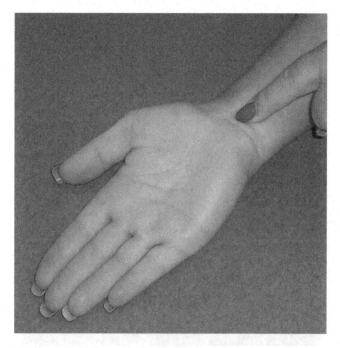

FIGURE 7.5. Median nerve percussion (Tinel's test).

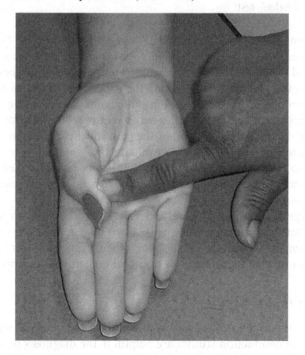

FIGURE 7.6. Thenar muscle strength test.

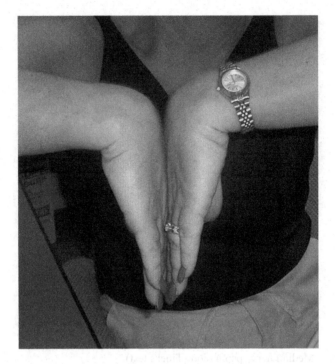

FIGURE 7.7. Phalen's test.

compartment over the radial styloid. These tendons form the floor of the anatomic snuffbox of the wrist (Figure 7.8). Palpate the tendons over the radial styloid and at the floor of the snuffbox for pain and tenderness. Perform Finkelstein's test (Figure 7.9) by asking the patient to ulnar-deviate the wrist with the thumb flexed and abducted into the palm places tension on the tendons and their sheaths. The examiner may have to provide an additional force to complete the test. Reproduction of the pain clinches the diagnosis.

Examination of the snuffbox to evaluate the scaphoid (Figure 7.10) is important to rule out a subtle fracture that has been overlooked from past trauma. How to do this examination will be explained when scaphoid fractures are discussed in Section 7 (Scaphoid Fractures).

This patient had positive Phalen's and Tinel's signs. She had no thenar atrophy and thumb opposition was not weak. Her Finkelstein's test is negative and there is no tenderness over the radial styloid (Figure 7.8). This history and physical examination makes the diagnosis of carpal tunnel syndrome most likely.

3.3. Additional Studies

No further studies are needed at this time unless a scaphoid fracture is suspected. Nerve conduction studies are helpful if the diagnosis is not clear or surgery is a therapeutic consideration.

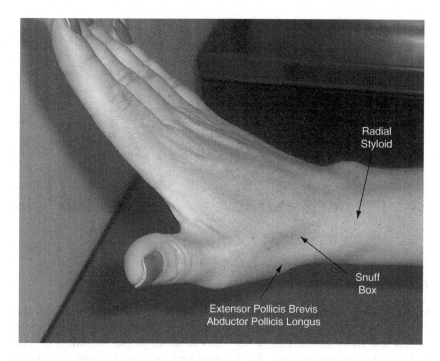

FIGURE 7.8. Anatomic snuffbox area.

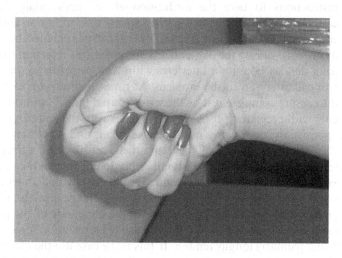

FIGURE 7.9. Finkelstein's test.

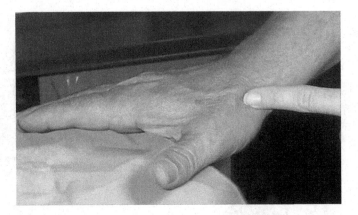

FIGURE 7.10. Examination of the snuffbox for scaphoid fracture.

3.4. Treatment for Carpal Tunnel Syndrome

Most cases will respond to conservative measures. First, identify and decrease the offending activity that is causing the problem. Workstation modifications to decrease wrist flexion can be very beneficial. Examples include adjusting keyboard height and supports for the wrist and forearm. Intermittent breaks from typing every few hours decreases fatigue. If none of these measures work, consider a change in occupation or sport technique. Writing a note to the patient's employer, coach, or teacher explaining how these changes will increase productivity helps patients obtain the cooperation of their superiors. If no contraindication exists, a short course (7 to 10 days) of nonsteroidal anti-inflammatory drugs (NSAIDs) or steroids will help. Be sure to provide the patient instructions to take the medication at the appropriate dose for 7 to 10 days, as described in Chapter 1. Wrist splints to limit flexion and extension are a mainstay of treatment (Figure 7.11). The splint should be worn at night and if needed during the day. Patients are sometimes reluctant to use the splint during the day because it interferes with work performance or they do not want to call attention to the problem. At times, a short-arm cast can be employed to assure complete rest of the wrist. Carpal tunnel syndrome sometimes occurs with pregnancy. It usually terminates with the end of pregnancy and is responsive to conservative measures like splints and steroid injections.

Steroid injections with 1 cc of local anesthetic and 1 cc of a long-acting corticosteroid can be of benefit to patients who do not respond to conservative measures. Use a sterile technique and a 3-cc syringe with a 25-gauge needle. Flex the wrist and identify the wrist flexion crease and the palmaris longus tendon. The needle will be inserted on the ulnar side of the palmaris longus about 1 cm proximal to the wrist crease (Figure 7.12). Some patients do not have a palmaris longus tendon. If this is the case use the ulnar side of the ring finger as a marker to direct the needle. Ask the patient to fully flex

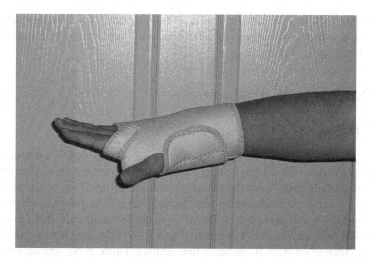

FIGURE 7.11. Wrist splints.

the fingers as noted in Fig. 7.12. Advance the needle at a 45° angle for about 1 cm until you feel resistance. Appropriate location of the needle can be accessed by moving the ring finger. This should produce movement of the needle. Ask the patient to now extend the fingers to bring the needle into the carpal tunnel and slowly inject 1 to 2 cc of the steroid–anesthetic solution. Advice the patient that there will be some mild soreness and it may require 24 h to feel the full effect.

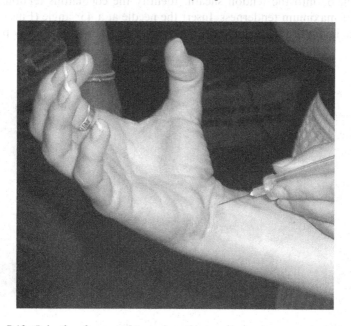

FIGURE 7.12. Injection for carpal tunnel syndrome.

Indications for consultation include no response to treatment after 3 months, persistence numbness or weakness, and thenar atrophy. Surgery may be indicated at this point.

4. De Quervain's Tenosynovitis

4.1. Diagnosis and Treatment

If the patient complains of pain over the radial styloid that is aggravated by attempts to move the thumb or make a fist, suspect de Quervain's. Tenderness will usually be present over the radial styloid and at the floor of the snuffbox (Figure 7.8) and the Finkelstein's test (Figure 7.9) will be positive. The history and physical examination are sufficient to make the diagnosis and usually no additional tests are needed. Attempt to discover the offending activity and work with the patient on ways to decrease that activity. Think about any activity that involves repeated wrist ulnar deviation and thumb flexion. If no contraindication exists, a short course (7 to 10 days) of NSAIDs or steroids should be started.

Splinting of the wrist and the thumb speeds recovery. Use a thumb spica cast if needed. The key is to use a splint that limits thumb movement. The most important motion to prevent is thumb flexion and abduction.

Consider a steroid injection if splinting and medications do not help. Similar to the carpal tunnel use sterile preparation and injection with a 3-cc syringe and 1 to 2 cc of a mixture of lidocaine–steroid. Remember the injection will be into the tendon sheath. Identify the edematous tendon at the point of maximum tenderness. Insert the needle at a 45° angle (Figure 7.13) into the involved tendons. Do not inject into the tendon but slowly pull the

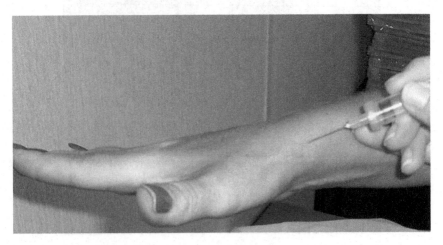

FIGURE 7.13. Injection for de Quervain's tenosynovitis.

needle back and attempt to inject the solution. As soon as the needle comes out of the tendon into the sheath the fluid will flow freely. It is difficult to inject into the tendon when using a 27-gauge needle. Short-term relief occurs because of the local anesthetic but it will take 24 to 36 h for full relief. Some patients may experience a rebound increase in pain for the first day. Ice and Tylenol help reduce this discomfort. Some patients may require more than one injection and in rare cases surgical release is needed.

5. Other Tendonitis

The flexor carpi ulnaris and the flexor carpi radialis can be involved in overuse syndromes. Crepitus and pain with passive wrist extension and resisted flexion are usually noted. The above examinations for carpal tunnel syndrome and de Quervain's disease will be negative and tenderness over the insertions of the tendons on the fifth metacarpal and the second metacarpal respectively will be noted. The patients will respond to splinting, NSAIDs, and a reduction of the offending activity.

6. Case

6.1. History

A 33-year-old healthy man presents to your office with right wrist pain for the last 5 days. Five days ago he fell while taking his daily run. He sustained a laceration to his knee so he went to the emergency room for care of the laceration. He did not notice much pain in the wrist at the time but the next morning he began to note swelling and limited motion of the right wrist. The pain is increasing and he has difficulty shaking hands and gripping is difficult. His past history is negative for wrist problems or any chronic disease. He notes that he broke his fall with his outstretched right hand.

6.2. Thinking Process

Overuse syndromes and medical disease are not likely, given the recent onset of the pain and the history of a fall. The history of falling on the outstretched hand makes scaphoid fracture or scapholunate ligament disruption (SLLD) most likely. Wrist sprain is a diagnosis of exclusion and should not be diagnosed until all other specific diagnoses have been excluded. Many so-called wrist sprains are missed scaphoid fractures or ligamentous disruptions. The examination will help differentiate one from the other and X-rays are needed to confirm the diagnosis. The examination should focus on palpation of the scaphoid (Figure 7.10) with the index finger in the anatomic snuffbox. This will be painful in both scaphoid fracture and SLLD. Ulnar deviation will bring the scaphoid closer to the examining finger and enhance the sensitivity and specificity of the test. Movement of the thumb against resistance will also be painful in scaphoid fractures. When attempting to shake hands patients with a scaphoid fracture are reluctant to grasp with their thumb. The patient with de Quervain's tenosynovitis will also have pain in the snuffbox area that will be aggravated by ulnar deviation but the tenderness is on the radial styloid or the ligaments of the floor of the snuffbox. All these landmarks are noted in Figure 7.8.

The examination in SLLD is positive for discomfort in the snuffbox and pain in the midportion of the wrist. Follow the third metacarpal proximal toward the wrist until you find a depression (Figure 7.14). Place your index finger in the depression and attempt to elicit pain. If no pain is noted, have the patient flex the wrist while your index finger remains in the depression. A portion of the lunate will become palpable and will be tender if a ligamentous disruption is present. The Watson test also helps make the diagnosis of SLLD. This test requires that the examiner stabilizes the scaphoid by placing his or her thumb over the volar pole of the scaphoid (Figure 7.15) while the wrist is held in ulnar deviation. As the hand is brought into radial deviation, pain is produced.

X-rays are indicated in this patient to rule out a fracture and ligamentous disruption. Plain films should be done first and usually make the diagnosis. More than the usual wrist films are needed and my routine is to let the X-ray technician know what I am looking for and request a scaphoid series and/or ligamentous series of films. If the technician is not sure, the radiologist will know what you are requesting.

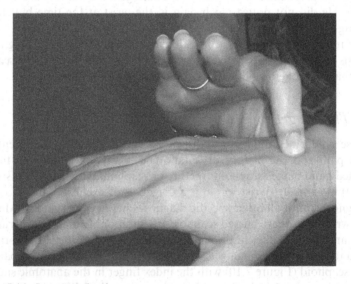

FIGURE 7.14. Lunate palpation.

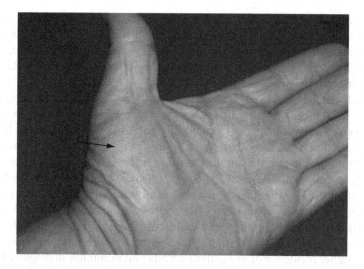

FIGURE 7.15. Volar pole of scaphoid.

This patient had pain in the snuffbox that was aggravated by ulnar deviation. The Watson test was negative and no pain was noted over the lunate. The patient complained of thumb pain with a weak attempt to shake hands. A scaphoid series and a ligamentous series of X-rays were negative at 5 days. The patient was placed in a thumb spica short-arm cast for 2 weeks and re-X-rayed. At that time a fracture of the midportion of the scaphoid was noted. After 8 additional weeks of immobilization the X-ray revealed adequate healing. The patient started a rehabilitation program to regain strength and has returned to full activity with no loss of function.

7. Scaphoid Fractures

Fractures of the scaphoid are the most common fractures of the carpal bones. The patient may not seek medical attention initially because the problem seems minor. As time passes the patient experiences more pain and disability and seeks medical attention. It is not unusual for the diagnosis of sprain to be made and later it is found to be a fracture. The mechanism of injury is probably forced hyperextension with the wrist in ulnar deviation. Because of the unique blood supply to the scaphoid there is a high incidence of fracture nonunion and avascular necrosis. The distal and middle portions of the scaphoid have a direct vascular supply but the proximal portion does not have a direct supply. The proximal portion is the most commonly fractured with its anatomic location. The subtle nature of scaphoid fracture, clinical presentation, and the high incidence of nonunion and avascular necrosis demand careful evaluation and judgment when dealing with wrist trauma.

Prudent clinicians usually consider any patient who has snuffbox tenderness after a fall to have a scaphoid fracture and will immobilize until a definitive diagnosis can be made. Nothing is lost with a few weeks of immobilization. Bone scans and magnetic resonance imaging (MRI) may help but are usually not needed.

Nondisplaced scaphoid fractures (less than 1-mm displacement) are treated in a short-arm thumb spica cast. Some clinicians prefer long-arm thumb spica casts. The patient can usually participate in all activities including sports if the rules of that sport permit participation with a protected cast. Immobilization is continued until healing is demonstrated by radiograph, usually within 3 months. Uncomplicated scaphoid fractures have a union rate of 95% when diagnosed early and immobilized. If healing is not obvious in 3 months, request an orthopedic consultation. If the patient will be participating in work or sport that involves wrist stress, protect the wrist for 6 to 8 weeks with a rigid splint. Rehabilitate any atrophied muscles.

The higher incidence of avascular necrosis and nonunion in displaced fractures and proximal third fractures drives some primary care clinicians to obtain consultations for these fractures. Consultation is also advised for patients who have had their diagnosis delayed for longer than 4 weeks and no immobilization. Operative management may be required for nonunion.

8. Scapholunate Ligamentous Disruption

This is the most common of the wrist ligament injuries. There are three ligaments between the scaphoid and lunate bones. They are the interosseous, the dorsal, and the volar. At least two of ligaments must be disrupted for disruption and dissociation to occur. The volar scapholunate is the strongest ligament and it must be ruptured for complete subluxation to occur. Depending on the severity of the injury, all types of variants may occur. Most of the time these patients do not present acutely and are seen after a nagging minor problem persists or becomes worse.

The usual history involves hyperextension of the wrist caused by a fall or direct blow. Pain, swelling, and tenderness is present over the dorsoradial aspect of the wrist in the area of the anatomic snuffbox. In addition to the pain upon palpation, the Watson test, as noted above, may be positive. X-rays that are specific for ligamentous injury should now be ordered. Characteristic radiographic signs of scapholunate dissociation are usually present and include a gap or widening of the interval between the scaphoid and the lunate; the scaphoid appears shorter; and because the scaphoid is rotated, a more radiopaque line or ring will be seen in the distal pole. Comparison with the films of the opposite wrist is needed to help make the diagnosis. Discussion with a radiologist who is experienced in reading wrist films will also be a big help.

If the X-ray is negative for ligamentous disruption, conservative treatment with a splint and reevaluation in 1 or 2 weeks is indicated. Obtain an orthopedic consultation if disruption is present on the X-ray or the Watson test is positive. Many of these patients will require surgery or prolonged immobilization with close follow-up.

Chronic scapholunate instability (lasted longer than 3 months) is a greater challenge in management. Degenerative changes may be noted on radiographs with loss of the interosseous space as well as with osteophyte formation. Early diagnosis and treatment is the best way for the primary care clinician to think about chronic instability. Once the problem becomes chronic it is a source of frustration for all the caregivers and the patient.

9. Wrist Sprain

Wrist sprain is a diagnosis of exclusion and the clinician should be reluctant to call any wrist pain a wrist sprain until the patient has completely recovered and no other diagnosis was made. Patients who sustain trauma to the wrist that produces enough discomfort to seek medical attention deserve a thorough evaluation. X-rays to rule out fracture or ligamentous disruption should be done. If the films are negative some type of splinting to reduce flexion and extension and short-term appropriate medication should be initiated. Meticulous follow-up to rule out fracture or ligamentous disruption is required. Most of the patients I diagnose with a sprain indeed turn out to have that, but I also have seen a fracture or ligamentous disruption masquerade initially as a sprain and only with follow-up does the diagnosis become obvious.

10. Medical Problems

Wrist arthritis associated with other diseases is usually not a difficult diagnosis. The patient has a known reason like gout or psoriasis, has other musculoskeletal complaints, and now develops wrist pain. The only exception to this rule of thumb is rheumatoid arthritis. Wrist pain can be the first major complaint that brings the patient with rheumatoid arthritis to the physician.

The patient, usually a young female, but can be older, often has swelling and redness of the wrist, severe pain, and limitation of flexion and extension. Carpal tunnel syndrome may have developed as the disease progressed. Other tips to the diagnosis of rheumatoid arthritis may be ulnar deviation of the wrist, swelling of the proximal interphalangeal (PIP) joints of the fingers, and the metacarpal phalangeal (MCP) joints. Also, ask about forefoot pain as the metatarsophalangeal (MTP) joint is one of the early joints to be involved.

Morning stiffness lasting more than 45 min and severe fatigue may also be present. Women in their first year postpartum are at increased risk of autoimmune disease so wrist pain in that group should make you suspicious. Laboratory confirmation is nice to have but only 50% of patients will have a positive rheumatoid factor early in the disease. Radiographic signs like bony erosions are not usually present for one year.

In the past, symptomatic treatment to make the patient comfortable was acceptable. Oral steroids were often given and gave great relief but the destruction of tissue continued. Disease-modifying antirheumatic drugs (DMARDs) are now available. These drugs prevent destruction. Joint destruction can begin as early as 4 months after the onset of symptoms. Early drug treatment preserves function. If the primary care clinician suspects rheumatoid arthritis, a consultation with a physician who understands how to administer DMARDs is indicated.

11. Wrist Exercises

Tell the patient to rotate from one exercise to the other. Do one set of one exercise and then rotate to another exercise and do a set. Do not exercise past the point of pain. Pain means stop.

1. **Extension**: With your palm toward the floor, bend your wrist up toward the sky, as noted in Figure 7.3. Hold for 5 s and repeat five times.
2. **Flexion**: With your palm toward the floor, bend your wrist down toward the floor, as noted in Figure 7.4. Hold for 5 s and repeat five times.
3. **Side to side (Figure 7.16)**: With your hand placed in a position to shake hands move your wrist from side to side like you are shaking hands. Hold each movement for 5 s and repeat five times. The remaining exercises are taken from the elbow chapter starting on page 112.
4. **Wrist flexion stretch (see Figure 6.14)**: With the injured hand in 30° of flexion begin to flex the wrist against the resistance of the other hand. Resist the movement for 15 s and repeat five times.

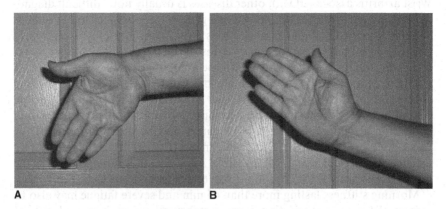

A   B

FIGURE 7.16. (A and B) Side-to-side hand movement exercise.

5. **Wrist extension stretch (see Figure 6.15)**: With the injured hand in 30° of extension, begin to extend the wrist against the resistance of the other hand. Resist the movement for 15 s and repeat five times.
6. **Wrist flexion exercise (see Figure 6.16)**: Hold a weight such as a can of soup with your palm facing up. Flex the wrist (bend it upward) and hold wrist in maximum flexion for 15 s. Return to the starting position slowly and repeat five times.
7. **Wrist extension exercise (see Figure 6.17)**: Hold weight like a can of soup with your palm facing down. Extend the wrist (bend up) and hold in maximum extension for 15 s. Return to the starting position slowly and repeat five times.
8. **Wrist radial and ulnar deviation strengthening (see Figure 6.18)**: Hold a weight like a can of soup in your hand with your thumb facing up and your wrist sideways. Rotate the wrist up and down through radial and ulnar deviation. Hold each position for 15 s and repeat five times.

Some patients may wish to use hand weights for some of the previously mentioned exercises. The amount of weight can be gradually increased to regain full strength.

Suggested Readings

Family Practice Notebook Wrist Injury accessed on Internet June 10, 2005 at http://www.fpnotebook.com/ORT388.htm.
Daniels JM, Zook EG, Lynch JM. Hand and wrist injuries: Part I. Nonemergent evaluation. *Am Fam Physician*. 2004;69:1941–1948.

8

Hand Problems

Edward J. Shahady

The primary care clinician's office will care for a significant number of hand injuries. The age, leisure time activities, and occupations of the patients in the practice will determine the type and frequency of problems encountered. Some studies indicate that fractures are the most common injury to the hand; others indicate that strains, contusions, dislocations, and ligamentous injury are more common. Hand injuries occur more frequently in adolescents, individuals participating in throwing and catching sports, and patients whose occupations involve repeated use of their hands.

Hand injuries can be intimidating because of the complex anatomy and concern for potential long-term disability. Overcoming the fear and frustration of caring for hand injury becomes possible with a few simple organizational steps:

1. Step 1 is to realize that 95% of patients seen in the office with hand complaints can be classified into three categories. The most common types of hand problems encountered in primary care are listed in Table 8.1. There are two major categories (trauma and arthritis), five anatomic areas in trauma, and two major categories of arthritis to consider when evaluating the patient with hand problems.
2. Step 2 is to take a focused history that segments the categories into acute trauma, overuse trauma, and medical disease. You now have a manageable list (Table 8.1) to begin further investigation.
3. Step 3 is to perform a focused thorough hand examination. With a focused history and a thorough hand examination you most likely now have the diagnosis. Your knowledge of the usual history and examination associated with the most common problems has facilitated the diagnostic process.
4. Step 4 is ordering confirmatory studies if needed (many times they are not).
5. Step 5 is to start treatment. (This may include appropriate consultation.) Five percent of the time, the diagnosis will not be so obvious. However, not being one of the 95% is usually obvious. That is when additional studies and/or a consultation becomes necessary.

TABLE 8.1. Classification of hand problems.

Trauma

Metacarpal problems
- Fractures

Metacarpal phalangeal joint
- Dorsal Dislocations

Thumb problems
- Ulnar collateral ligament tears—gamekeepers or skier's thumb
- Bennett's fracture

Proximal interphalangeal joint
- Dislocations
- Extensor mechanism injury (Boutonnière deformity)
- Volar plate injury

Distal interphalangeal joint
- Extensor injury (mallet finger)
- Flexor injury (Jersey finger)

Medical problems

Osteoarthritis
- Heberden's nodes of the DIP
- Bouchard's nodes of the PIP
- Thumb carpal metacarpal joint arthritis
- Erosive osteoarthritis

Rheumatoid arthritis
- PIP swelling

Some hand injuries are subtle and insignificant and others may lead to significant disability. Early recognition and treatment will decrease the chance for disability. A thorough knowledge of the anatomy, mechanism of injury, and epidemiology will help guide the process.

1. Focused History

The first question is usually related to the acuteness of the problem. Did it just start or has it been present for a long period of time. The next questions would depend on the answer to the first. Ask about recent trauma or significant past trauma. Some injuries are not thought to be significant by the patient or the clinician who initially evaluated the patient but they turn out to be important clues to the diagnosis. Occupations, hobbies, or sports that involve extensive use of the hands are more likely to cause injury. Certain injuries are more common with a specific activity or sport. For example, skiers have a higher incidence of tears to the ulnar collateral ligament (UCL) of the thumb metacarpophalangeal joint. Accidents associated with the ski pole can produce a forceful radial and palmar abduction of the thumb and subsequent ligamentous disruption. Sports like basketball, football, and baseball that involve a high-speed moving object are associated with distal interphalangeal (DIP) and proximal interphalangeal (PIP) joint dislocation and ligamentous tears as well as fractures of various bones. Ask about osteoarthritis (OA) and rheumatoid arthritis (RA) in other joints of the body as both diseases can produce some characteristic hand problems that need to be recognized and treated. Trauma no matter how insignificant can produce significant injury to an arthritic joint.

2. Focused Physical Examination

Start by observing for deformities, swelling, and discoloration. Do this on both the palmar and the dorsal surfaces of the hands and fingers. The usual position of the hand is a flexed position as the flexors of the metacarpals and fingers are stronger than the extensors (Figure 8.1). Observe for any deviation from the usual anatomic position. Next, ask the patient to extend and flex the metacarpal phalangeal (MCP) joints (Figures 8.2 and 8.3), the PIP joints (Figures 8.2 and 8.4), and the DIP joints (Figures 8.2 and 8.5).

3. Case

3.1. History

A 30-year-old male construction worker comes to your office after being hit on the dorsum (top) of his hand with a piece of machinery 1 day ago. He noted immediate swelling and some tenderness on the dorsal side of hand. He

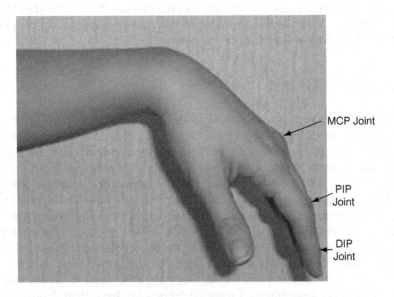

FIGURE 8.1. Flexion as the dominant hand position.

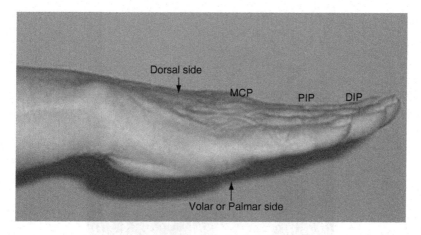

FIGURE 8.2. Extension of the MCP, PIP, and DIP joints.

placed some ice on it and the discomfort subsided. He was able to work a few more hours but was then sent home because of the pain. The next day he went to work but was unable to use the hand without pain. The examination reveals some swelling over the dorsum of the hand and early ecchymosis. Most tenderness is over the shaft of the third metacarpal. You ask him to flex his fingers into his palm and note that the middle finger is in an unusual position (Figure 8.6). The fingers should all point in a similar direction as noted in Figure 8.7.

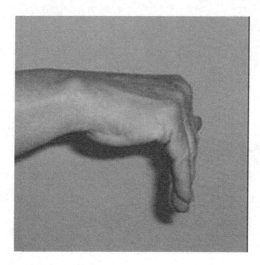

FIGURE 8.3. Flexion of MCP joint.

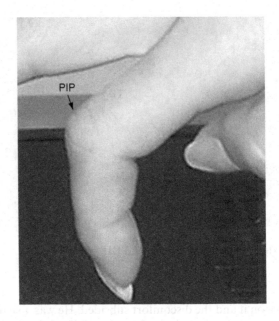

FIGURE 8.4. PIP flexion.

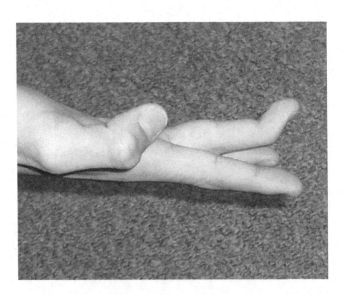

FIGURE 8.5. Flexion of the DIP joint.

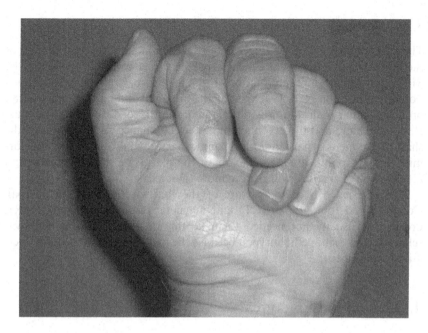

FIGURE 8.6. Abnormal finger alignment.

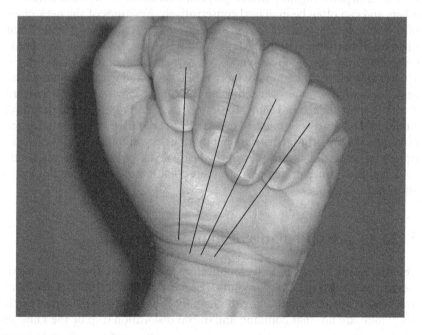

FIGURE 8.7. Normal finger alignment.

3.2. *Thinking Process*

The unusual position of the finger in the flexed palm indicates malrotation of the bone. If a fracture of the metacarpal shaft has occurred, flexion at the MCP joint will produce malrotation of that metacarpal and the unusual position noted in Figure 8.6. Fractures of the proximal and middle phalanx can produce similar malrotation with flexion at the PIP or DIP joint. The muscles of the hand and fingers function in perfect balance and fractures of the shaft of the metacarpals and/or phalanx can cause malrotation and a deformity. The key points are (1) a fracture of the shaft is most likely present and (2) this type of fracture will require more than a cast.

X-rays revealed a spiral fracture of the shaft of the third metacarpal. Computerized tomography (CT) and magnetic resonance imaging (MRI) ordering is usually not needed to make this diagnosis. This patient was referred to an orthopedic surgeon because the malrotation may require operative management.

4. Metacarpal Fractures

Fractures of the metacarpals can occur at the base, shaft, and neck. The management of metacarpal fractures depends upon the location on the metacarpal of the fracture and which metacarpal is fractured. The fourth and fifth metacarpals (ring and little finger) can tolerate more angulation than the others and can often be managed conservatively. Fractures of the neck of the fifth metacarpal are called boxer's fracture because they commonly occur when the fist strikes an object. Metacarpal fractures of the index and middle fingers tolerate less angulation and may require operative management. Thumb metacarpal fractures are more problematic and usually require orthopedic evaluation. Primary care clinicians can manage many of these fractures if they fully understand how to immobilize and protect the fractures. Additional reading, training, and experience are required to understand these principles. Many orthopedists are happy to help you understand these principles and respond to your questions when you are not sure. This allows the orthopedist to concentrate on the fractures that require more complex evaluation and treatment.

5. Metacarpal Phalangeal Joint Dislocations

The MCP joint, because of its architecture, allows more freedom of movement than the interphalangeal joints. The surrounding soft tissues are therefore more critical in maintaining the stability of the joint. Dislocations of the MCP joint are not that common and dorsal dislocation (top of the knuckle) is the rule. Volar dislocations are rare and often require operative treatment. Dorsal dislocations usually respond to reduction. Some simple rules help with understanding how to reduce the dislocation. First, provide adequate anesthesia with 1% or 2% lidocaine infusion into the joint. This not only reduces pain and spasm but will assure that any volar tissue torn during the dislocation will appropriately move to allow an easier reduction. Next, have the patient flex the wrist and digits. This relaxes the dominant flexor system. Reduction is now accomplished by hyperextending the MCP joint while pulling the proximal phalanx forward, maintaining the tension of the pull and flexing the MCP joint. Figure 8.8 demonstrates a simple dorsal dislocation with the volar plate tissue in an appropriate place and directions on how to relocate the dislocation. Figure 8.9 demonstrates a complex dislocation with the volar plate tissue blocking the relocation. The ability to flex and extend the joint actively and passively indicates a successful relocation. Inability to do this indicates the possibility of a complex dislocation and the patient should be referred. X-rays should be taken to assure that reduction is complete. Splinting in full flexion for 1 week followed by buddy taping (tapping one finger to the one adjacent to it) for two additional weeks to prevent hyperextension is indicated. The MCP joint is more stable in the flexed position and this position is known as the *safe position* because of its stability. More than 1 week in this position may lead to stiffness and an increased need for rehabilitation. Return to activity is permitted as long as the joint can be protected from hyperextension.

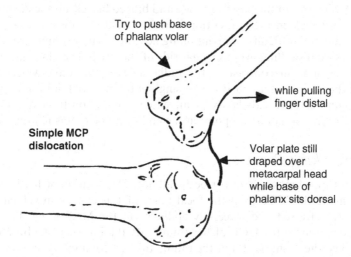

FIGURE 8.8. Simple MCP dislocation and relocation. (Reproduced from Richmond J, Shahady E, eds. *Sports Medicine for Primary Care*. Cambridge, MA: Blackwell Science; 1996:354, with permission.)

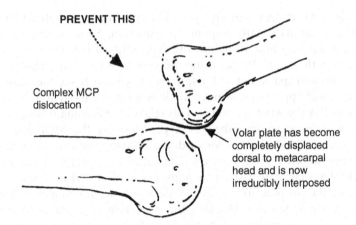

FIGURE 8.9. Complex MCP dislocation and relocation. (Reproduced from Richmond J, Shahady E, eds. *Sports Medicine for Primary Care*. Cambridge, MA: Blackwell Science; 1996:354, with permission.)

6. Case

6.1. History

A healthy 35-year-old woman comes to your office complaining of left thumb pain. She was involved in a minor automobile accident 2 days before the visit. She was on the passenger side and braced herself on the dashboard. She did not seek medical attention initially but does now because of left thumb pain and difficulty in maintaining her grasp. Her examination reveals tenderness and swelling over the ulnar side of the MCP. The ulnar side points toward the ulna in contrast to the radial side of the joint, which points toward the radius (Figure 8.10). Stressing the thumb MCP joint into abduction (Figure 8.10) reveals laxity or increased opening on the left compared with the right. No good end point at the end of abduction is felt on the left.

6.2. Thinking Process

The car stopped moving but her body did not. The position of her hand and thumb made the MCP joint the focal point of this change in velocity. The thumb was stressed and forcefully abducted at the MCP joint. This force most likely injured the UCL of her thumb MCP joint when she braced herself against the dashboard. For the thumb this is a common type of injury. It occurs in sports that predispose to thumb abduction stress like football and skiing. The best name for the injury is UCL injury but names like skier's or gamekeepers' thumb are commonly used. The term gamekeepers' thumb comes from an injury suffered by gamekeepers in England when they twisted

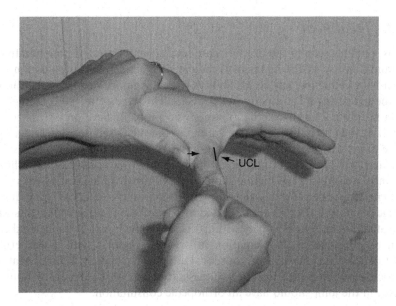

FIGURE 8.10. Test for UCL integrity.

the neck of the game they caught. This maneuver would injure the UCL ligament and cause a chronic instability. Skiing accidents associated with the ski pole can produce a forceful radial and palmar abduction of the thumb and subsequent disruption of the UCL. This injury can lead to significant disability because of the importance of the thumb. If a fracture is present and/or the UCL has migrated into the joint space a more complex injury is likely. The physical examination helps access the extent of the damage. Perform abduction stress (Figure 8.10) in both neutral and flexed positions. The flexed position is usually more stable and weakness in this position indicates a more serious problem.

Some patients will resist attempts to assess for instability because of the pain. Lidocaine can be infused into the joint to allow for a more complete examination. Once adequate anesthesia is accomplished, the examination can be easily performed. It is important to perform thumb abduction in both the neutral and the flexed positions to assess for stability in both positions.

A plain film X-ray is indicated in most cases especially if instability in flexion is demonstrated. Fractures may be present and the fracture fragment or tissue may become lodged in the joint. This fragment or tissue must be removed surgically for proper healing to occur. The X-ray in this patient revealed no fracture or indication of tissue in the joint. Magnetic resonance imaging may be indicated to access the amount of tissue that has been displaced into the joint. Save the ordering of the MRI for the orthopedic or hand surgeon.

6.3. *Treatment*

Most patients seen in the primary care setting can be treated nonoperatively. Minimal injury to the ligament is indicated by tenderness to palpation and pain with abduction but no instability. Treat this injury by taping the thumb to the index finger for a period of 3 weeks. This type of injury is commonly seen in football and basketball players who probably have only strained the UCL. Instability in the neutral position but not the flexed position and a negative X-ray can be treated with a thumb spica cast or splint. The initial splint is placed for 3 weeks. An additional splint that allows wrist flexion but limits thumb extension and abduction should be used for an additional 2 weeks. This patient was treated like this and did well. Exercises to regain lost strength and range of motion (ROM) are indicated as part of the treatment. Patients who are athletes can return to play within 1 week of the injury. A rubberized cast can be constructed. Participation in organized sports with a rubberized cast depends on the rules of your local athletic association. Injuries that are associated with thumb flexion weakness, fractures, or suspicion of bone or tissue in the joint should have an orthopedic consultation.

7. Bennett's Fracture

About 25% of metacarpal fractures involve the base of the thumb. These are common when someone falls and the thumb takes the brunt of the force in breaking the fall. The names Bennett and Rolando are attached to comminuted (more than one piece of bone) fractures of the thumb base. The strength of the thumb abductors produces a deformity that most of the time will require a surgical solution. All thumb metacarpal fractures are best treated by an orthopedic surgeon.

8. Case

8.1. *History*

A 25-year-old female softball player comes to your office after being hit in the hand by a softball 2 h previously. She says her middle finger was pushed back by the ball and came out of place. The coach tried to push it back in place but was not successful. Your examination reveals the middle phalanx is displaced dorsally above the proximal phalanx at the PIP joint. The patient is unable to extend or flex the finger. You reassure the patient and do a digital block with lidocaine to obtain adequate anesthesia. Once the pain has disappeared, you grasp the finger firmly over the middle phalanx and gently hyperextend the joint while at the same time applying longitudinal traction and then flexion similar to the MCP joint dislocation. The middle phalanx nicely came back into place. The patient was now able to flex and extend the finger at the PIP joint. A postreduction X-ray revealed no fracture and good alignment of the middle and proximal phalanx at the PIP joint. A splint to limit extension of the PIP joint only was placed for 1 week and this was followed by 2 weeks of buddy taping the third finger to the index finger. There was some residual swelling and minor discomfort for the next 2 months but the patient completely recovered. She went back to playing softball after the splint was removed.

8.2. *Thinking Process*

Proximal interphalangeal joint dislocation is the most common joint dislocation in the hand. Almost all of them occur in a dorsal direction. They are usually easily reduced and many are reduced on the field by the coach, trainer, or the athlete. Thus, the name "coaches finger." The sooner it is reduced the easier the reduction. On-the-field reduction is ideal. An X-ray is not needed before reduction unless the reduction cannot be accomplished with the usual means. This may indicate that either bone or tissue is in the joint space, limiting the ability to reduce the dislocation. The key to preventing complications with dislocations is the postreduction care. An X-ray is always indicated after the reduction to assure that the reduced bones (middle phalanx and proximal phalanx) are now aligned/congruent. The radiologist will be attentive to this if the request is marked "after reduction." If it is not aligned/congruent, an orthopedic consultation is indicated. The other complication that should concern you is the boutonnière deformity. This results from a disruption of the extensor mechanism over the PIP joint (Figure 8.11B). This deformity is not noted immediately but weakness or absence of extension will be noted immediately. Discussion of this injury occurs in Section 9.

The vast majority of the time, PIP dislocations relocate easily and after a reassuring X-ray and demonstrating the extensor mechanism is intact, buddy taping is all the treatment that is needed.

Injury can also occur to the collateral ligaments of the PIP joint with the dislocation. The ligaments known as the radial and UCLs of the PIP joint should be tested for stability. Test for stability with the finger flexed (bent to 90° at the PIP joint) and also when it is extended (completely straight at 0°). Place both an ulnar- and a radial-directed force on the joint to see if it opens. Any opening would be abnormal. This is similar to testing the medial and lateral collateral ligaments of the knee. Significant opening indicates a need for longer splinting and letting the patient know that this enhances the chances of chronic deformity and arthritic changes. An orthopedic or hand surgeon should evaluate significant laxity.

Plain film radiographs are usually all that is needed. Additional imaging may be needed for more complex fracture dislocations but this will usually be ordered by the orthopedic or hand surgeon.

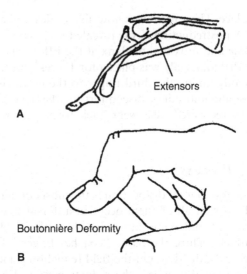

FIGURE 8.11. (A) Mechanism of the deformity in a boutonnière injury. (B) Clinical appearance of the boutonnière deformity. (Reproduced from Shahady E, Petrizzi M, eds. *Sports Medicine for Coaches and Trainers*. Chapel Hill, NC: University of North Carolina Press; 1991:83, with permission.)

8.3. Treatment

As previously mentioned, the dislocations without significant fractures or ligamentous injury will require 2 to 3 weeks of buddy tapping only. Significant fractures should be managed by the orthopedists and will require dorsal extension splints that are gradually straightened over a 4-week period. Remember to evaluate the ability to extend the joint before splinting in flexion. If a tear in the extensor mechanism exists, treating flexion will increase the chances of the boutonnière deformity. If a splint is used it should only involve the PIP joint. Limiting the movement of the DIP and MCP joints will create stiffness in these joints and increased recovery time.

9. Boutonnière Deformity

This deformity although not common is usually preventable. Unfortunately, it is not recognized early enough to prevent it. It is up to the primary care practitioner to recognize and treat this injury in its early stages. The mechanism of the deformity is a disruption of the central extensor slip that inserts on the middle phalanx. This injury makes it impossible to extend the finger at the PIP joint (middle knuckle). The head of the proximal phalanx migrates (buttonholes) through the torn extensor mechanism and the two lateral bands of the extensor slip now migrate down or volar. This now turns the extensors into flexors of the PIP joint (Figure 8.11A). The joint can still be passively moved into extension but only with assistance. This also leads to hyperextension of the DIP joint. In most cases it takes several weeks for the classic deformity (Figure 8.11B) to develop, leading to high number of missed or delayed diagnosis.

A well-conceived examination early in the injury will help with prevention of this deformity. Dislocations and jammed fingers are predisposing injuries. Evaluate any patient with either one of these injuries for weakness or inability to extend the finger at the PIP joint. Start the evaluation by assessing for the point of maximum tenderness. Extensor injury will be most tender on the dorsal surface (top) of the PIP joint (Figure 8.12) in contrast to the volar plate injury that is most tender on the volar surface (bottom) of the PIP joint (Figure 8.12). If maximum tenderness is elicited over the dorsal surface of the joint, the chances of an extensor injury are likely. The next step is to access the ability of the patient to actively extend the PIP joint. Pain may limit extension. Infusing the joint with a local anesthetic will assess the influence of pain on the ability to extend. Do not be fooled by the ability of the patient or yourself to place the finger in extension and its ability to remain extended. As soon as the patient flexes the finger it will remain that way until passively extended again.

Treatment in the initial phase of the injury is a splint that immobilizes the PIP joint in full extension for 4 to 5 weeks followed by nighttime splinting for another 2 weeks. Do not involve the MCP and DIP joints in the splint. This will result in unnecessary stiffness in these two joints. Instruct the patient to flex and extend the MCP and DIP joint while the PIP joint is splinted to prevent stiffness.

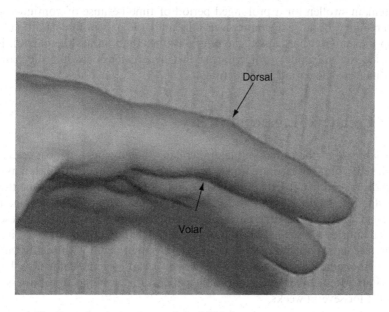

FIGURE 8.12. Dorsal volar surfaces of the PIP joint.

If the diagnosis is delayed and the classic deformity of fixed PIP flexion and DIP hyperextension is present, refer the patient to an orthopedic surgeon. Surgical reconstruction is reserved for the patients that fail nonoperative measures.

10. Proximal Interphalangeal Volar Plate Injury

This injury is common and results from hyperextension of the PIP joint by a ball or another object that causes hyperextension. This is commonly called the jammed or stowed finger. The initial injury does not usually cause significant concern or discomfort but within 24 h, the joint is swollen and tender to motion. Tenderness is noted on the volar side (Figure 8.12) and hyperextending the joint will reveal laxity. Collateral ligament injury often accompanies volar plate injuries. Be sure to test these ligaments for stability. Collateral ligament stability examination is discussed under PIP dislocation additional examinations. Order X-rays if there is significant instability or the patient is a child with a growth plate that has not closed. Small avulsion fractures are common and do not require different treatment. An orthopedic surgeon should evaluate fractures that involve over 30% of the articular surface.

Almost all jammed fingers seen in the primary care setting will have minimal instability and not require an X-ray. Splinting the PIP joint in slight flexion for 1 to 2 weeks followed by 2 weeks of buddy taping is sufficient. For the mild injuries, buddy taping is all that is needed. It is not unusual for the joint to remain swollen for a prolonged period of time because of continued use and reinjury. Because the injury is usually mild, the patient finds it difficult to stop the activity that caused the injury. Rather than harass the patient, just provide the maximum protection against hyperextension while the patient continues participating in the activity.

11. Collateral Ligament Injury

Partial tears of the radial and lateral collateral ligaments are most common at the PIP joint but also are noted at the DIP and MCP joints. With jammed and dislocated MCP, PIP, and MCP joints, these ligaments should be tested for stability. Testing should be done in full extension and 30° of flexion. The great majority of the time partial tears and minimum instability is present. These injuries are treated with 2 to 4 weeks of buddy taping. Marked instability secondary to complete tears is also usually treated with buddy taping but orthopedic surgeon advice is suggested because of the deformity that is inevitable. Remember to explain to the patients that swelling and stiffness can persist for several weeks.

12. Distal Interphalangeal Joint

12.1. Extensor Injury (Mallet Finger)

Another common finger injury it is also sometimes called baseball finger or
drop finger (Figure 8.13). Get a group of 50- to 70-year-old men in a room
and look at their hands and you are likely to find someone with a drop finger. In the past both patients and physicians neglected this type of injury.
Many young boys and recently girls injure their fingers when a ball strikes the
DIP and forces the joint into flexion while they were trying to extend the finger. This causes a rupture of the extensor mechanism. The young man or
woman will complain of pain and swelling on the tip of the finger. Testing for
the ability to extend the finger at the DIP joint is important but sometimes
difficult because of the pain.

Often, the patient does not seek medical attention until the finger "drops."
The initial swelling made the deformity difficult to appreciate and once the
swelling decreases patients then realize they have a more problematic lesion.

Treatment is usually by a splint that provides 5° to 10° of hyperextension for
6 to 8 weeks. Commercially available splints can be purchased. Patients will want
to remove the splint to clean it and wash their hands. Tell them how important it
is to keep the distal phalanx extended when the splint is removed. Some practitioners will have the patients return for a clean replacement splint to their offices
so they can demonstrate how to maintain extension while performing the cleansing. No matter how late the patient presents for treatment, always try to splint the
finger. It may not help after 2 to 3 months but nothing is lost in the effort.

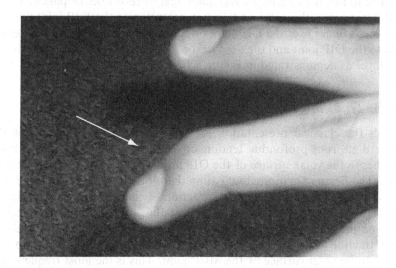

FIGURE 8.13. Drop or mallet finger.

X-rays should be obtained to see if a fracture is present and how much of the articular surface is involved in the fracture. If 50% or greater of the articular surface of the joint is involved consult an orthopedic surgeon. The treatment will still probably be a splint but let the orthopedist make this decision. Surgery has little place in the treatment of this type of extensor tear unless there is significant instability.

13. Case

13.1. History and Exam

A right-handed high school football player comes to your office 3 days after injuring his right ring finger. The injury occurred when he was trying to tackle another player by grabbing his shirt. The other player was able to pull away from him and he noticed immediate pain in his ring finger. He did not feel the injury was significant so he did not seek attention immediately. That evening he noted difficulty grasping objects, and increased swelling and pain. He made a trip to the emergency department. An X-ray was obtained that was considered normal. He was informed that he had a strained finger and should follow up with you as his primary care clinician. The discomfort and disability have increased and his grasp strength has decreased. Examination reveals tenderness on the volar aspect of the DIP joint and swelling and tenderness over the volar surface at the MCP joint and a feeling of a lump on the volar surface of the MCP joint. Extension of all the joints is normal and flexion is normal at the MCP and PIP joints. He was not able to flex the ring finger DIP joint against resistance or passively. Test DIP flexion with the patient's finger in extension at the DIP joint and the examiner's finger over the DIP joint on the volar surface. This limits flexion only to the DIP joint and the deep flexor. The patient is asked to flex (bend) the finger as demonstrated in Figure 8.14.

13.2. Thinking Process

This is the classical presentation for "Jersey finger," an avulsion of the flexor digitorum profundus tendon or deep flexor tendon. This tendon attaches to the volar surface of the DIP joint and functions to flex the DIP joint. The flexors are more dominating than the extensors in the hand so a tear of a flexor tendon results in retraction of that tendon. The retraction can be minimal or go all the way to the palm. If there is a large piece of bone on the end of the tendon the retraction will be minimal. In this case the retraction was more extensive. The retracted tendon is the lump palpated at the volar surface of the MCP joint. This is the most frequent and most worrisome of the tendon ruptures because the loss of usual blood supply and quick occurrence of contractures make reinsertion more diffi-

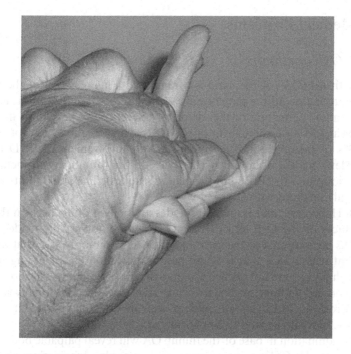

FIGURE 8.14. Test for the deep flexor.

cult. Quick diagnosis and surgical treatment produces the best results. After 10 days reinsertion is not as successful.

X-rays are not needed to make the diagnosis. In fact, they may confuse the situation. The diagnosis is purely clinical and once the primary care practitioner discovers loss of deep flexion the next move is calling the hand surgeon. The surgeon may want some imaging studies but leave the decision to the surgeon.

13.3. Treatment

The best option is early recognition and repair. Ten days is considered the magic window, anything after that is less likely to be successful. Later repair may not be successful because of the lack of adequate blood supply and tendon contracture. If you are faced with a delayed diagnosis, it is still worthwhile asking the patient to discuss it with a hand surgeon. There may be procedures that will allow some increased function. If the loss of function is acceptable to the patient there may not be any indication for surgery but at least the patient is fully informed of options.

14. Medical Problems

14.1. Osteoarthritis

Osteoarthritis (OA) of the hand is common with aging. Most of the time it is asymptomatic and the patient only seeks care because of appearance and concern about cause and further deformity. Seventy-five percent of individuals over age 65 have some form of OA. It is symptomatic in 26% of women and 13% of men. The most common area of involvement is the DIP joint (Heberden's nodes), followed by the base of the thumb carpal metacarpal (CMC) joint and the PIP joint (Bouchard's nodes). The MCP joints are not commonly involved with OA.

Both Heberden's and Bouchard's nodes are bony prominences on the dorsal surfaces of the DIP and PIP joints. They are not usually tender unless there has been trauma to the area. Patients will commonly ask what they are and want reassurance that they are not an indication of something serious. Although X-rays are not needed to make the diagnosis, they will show osteophytes formation, joint space narrowing, sclerosis, and occasionally subluxations. Erosions and cysts are seldom seen in OA and if present another diagnosis like gout should to be considered.

The examination in base of the thumb OA will reveal palpable bony prominences over the CMC joint secondary to osteophyte formation and occasionally radial deviation of the joint secondary to subluxation. The base of the thumb CMC joint has four articulations. Osteoarthritis involves only one of the articulations of the trapeziometacarpal joint and occasionally the trapezioscaphoid joint. X-rays should be taken to make the diagnosis of OA in this location. Isolated degenerative changes in the trapezioscaphoid joint suggest other causes of arthritis like rheumatoid arthritis.

Treatment of hand OA in the asymptomatic patients consists of explaining the process and excellent prognosis. Patients should be encouraged to stay active and use their hands but protect them against trauma. Symptomatic patients also require appropriate explanation of the process and good prognosis. Exercises and continued protected movement is important and occupational and physical therapy may be appropriate. Tylenol in doses up to 4 g a day is helpful. Cautious use of appropriate nonsteroidal anti-inflammatory agents (NSAIDs) will also help (see Chapter 1). If exercises and medications do not relieve symptoms, consider injecting the joint with steroids and/or splinting and protecting joints.

For the patients with more severe disease, consultation with an occupational therapist (OT) and/or physical therapist (PT) may provide other suggestions to preserve function and decrease discomfort. Surgery may be helpful to some patients and consultation with an orthopedic or hand surgeon may be indicated in the patients with more severe disease.

Other keys to making the diagnosis of OA of the hand include arthritis of the other joints commonly afflicted by OA like the neck, back, hip, and knee, and the classic symptoms of little to no pain at rest, increased pain during and immediately after movement, and minimal morning stiffness. Examination usually reveals bony prominences over the joints, and crepitations with joint movement. Routine laboratory tests are negative and only serve to rule out other diseases. X-rays are diagnostic but not prognostic. Do not let an X-ray make the decision about the diagnosis. Osteoarthritic radiographic changes are common in any patient after age 50. Symptoms are not caused by the bone pathology but the surrounding soft tissue, ligaments, and cartilage damage.

14.1.1. Erosive Inflammatory Osteoarthritis

Osteoarthritis is not usually associated with acute inflammatory episodes like swelling, painful joints, erythema, warmth, and limitation of motion. But, occasionally it can be and this is called erosive inflammatory OA. Some investigators feel this is a separate entity but most feel it is an extension of noninflammatory OA. This entity is most common in postmenopausal women and involves primarily their hands and not the other joints commonly involved with OA. The DIP and thumb base are the most common joints involved and can be quite painful. Most clinicians when first faced with this entity think it is infectious or due to RA. Knowing this entity exists and including it in the differential diagnosis is helpful to both the patient and the physician.

X-rays reveal erosions. Rheumatoid factor and serum uric acid should be obtained to rule out these entities. If the patient has all the signs and symptoms of OA and nothing else to suggest another disease process treat the patient symptomatically. The joints need to be protected and pain relief should be sought with NSAIDs and, if needed, short-term narcotics. Joint injection with lidocaine and steroids can also help. As with noninflammatory OA splints, consultations with PT, OT, and an orthopedic surgeon may be of benefit.

14.1.2. Rheumatoid Arthritis

Swelling and tenderness of one or two PIP joints in the absence of any signs of OA like Heberden's or Bouchard's nodes is suspicious for RA. The age of the patient is also a tip. It is unusual for patients to have significant OA before their 50s. Arthritic hand symptoms before age 50 should alert you to the diagnosis of RA. Erosive inflammatory OA, gout, and psoriatic arthritis are part of the differential diagnosis. Once they are ruled out a preliminary diagnosis of RA can be made. Medications that prevent loss of function in RA if given in the first 4 to 6 months of the disease are now available. Early diagnosis decreases the disability that accompanies RA.

Additional tips to aid in the diagnosis of RA, as noted in Chapter 7, may be ulnar deviation of the wrist, swelling and pain of the MCP joints, and forefoot pain secondary to involvement of the metatarsophalangeal (MTP) joint.

Morning stiffness lasting more than 45 min and severe fatigue may also be present. Women in their first year postpartum are at increased risk of autoimmune disease, so suggestive symptoms in this group should be given appropriate attention. Laboratory and radiographic confirmation is nice to have but only 50% of patients will have a positive rheumatoid factor early in the disease and radiographic signs of bony erosions are not usually present during the first year.

In the past, symptomatic treatment to make the patient comfortable was acceptable. Relief with steroids was significant but the destruction of tissue continued. Diseases-modifying antirheumatic drugs (DMARDs) are now available. These drugs prevent joint destruction. Joint destruction can begin as early as 4 months after the onset of symptoms and early drug treatment preserves function. The drugs are expensive and have significant side effects.

If the primary care clinicians suspect RA a consultation with a physician who understands how to administer DMARDs is indicated. Primary care clinicians should familiarize themselves with all the side effects and interactions of all these drugs as these patients will still rely on their primary care clinician to provide other aspects of their care.

Suggested Readings

Sorock GS. Acute traumatic occupational hand injuries: type, location, and severity. *J Occup Environ Med.* 2002;44(4):345–351

Daniels JM. Hand and wrist injuries: Part II. Emergent evaluation. *Am Fam Physician.* 2004;69(8):1949–1956.

Part III

Spine

9

Neck Problems

Edward J. Shahady

Neck pain is a common complaint in the general population. Forty to seventy percent of adult patients will experience a least one significant episode of neck pain during their lifetime. Most of the time it is mild and not a source of concern for the patient. Although not as common as back pain, the prevalence is great enough in primary care to warrant attention, particularly in the geriatric population.

Multiple diseases can cause neck pain. Medical problems like angina or myocardial infarction refer pain to the neck, meningitis produces neck stiffness, and migraine headache can be associated with neck pain. Whiplash injuries after an auto accident, osteoarthritis (OA), and herniated cervical disk are probably the most common causes of neck pain in primary care. A good working knowledge of the epidemiology, anatomy, associated symptoms, and examination reduce confusion and enhance the diagnostic and therapeutic process when evaluating the patient with neck pain.

Remember the neck supports a 20- to 25-lb weight (the head) that is constantly moving around and places stress on the cervical spine and surrounding musculature. This stress will never be eliminated but it can be reduced.

Caring for neck problems is easier if a few simple organizational steps are followed:

1. Step 1 is to realize that 95% of patients seen in the office with neck complaints can be classified into the categories of problems noted in Table 9.1.
2. Step 2 is to take a focused history that segments the categories into acute trauma, degenerative disease, and medical disease. This process reduces the number to a manageable list to initiate further investigation.
3. Step 3 is to perform an examination that focuses on the most likely causes suggested by the history. With a focused history and examination you now have a likely diagnosis. Your knowledge of the usual history and examination associated with the most common problems has facilitated this process.
4. Step 4 is ordering confirmatory studies if needed (many times they are not).

TABLE 9.1. Common neck problems.

Neck pain of no specific cause (cervical strain)

Acute trauma
- Fractures
- Whiplash

Degenerative disease
- Herniated disk
- Spondylosis

Medical problems
- Cardiac disease
- Other types of arthritis

Other
- Torticollis

5. Step 5 is to start treatment. (This may include appropriate consultation.) Five percent of the time, the diagnosis will not be so obvious. However, not being one of the 95% helps the examiner now think of the 5%.

Some clinicians feel that ruling out the rare is our first responsibility based on the old theory "I got burned once and it will not happen again." Unfortunately, this theory leads to unneeded testing, loss of treatment time, and missed diagnosis of common problems. Unless the situation is life-threatening or a red flag is present, ruling out the common is the most effective way to care for neck pain. If the common is not present, additional confirmatory studies and/or a consultation will be required to discover the rare causes.

1. Focused History

Inquiring about general health and constitutional symptoms should start the process. Questions about chills, fever, and malaise will help rule out the diagnosis of meningitis. Pain with exertion is suggestive of angina. Angina pain may start in or radiate to the neck, face, and arms. Myocardial infarction pain is usually accompanied by sweating and may radiate or start in the neck and face. Osteoarthritis of the neck is more common in older patients. If you suspect OA of the neck, attempt to elicit other symptoms of OA in the hands, hips, and knees. A history of acute blunt trauma should make you suspicious for a fracture. If the patient was involved in a car accident, think about whiplash. Burning radiating pain down to the arms and hands suggest nerve root compression and a herniated cervical disk. Since cervical root, compression may cause shoulder pain without neck pain it is important to ask questions to rule out rotator cuff problems. Rotator cuff disease produces pain with shoulder abduction and cervical root compression usually does not. Patients with rotator cuff problems have great difficulty raising the involved arms above their heads. Questions about gait, coordination, bowel and bladder control, and balance are important to rule out myelopathy (severe cord compression) that can occur with cervical root compression. Questioning about the patient's past treatment successes and failures will help develop an effective treatment plan.

2. Focused Physical Examination

The examination should focus on what the history suggests. A more extensive examination may be indicated if the symptoms suggest a systemic disease. First, observe for reduced spontaneous head movement, head tilt, and neck deformity. Next, palpate and percuss over the cervical spine checking for the presence of tenderness. Have the patient move the neck through the motions of forward flexion and backward extension (Figure 9.1), left and right lateral rotation (Figure 9.2), and left and right lateral bending (Figure 9.3). Measure the degrees of movement and compare one side to the other. Differences from one side to the other are diagnostic and can be used to judge treatment success at follow-up visits. The neurological examination includes testing the strength of the deltoid and rotator cuff muscles (see Chapter 5), biceps and triceps muscle strength (Figure 9.4), and wrist flexion and extension (see Chapter 7). Sensory examination concentrating on the dermatomes of the upper extremities also helps discover specific cervical root deficits as noted in Figure 9.5. C5 and C6 are the most common cervical roots compressed. Conclude the neurological examination with upper extremity deep tendon reflexes. If lower extremity symptoms are present neurological examination of the lower extremity as outlined in Chapter 10 should be performed.

Provocative tests to increase the pain in cervical root compression include the Spurling's, axial loading, Adson's, and elevated arm tests. Spurling's test is performed by asking the patient, while seated, to extend the neck while the examiner assists with tilting the head to the side (Figure 9.6). If this induces radiating pain and numbness into the symptomatic extremity, it suggests underlying nerve root compression usually secondary to disk herniation. The axial loading test is performed with the patient standing and the examiner pushes down on the patient's head (Figure 9.7). This may provoke neck pain if disk pathology is present.

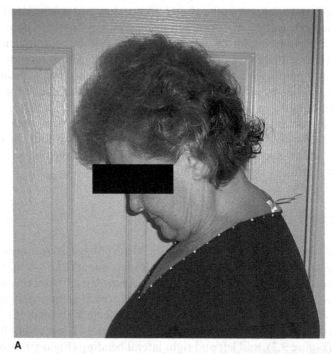

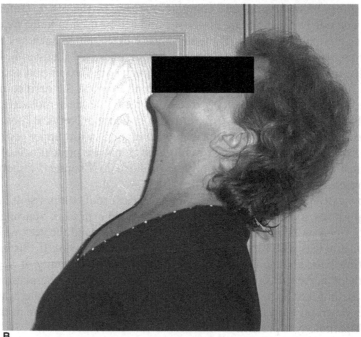

FIGURE 9.1. (A) Forward flexion. (B) backward extension.

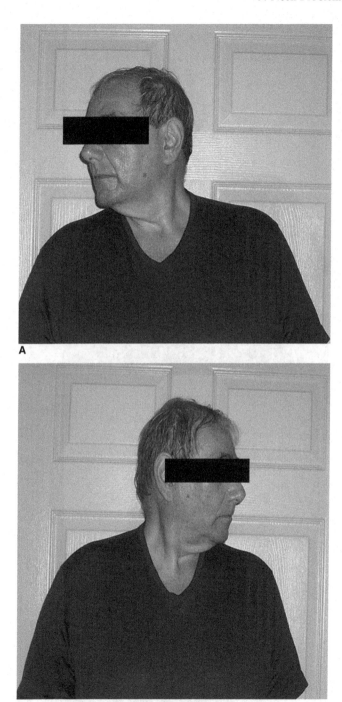

FIGURE 9.2. (A) Right and (B) left lateral rotation.

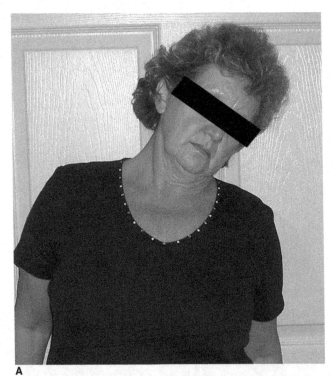

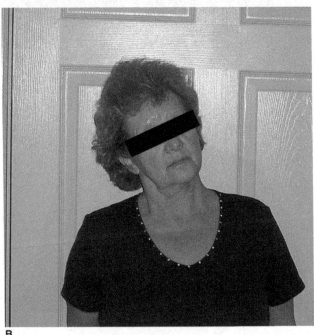

FIGURE 9.3. (A) Left and (B) right lateral bending.

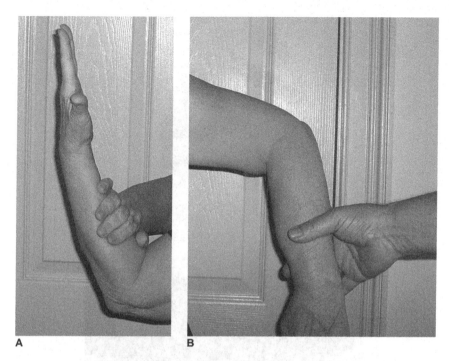

FIGURE 9.4. (A) Biceps and (B) triceps muscle strength.

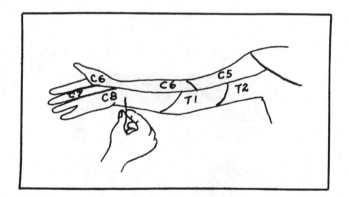

FIGURE 9.5. Cervical root deficits (dermatomes). (Reproduced from Shahady E, Petrizzi M, eds. *Sports Medicine for Coaches and Trainers.* Chapel Hill, NC: University of North Carolina Press; 1991:33, with permission.)

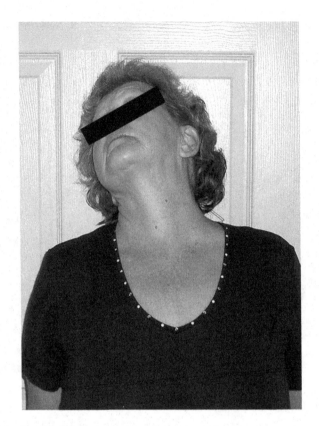

FIGURE 9.6. Spurling's test.

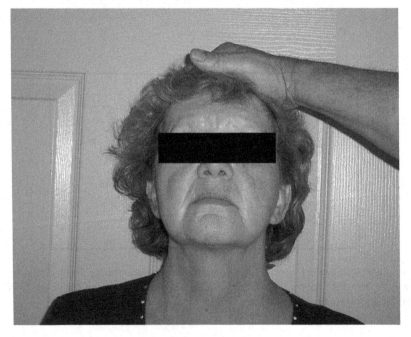

FIGURE 9.7. Axial loading test.

3. Case

3.1. History and Exam

A 35-year-old woman presents to your office with neck pain of 3 days' duration. She is in good general health and there is no history of trauma. She has a past history of posterior neck pain and headaches that have responded to Tylenol and ibuprofen in a few days. This pain is usually confined to the posterior neck but will sometimes radiate to the upper back and occiput. There is no history of pain radiating to the arms or weakness in the arms or lower extremities. Her sleep is not disturbed and the discomfort improves after a good night's sleep. She is concerned about the recurrent nature of the problem and wonders if further studies are needed. She has no complains of chills and fever and is afebrile. Examination reveals 15° of limited motion with lateral bending and rotation on the left compared with the right. This motion also increases the pain. There is no tenderness over the spinous processes. She does have some trapezius muscle tenderness with palpation but no trigger points. Spurling's and axial loading tests are negative. Neurological examination reveals no loss of muscle strength in the upper and lower extremities and sensory evaluation is normal.

3.2. Thinking Process

This is a common patient scenario for all primary care clinicians. The lack of a history of trauma rules out fracture and whiplash syndrome. There is no spinous process tenderness. Cervical spine fractures usually have tenderness over the spines. Herniated cervical disk is always a possibility and needs to ruled out with a careful neurological examination and provocative testing. The lack of radiation of the pain, negative Spurling's and axial loading tests, and no signs of motor or sensory deficit make a herniated disk with root compression unlikely. The absence of trigger points and lack of sleep disturbance rules out fibromyalgia. No complaints of chills and fever make an infectious cause unlikely. Osteoarthritis is a possibility but the patient's young age is against that diagnosis.

The most likely diagnosis is recurrent neck pain of uncertain etiology or cervical strain. This is a diagnosis of exclusion that is made after the other causes are ruled out by history and physical. Diagnostic studies, like magnetic resonance imaging (MRI), are not needed unless the pain does not respond to treatment or signs of root compression appear (like radiation of the pain to the arms, a positive Spurling's test, sensory or motor deficits). The patient responded very well to conservative measures that included Tylenol, a cervical pillow and the neck exercises included at the end of this chapter.

3.3. Treatment

Cervical strain is the most common cause of neck pain and has a high rate of spontaneous resolution. Eighty percent will have complete or partial relief after 3 months of conservative care. Cervical disk compression and cervical stenosis in the early stages will mimic cervical strain. If the symptoms of strain recur, it is important to keep evaluating the patient for root compression.

The treatment of nonradiating neck pain may include the following.

- A cervical pillow or towel rolled up and placed under the neck when reclining or sleeping.
- Tylenol in full doses of 3 to 4 g a day for at lease 10 days. Nonsteroidal anti-inflammatory drugs (NSAIDs) also in full doses for 10 days but not chronically. Muscle relaxants may help. Resist the temptation to use narcotics of any type as the chances for addition are increased.
- Local application of heat or cold often helps.
- Short-term use of a soft cervical collar often worn in reverse to allow for neck flexion may help especially with necessary activities of daily living (ADL), such as driving. As previously stated, the neck supports a 20- to 25-lb weight that is constantly moving around and places recurrent stress on the cervical spine and surrounding musculature. Minimizing the movement with a collar or towel may be very beneficial. The collar should not be worn for more than 3 to 4 days. Neck muscle weakness can result from prolonged use.
- Because the problem will most likely be recurrent, provide a ton of support and understanding. This helps empower the patient to self-manage the problem.

4. Fractures

Cervical vertebral fractures are usually associated with some type of trauma. Unless you work in the emergency department or the urgent care center these problems will not come to your attention too often. There are a few subtle fractures like isolated spinous process fractures that may present more commonly to the primary care practitioner. The most common etiology involves a strenuous contraction of the trapezius and rhomboid muscles, which avulses the spinous process. Another mechanism resulting in spinous process fractures is a hyperflexion or hyperextension injury to the neck that also results in avulsion of the spinous process. Direct blows to the spinous process from sports such as football or hockey can also produce this type of fracture. Spinous process fractures take 2 to 3 months to heal and become pain-free. Treatment is symptomatic. Protection against reinjury is important and return to a contact sport is discouraged until the fracture is healed.

5. Whiplash

Whiplash-associated disorder (WAD) is associated with acute or subacute neck pain that is preceded by an injury that combined acceleration and deceleration. It commonly occurs in rear-end motor vehicle accidents but other causes like diving that produce the same mechanism can produce WAD. The Quebec Classification of WADs identifies four categories of injury: grade I symptoms consist of general, nonspecific complaints regarding the neck, such as pain, stiffness, or soreness without objective physical findings; grade II symptoms include the grade I neck complaints plus objective findings limited to musculoskeletal structures; grade III injury consists of all the prior signs and symptoms and neurological signs; and grade IV injury now adds fracture or dislocation. Grade III and IV are not common and are usually not seen in the primary care setting. Grade I and II are more common and will be seen in the primary care setting. The discussion that follows is about patients with grade I and II.

Patients with WAD typically seek medical care a day or two after the injury because the discomfort is increasing. If involved in an auto accident the patient may have visited the emergency department and had X-rays that were "normal." They were told to see their physician if they became worse. The pain or soreness is usually in the posterior neck muscles, with radiation to the occiput, shoulder, or scapula. Stiffness in one or more directions of motion and headache are common. Localized areas of muscle tenderness (trigger points) in the posterior musculature may develop.

Treatment is similar to cervical strain. Tylenol, NSAIDs, cervical collars, and lots of support as outlined above are key. A physical therapy referral for use of other modalities and exercises is usually advisable.

Unfortunately, many of these patients have been informed that they should not settle with the insurance company until they have completely recovered. In addition, some of the patients may not recover until a settlement is made. It is important to extensively document all of your findings, as you may need to write a detailed report later. The request, usually from an attorney, will ask for an estimate of temporary and permanent disability. In addition to the history and physical examination, as noted previously, it may be advisable to have other evaluations in addition to yours. Some physical therapists can provide excellent assessments of degrees of disability and can document their findings. Orthopedic or physical medicine specialists can also provide helpful evaluations.

Chronic neck pain like chronic back pain is physically and psychologically disabling. These patients will get well but not as rapidly as clinicians desire. Some patients lose trust and confidence in the clinician because they feel the clinician does not believe they have pain and disability. This lack of trust may lead to seeking out of nontraditional or alternative methods of treatment. Alternative therapists are many times more patient and understanding of the patients. Continue to be supportive and encouraging, being careful not to overmedicate especially with narcotics. Low-dose antidepressants may help reduce the pain.

6. Case

6.1. History and Exam

A 52-year-old man presents to your office with a 3-week history of neck pain that radiates to his right shoulder, lateral aspect of his arm, his thumb, and index finger. He awoke with the pain in his neck 3 weeks ago. It has become worse over the past 10 days and the pain has started to radiate. His symptoms increase when he moves his head to acknowledge a fellow worker. He has difficulty holding his coffee cup and notes some numbness and tingling in his thumb. His general health is excellent. He works on construction and recently has had to lift 100-lb objects. The last 2 days he has not been able to work because the lifting produces severe pain and he notes a decrease in his strength. He reports no loss of bowel or bladder control and no weakness of his lower extremities. On examination, his temperature is normal. When asked to move his neck he limits all motions especially right lateral bending and right lateral rotation. Spurling's maneuver to the right is positive. His right biceps and wrist extensor strength is 2/4 compared with 4/4 on the left arm. He has diminished sensation on his right thumb compared with the left. He is able to elevate the right arm above his head without discomfort. He has no weakness of the lower extremities on examination.

6.2. Thinking Process

The above patient's story is worrisome and requires immediate evaluation. Radiating neck pain, decreased ability to lift and trouble holding a coffee cup suggests compression on a nerve root. A positive Spurling's maneuver accompanied by decreased bicep and wrist extensor strength and sensory loss on the thumb is diagnostic for compression of the C6 cervical root. This compression may lead to a permanent loss of function if it continues for a prolonged period of time. Rotator cuff problems are probably ruled out by the patient's ability to (abduct) lift his right arm above the head with minimal discomfort. Shoulder abduction is decreased and painful when rotator cuff problems are present. Spondylosis (cervical canal stenosis) is usually more chronic and appears in older individuals with recurrent neck pain. Spondylosis is many times accompanied by weakness in the lower extremities, which he does not report. This is still a possible diagnosis and imaging studies will need to done to rule this out if he does not improve.

A tentative diagnosis of a cervical disk herniation with C6 nerve root impingement was made. Plain films of the neck revealed no fractures and some mild cervical arthritis. He was treated with cervical traction, physical therapy, and a 14-day course of steroids. For the first 3 days, he used a cervical collar at bedtime and as needed during the day. He rested and did not to work for 7 days. He responded very well to the treatment. He returned to work with some restrictions on heavy lifting for the first 4 weeks. The patient was counseled about the possibility of recurrence and asked to return for follow-up if the symptoms recurred.

6.3. Discussion

Intervertebral disk herniation is a common cause of radiating neck pain. People in their 40s and 50s are particularly at risk for disk herniation. The annual incidence of disk herniation is reported to be 83.2 per 100,000. Risk factors include heavy manual labor, operation of vibrating equipment, lifting heavy objects, frequent automobile travel, smoking, and coughing. There is a history of trauma in 15% of cases, back problems in 41%, and a prior history of neck discomfort in most. Most patients wake up with neck pain in the morning and no recall of an associated precipitating event. C6 and C7 are the most common cervical roots compressed. C7 compression is present in 55% of patients, C6 in about 30% of patients, and C5 in about 10%.

The initial symptoms after disk herniation are neck pain and stiffness. Within a week or two, the pain begins to radiate into the shoulder, scapular region, and upper extremity depending on which nerve root is involved. Other symptoms include weakness and numbness along a dermatomal distribution. Table 9.2 lists some of the signs and symptoms noted with the different cervical roots compressed.

6.4. Imaging

In most cases, imaging is not required to make the diagnosis but anteroposterior (AP) and lateral radiographs are ordered to help rule out fractures and

TABLE 9.2. Signs and symptoms C5, C6, and C7 root compression.

Root	Pain distribution	Sensory loss distribution	Weakness	Reflex lost
C5	Posterior neck, shoulder, anterior lateral arm	Deltoid and lateral arm	Deltoid and biceps	Biceps
C6	Posterior neck, scapula, radial aspect forearm	Thumb and index finger	Biceps and wrist extensors	Biceps brachioradialis
C7	Neck shoulder dorsum of forearm	Middle finger	Triceps	Triceps

degree of degenerative changes. Degenerative changes do not mean a patient has "arthritis" as many asymptomatic patients especially young females have some changes. Magnetic resonance imaging is the study of choice to make the diagnosis of disk herniation. Similar to the lumbar area some patients may have asymptomatic disk herniation. Be sure the patient has a history and examination consistent with the radiographic findings. Table 9.2 helps relate the clinical signs with the radiographic findings. Magnetic resonance imaging studies are expensive and some patients are unable to tolerate the procedure because of claustrophobia. The open MRI and pretest treatment with an anxiolytic helps some.

7. Spondylosis

Cervical spondylosis is a narrowing (stenosis) of the cervical spinal canal. Degenerative changes of the spine occur with aging. Vertebral height decreases because of the shrinkage of the intervertebral disks. The disks are weaker and begin to bulge into the spinal canal. Other osteoarthritic changes produce osteophytes and spurs that further increase compromise of the cervical canal. The accumulation of degenerative changes produces gradual narrowing of the cervical canal, cervical spondylosis, and eventually compression of the spinal cord and neurological symptoms. The same process occurs with spinal stenosis in the lumbar region. No treatment is required until neurological symptoms are produced. Trauma may contribute to the problem but it is a rare cause. The major risk factor is aging but occupations that require heavy lifting and exposure to vibration increase the risk. Prior disk herniation and underlying systemic arthritic disorders may also predispose the patient to spondylosis.

The usual clinical picture is a patient over 55, with other signs of OA, who complains of chronic neck pain and pain radiating into the arms. The onset of symptoms is usually insidious. Upper extremity weakness and loss of sensation are common presenting symptoms. Leg weakness and loss of sensation may also be present. Elderly patients may present for gait problems and falling and not realize they have leg weakness. Rarely, the patient may present with acute onset of paralysis after a fall.

The examination usually reveals some limitation of neck mobility. Weakness of the upper extremity is more common than lower extremity weakness. Biceps, triceps, and wrist extensors may be weak. Atrophy and fasciculations mimicking amyotrophic lateral sclerosis may be present. Weakness of hip flexion (iliopsoas muscle), lower leg flexion (hamstrings), and extensors (anterior tibial muscles) of the feet and toes may also be present. Muscle tone may be spastic and clonus will be present along with a Babinski's sign. Sensory loss to light touch, vibration, and joint position may be present. The sensory loss may follow a dermatome or be patchy because of multiple root involvement.

Perform an MRI to assess the adequacy of the spinal canal. The issue of differential diagnosis is important because of the incidence of a radiological finding that may not be causing the symptoms. Slowly progressive spastic weakness of the extremities, worse in the lower than in the upper extremities, may be produced by a variety of conditions. Obtain a neurological consultation to help sort out the differential diagnosis.

Treatment is usually surgical if significant neurological findings are present. If the neurological deficit is minimal use nonsurgical treatment, similar to that used for a cervical disk.

8. Medical Causes

The pain associated with angina and myocardial infarction can occasionally be isolated to the neck but the associated symptoms and risk factors should help the clinician focus on these problems. Angina is exercise-induced and relieved by rest. If the patient has high-risk characteristics like diabetes, hyperlipidemia, and smoking, consider angina and myocardial infarction in the differential diagnosis.

The neck is not a common site for rheumatoid arthritis (RA). If RA is the cause it will be late in the course of the disease. Remember RA is a symmetrical disease that attacks the small joints of the hand and the wrist. If other signs of RA are present then consider RA as a cause of the neck pain. Ankylosing spondylitis is another unusual cause of neck pain. This disease usually begins with back pain that is improved by exercise and not relieved by rest. There is usually a loss of lumbar lordosis, radiographic sacroliitis, and HLA-B27-antigen-positive. The same thing can happen to the neck but usually after the back is already symptomatic.

9. Torticollis

Torticollis or tilting of the head to one side can be secondary to trauma or an infectious process. It is usually self-limited and when the condition that caused the pain subsides, the torticollis will do the same. It can be a congenital condition secondary to a contracture of the sternocleidomastoid muscle. The contracture comes from birth trauma and a resulting scar in the muscle. The scar contracts and the head tilts toward the affected side and rotates toward the unaffected side. Flattening of the face on the affected side occurs if it is not treated early.

At 4 to 6 weeks of age, the parents will usually note a difference in head position. A lump may be felt in the sternocleidomastoid. Stretching exercises that tilt and rotate the head in a direction away from the deformity will help. A physical therapist can help with this. If the deformity persists past 18 months, surgery may be indicated.

10. Neck Exercises

Tell the patient to stop doing any of these exercises if they produce numbness or tingling. Do three sets of each exercise two times a day. Rotate from one exercise to the other. Do one set of one exercise and then rotate to another exercise and do a set. Do not exercise past the point of pain. Pain means stop.

A. **Neck flexion (Figure 9.8)**: Place the palm of your hand against your forehead and push your forehead into your palm while exerting some resistance with your palm. Hold for 5 s and repeat five times in one set.

B. **Neck extension (Figure 9.9)**: Place your clasped hands behind your head and press the back of your head into your hands while exerting some resistance. Hold for 5 s and repeat five times in one set.

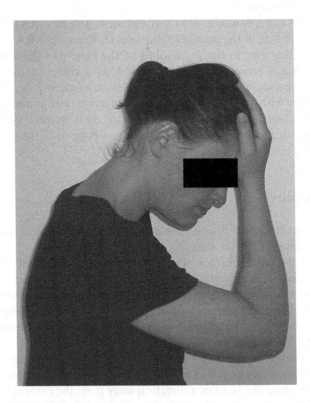

FIGURE 9.8. Neck flexion exercise.

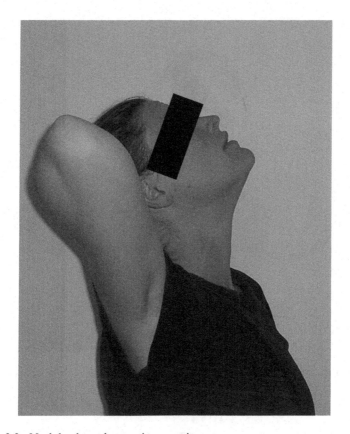

FIGURE 9.9. Neck backward extension exercise.

C. **Neck side bend (Figure 9.10)**: Place the palm of your hand on your temple and press into the hand while exerting some resistance. Hold for 5 s and repeat five times in one set.
D. **Neck lateral rotation (Figure 9.11)**: With the neck in a neutral position rotate the head to each side against the resistance of a clinched fist against the mandible. Hold for 5 s and repeat five times in one set.
E. **Shoulder shrugs (Figure 9.12)**: Stand with your neck in a neutral position and shoulders thrown back. Shrug your shoulders up and then relax. Do three sets of 10.

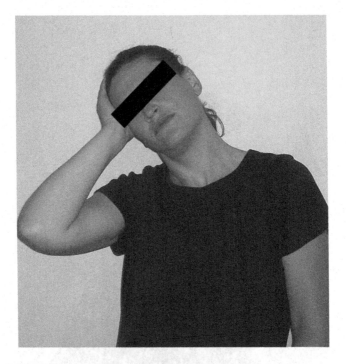

FIGURE 9.10. Neck sidebend exercise.

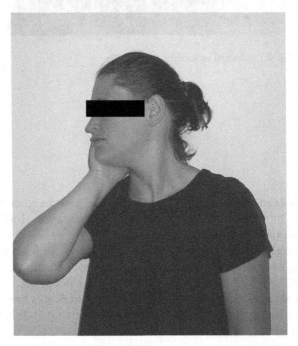

FIGURE 9.11. Neck lateral rotation exercise.

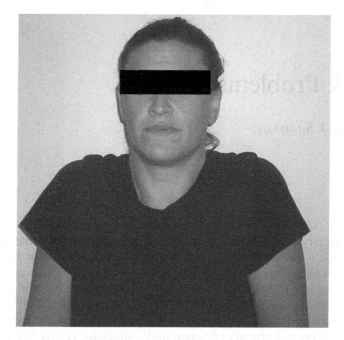

FIGURE 9.12. Shoulder shrug exercise.

Suggested Readings

Slipman C, et al. Chronic neck pain: mapping out diagnosis and management. *J Musculoskelet Med.* 2002;19:242–255.

Rao R. Neck pain, cervical radiculopathy, and cervical myelopathy: pathophysiology, natural history, and clinical evaluation. *J Bone Joint Surg Am.* 2002;84:1872–1881.

10

Back Problems

Edward J. Shahady

Low back pain (LBP) is the fifth most common reason for outpatient visits in the primary care setting. It is also a leading cause of lost work time, disability, and is responsible for direct health care expenditures of more than $20 billion annually. Back pain can be a straightforward mechanical problem or it can be one of the most challenging problems seen by the primary care clinician. Studies of satisfaction with back pain care indicate 50% to 70% dissatisfaction with the care received. Chiropractors receive the highest satisfaction ratings and primary clinicians and orthopedist receive lower ratings. Lack of recognition and/or treatment of the behavioral or psychosocial issues account for most of the dissatisfaction.

Almost everyone experiences back pain at some time during his or her life and up to 50% of working adults have one bout of back pain each year. On average, 60% recover by 6 weeks and 90% by 12 weeks. Lifetime recurrence rates of back pain may be as high as 80%. Recovery and prognosis are influenced by the presence of depression, previous history of back trouble, reimbursement issues, and ongoing litigation. If the back pain is work-related and/or a lawyer is involved, recovery is delayed. Each year, about 2% of the American workforce has back injuries covered by workmen's compensation. The injuries covered by workmen's compensation usually take longer to recover, involve more nonspecific symptoms, and are a source of frustration for clinicians.

Low back pain secondary to serious pathology is rare. Mechanical problems are the usual diagnosis. It is most often a self-limited process lasting 6 weeks or less and complete recovery is the rule.

Satisfaction derived by patients with the care they receive for back problems is related to how well clinicians validate the patients' suffering, help them return to normal functioning, and act like they care. Keep the following words of wisdom in mind: The patient does not care how much you know until they know how much you care.

Simply stated, caring for the patient with LBP is exactly that: *caring*. The prudent clinician must realize that the psychosocial aspect of LBP is as important if not more important than looking for a biological cause of the pain. As the history and physical is performed, equal emphasis must be placed on collecting information that facilitates making the biological as well as the psychosocial diagnosis. It is not unusual to find data that indicate both types of diagnosis are present. This chapter, like others, will use epidemiology and anatomy to aid discovery of an anatomical cause of the problem as well as describe methods of data collection that will enhance making a psychosocial diagnosis (Table 10.1). Effective treatment addresses both diagnoses.

1. Focused History

Ask about any preceding events like lifting, bending over, twisting, or trauma. Many patients with an acute onset of back pain can remember an event within the past 24 h like repeated lifting that is not their usual activity or a significant twisting activity like dancing the twist the night before. The lifting may be with a heavy item or it may just be the way the lift was performed. Healthy ways to lift are described in the last part of the chapter. Acute onset of severe debilitating pain with no trauma or minimal activity suggests a fracture that may be seen with a malignancy or a compression fracture of osteoporosis. Radiation of the pain to the buttocks and/or down the legs is significant. This radiation is called "sciatica or lumbago." It does not always mean nerve impingement. In fact, the most common cause of radiation is hamstring tightness that usually accompanies back pain. Hamstring tightness pain is usually described as discomfort rather than the burning pain of nerve compression. Nerve compression pain usually radiates down to the lower leg and foot but it may not. The burning or stinging quality of the pain usually signifies nerve compression. What relieves the pain and what makes the pain worse is a helpful piece of history. Mechanical pain is relieved by bed rest and sitting and increased with rising from a chair and standing. The pain

TABLE 10.1. Classification of low back pain problems.

(1) Low back pain syndrome
- Mechanical back pain
- Psychogenic back pain

(2) Low back pain associated with loss of neurologic function
- Herniated disk
- Spinal stenosis
- Cauda equina syndrome

(3) Low back pain associated with red flags
- Pathological fractures
- Compression fractures
- Infections

(4) Other causes
- Ankylosing spondylitis
- Spondylolysis

of a herniated lumbar disk is better with lying down, worse with sitting, and better with standing. Spinal stenosis pain is worse with walking and bending backward and relieved by bending forward. The pain of a fracture or metastatic bone pain is characteristically worse at night and when lying down whereas almost all other types of back pain are relieved by lying down.

Asking about weakness or loss of strength and numbness in the legs is important. Herniated lumbar disks with nerve compression can lead to progressive leg weakness and numbness. These symptoms can also be present with spinal stenosis. The symptoms of stenosis are usually brought on by walking and relieved by stopping and bending over.

The cauda equina (CE) syndrome is a rare but devastating complication of disk herniation. The symptoms are inability to void and involuntary loss of stool. All patients with back pain should be asked questions about inability or difficulty voiding and involuntary loss of stool. Warn patients with any type of back pain to report any signs of bowel or bladder problems. The window of opportunity to prevent permanent loss of bladder or bowel function is 24 h or less. Loss of bladder or bowel function constitutes a surgical emergency.

Infections like tuberculosis (TB) or osteomyelitis rarely may be the cause of back pain. If signs of systemic illness like fever or weight loss are present, consider an infectious process.

Ask about past problems with back pain, how long it took to recover, satisfaction with the care for that episode, and similarity of this episode to the past episode. Recurrent back pain usually has some psychosocial issues involved. Depression may be present so a few questions about inability to concentrate, not sleeping well, crying easily, guilt, and depressive mood are indicated. If depression is present, the back pain will not get better unless the depression is also addressed. Both can be treated at the same time. Most primary care practitioners are well versed in the treatment of depression and this book is not intended to cover therapy for depression. The emphasis here is on the importance of recognizing it as a comorbid condition with back pain.

Always ask if the back pain is work-related. If workmen's compensation is involved some but not all of these patients may take longer to recover. Quick follow-up and use of a physical therapist helps hasten recovery with this group.

Progressive back pain for at least 3 months in a male under 40 that involves the sacroiliac (SI) and gluteal regions, and is accompanied by decreased mobility, should alert the clinician to the possibility of ankylosing spondylitis (AS). This is a rare but important cause of back pain in younger men.

2. Focused Examination

First obtain the vital signs to be sure the patient is not febrile and also evaluate the blood pressure (BP). Pain elevates BP and the patient (especially males who avoid seeking health care) may not be aware they are hypertensive.

The BP may be greater than 180/110 and require treatment or at least appropriate follow-up.

The history will be pointing you to a more specific diagnosis but here are some general tips for a focused examination. The position of the patient when you walk into the room may be diagnostic. If they are standing and even pacing the room this is characteristic of a herniated disk. Patients with mechanical back pain are sitting in a chair and when you ask them to get up they struggle and grimace because of the pain.

Next have the patient walk on their tiptoes and then their heels (Figure 10.1A and 10.1B). This is a good screening test for L5 and S1 nerve root compression. Weakness of toe walking is indicative of S1 root compression and heel walking of L5 root compression. If heel and toe walking are normal and there is nothing else to suggest root compression from the history or physical, no other tests for lower leg strength need be performed.

Range of back motion is a very helpful part of the examination. With the patient standing in front of you, have him/her perform forward flexion (Figure 10.2). If the patient can achieve 90° of forward flexion, it is unlikely

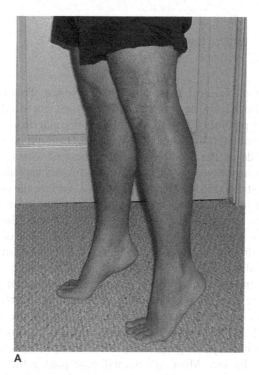

A

FIGURE 10.1. (A) Walk on toes.

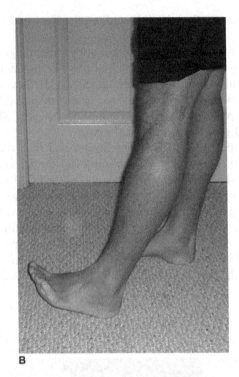

B

FIGURE 10.1. (B) Walk on heels.

that a disk or mechanical back problem is present. Backward extension (Figure 10.3) should now be performed. The patient can usually reach 30° to 40°. Limited or painful backward extension is characteristic of spinal stenosis. Left and right lateral movement (Figure 10.4) should now be attempted. Pain on one side or the other is usually associated with mechanical back problems. Twisting movement, discomfort or stiffness may also be indicative of mechanical strain or SI problems. Be sure to stabilize the pelvis when asking the patient to twist. Stand behind the patient and place your hands on both iliac crests to assure that the patient is not moving the pelvis but the back. Marked stiffness of all movements may be indicative of AS.

The patient should now be asked to lie on the examination table. Observe the patient's ability to get on the table. Patients who have no problems with the above movements and smoothly get on the examination table may have more of a psychosocial problem than an anatomic problem. Perform a straight leg raise as demonstrated in Figure 10.5. Be sure the opposite knee is flexed to 90°. If pain is present between 30° and 70°, be sure to ask where it radiates and what type of pain it is. Nerve compression pain is burning and goes in to the foot. Most patients will have pain in the posterior thigh, indicating hamstring tightness that is common with back problems. If pain is

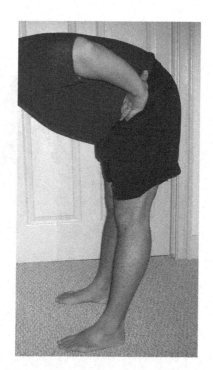

FIGURE 10.2. Forward flexion.

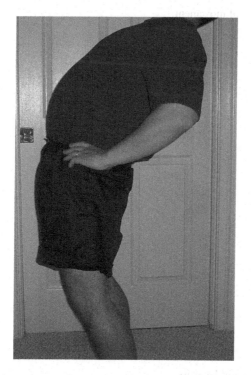

FIGURE 10.3. Backward extension.

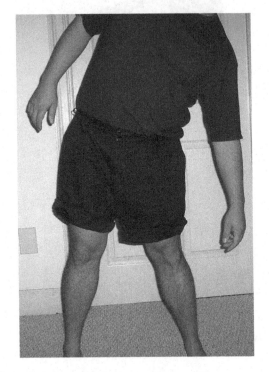

FIGURE 10.4. Lateral movement.

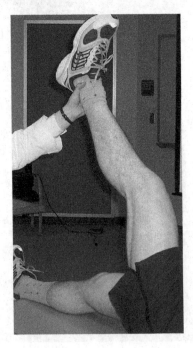

FIGURE 10.5. Straight leg raise.

not present at 70° of straight leg raising, dorsiflex the foot to elicit pain. This maneuver stretches the sciatic nerve and may help demonstrate nerve root compression. This maneuver will also stretch the hamstrings so again ask for pain location and type. Some patients may be very familiar with what you are looking for in an examination and have learned the right response to the straight leg test. If you are not sure of the results of your examination or want to confirm the results, do a distracting test (Figure 10.6). This test is performed with the patient sitting on the examination table. The affected knee is moved from 90° of flexion to complete extension. If patients have root compression, they will lean back and grimace to relieve the discomfort.

If you have a strong suspicion of nerve root compression or spinal stenosis, additional tests for muscle strength should be performed. Figure 10.7 demonstrates testing for the ability to dorsiflex the foot against resistance. Weakness of dorsiflexion indicates L5 root compression. Figure 10.8 demonstrates testing for plantar flexion against resistance. Weakness of plantar flexion indicates S1 root compression. Plantar and dorsiflexion of the big toe can also serve the same purpose. Sensory testing can also be done although it is less reliable because of the subjective nature of the response. Loss of sensation to pinprick over the outer lateral portion or fifth metatarsal portion of the foot is consistent with S1 root compression. L5 root compression is associated with sensory loss in the big toe area. Reflexes are usually not that helpful in making the diagnosis. The Achilles reflex may be diminished in S1 root compression. If the patient has symptoms of bladder or bowel problems, assess the patient for loss of sensation in the perineum and perform a rectal examination for anal sphincter tone.

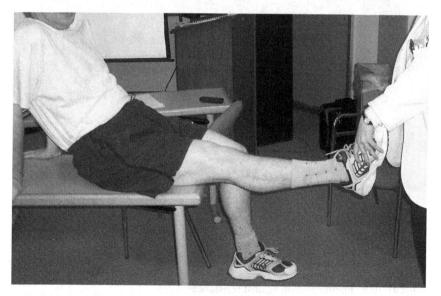

FIGURE 10.6. Distracting straight leg-raising test.

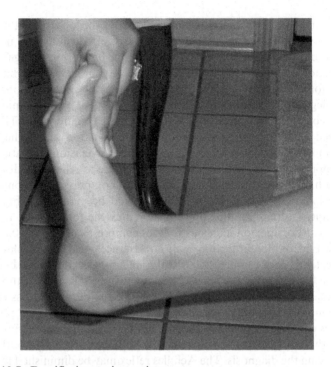

FIGURE 10.7. Dorsiflexion against resistance.

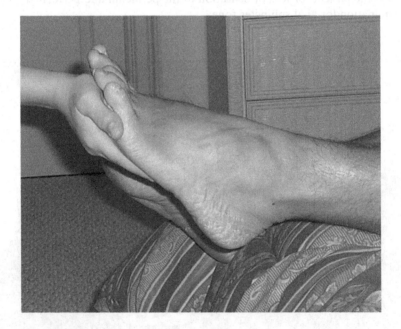

FIGURE 10.8. Plantar flexion against resistance.

Palpation may also yield valuable information. Trigger points that will respond to injections might be found. Tenderness over paraspinal muscles is common with mechanical pain and herniated disks. Tenderness over the vertebral bodies and/or the spinous processes may be associated with fractures and infectious process.

The FABER test, as demonstrated in Figure 10.9, helps diagnose SI pathology. FABER is an abbreviation for hip flexion, abduction and external rotation. This test can also indicate hip pathology, specifically osteoarthritis of the hip.

3. Case

3.1. History

A 45-year-old male executive comes to your office with a 1-day history of back pain. The pain is in his lower back and does not radiate. He has never experienced back pain before. He was doing some work in his garden yesterday and leaned over to pick up a rake and felt something "go" in his back. He had been lifting heavy items and working for about 3 h outside before this happened. He was unable to continue working and had to be helped back to

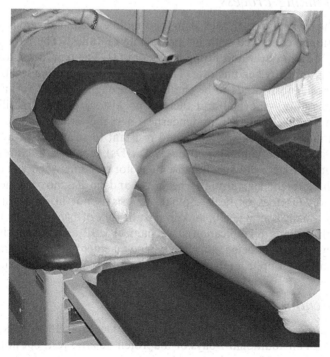

FIGURE 10.9. FABER (flexion, abduction, external rotation) test.

the house. He obtained some relief for his pain by placing a heating pad on his back and taking 600 mg of ibuprofen every 4 hours. The pain is not as severe today but he is unable to move around without difficulty.

He has gained about 10 lb over the last year and he is not as physically active as he once was. This was the first time this spring he had done any yard work. In fact, he says his weekends this past winter have been spent watching football games and enjoying indoor activities with his family with minimal exercise. His wife had to help him put his underwear, pants, shoes, and socks on this morning to come to your office. He has no other medical problems and a physical examination in your office 2 years ago was normal.

On examination, his BP is 155/88 and he is not febrile. He is sitting in a chair when you walk into the room. When asked to get up from the chair he grimaces and has difficulty getting up from the chair. He points to his lower back as the area of discomfort. He is able to walk on his toes and heels although it is uncomfortable to move. He can only forward-flex to 30°. Backward extension is to 45°. Left and right lateral movement and twisting maneuvers are all within normal limits although he is uncomfortable with both. There is minimal pain with palpation over the paraspinal muscles bilaterally. The straight leg test produced some mild hamstring pain but no burning pain down to the feet.

3.2. Thinking Process

This is the first episode of back pain for a middle-aged man who is probably deconditioned compared with his prior state of fitness. The pain was preceded by bending over and lifting heavy objects. The pain does not radiate and he has difficulty bending over. This is suggestive of mechanical back pain but other diagnosis needs to be eliminated through a focused examination. His temperature is normal and there is no history of systemic illness, so infection is unlikely. There is no tenderness over the vertebral bodies and the pain, although acute, is not severe and resistant to treatment with heat and nonsteroidal anti-inflammatory drugs (NSAIDs), making a fracture unlikely. A herniated disk is not likely because he is not standing when you enter the room, the straight leg raising is negative, and he has no weakness when walking on his toes or heels. Spinal stenosis is not likely given his age (patients usually over age 60), and no past history of back pain or lower leg pain with walking (claudication). Mechanical LBP as a diagnosis is supported by the patient being in a chair when you enter the room, grimacing in attempting to get up from the chair, and limitation of forward flexion.

3.3. Treatment

The diagnoses postulated for this patient was mechanical low back. He was treated with an additional 7 days of ibuprofen, relative rest, but not bed rest for 2 days. Stretching and strengthening exercises were started after the second day. (Exercises are described at the end of this chapter.) No imaging studies were ordered. After 1 week, he was feeling well enough to return to work. He was advised to do the exercises daily for an additional 14 days and then to do them two to three times a week to prevent a recurrence of his back pain for the rest of his life. He also was instructed in a program of back hygiene to prevent future back problems. (See description at the end of this chapter.) To increase his general fitness he began a walking program with his spouse and lost 15 lb. With the weight loss and the walking program his BP on return visits had decreased to 115/76. Follow-up 1 year later revealed no recurrence of the back pain and he was able to maintain his weight and normal BP. He continues to do his back exercises two times a week and follow the back hygiene suggestions.

4. Mechanical Low Back Pain

This is the most common cause of back pain. It is commonly preceded by an event like lifting a heavy object or trying to perform an activity that requires the use of back muscles that have not been used for some time. The patients are usually not as conditioned as they once were and have lost abdominal tone either through childbirth or through increased abdominal girth. They usually have had a few self-limited bouts of back pain that were self-treated prior to seeking medical advice. The usual reason for seeking your advice is difficulty with performing occupation-related activities. The pain is usually nonradiating or if it radiates it is usually not below the knees. Difficulty rising from a chair and bending over to pick up items and putting on shoes and socks are usual complaints. Extremity weakness is rarely a complaint.

The examination is characterized by the absence of neurological deficits so the patients are able to walk on their toes and heels (see Figure 10.1A and 10.1B), difficulty with forward flexion (Figure 10.2), normal backward extension (Figure 10.3), and some problems with lateral movement and twisting (Figures 10.4 and 10.5). Trigger points may occasionally be found but they are not numerous.

4.1. Imaging

Multiple studies of back pain indicate that unless red flags or persistent neurological deficits are present, imaging harms rather than aids care in the first 6 weeks of treatment. Unfortunately, clinicians have trained patients to think images are needed to make the diagnosis. Keep in mind that we are discussing the need for images when no red flags are present and there is not persistent neurologic deficit. Some clinicians argue that they obtain the films for medical or legal reasons. The data reviewing the reason why most physicians obtain unneeded X-rays and laboratory tests reveal that clinician ignorance about the clinical aspects of the presenting problem is more predictive of obtaining unneeded studies than their fear of malpractice.

Another problem with diagnostic imaging is the high incidence of abnormalities that are not related to the clinical symptoms. Autopsy results reveal that by the age of 50, 95% of patients show age-related changes including disk narrowing, osteophytes, and sclerosis in their spinal columns. Patients, both with and without symptoms, have the same amount of radiographic changes. The same is true with magnetic resonance imagings (MRIs). Herniated disks are found radiographically in patients with and without symptoms. X-Rays are of value to diagnose a fracture and MRI is of value to confirm clinical impression. If the MRI is negative and the clinical picture indicates persistent localized nerve deficit refer the patient to a neurosurgeon for further diagnostic evaluation.

4.2. Treatment

Back pain is difficult to treat. Many studies indicate that 40% to 50% of patients are not satisfied with their treatment because they do not respond rapidly to treatment. Treatment for back pain starts, ends, and restarts with back exercises. Unfortunately, most clinicians think of some type of oral medication as their first option. Mediations are not as effective as exercises. Back pain may lead to overreliance on medication and addiction because of this tendency to medicate. Clinicians who understand how to encourage patients to use exercise usually transmit confidence and enthusiasm to their patients for exercise and decrease reliance on medication. Back pain in many patients is a chronic problem and exercises provide the best means for the patient to live with the pain. Tricyclic antidepressants in low doses help chronic pain. All patients with chronic back pain should be evaluated for depression. All patients with back pain should be advised about back hygiene to prevent recurrence, in addition to being advised about back exercises. Back hygiene and back exercises are described at the end of the chapter.

5. Herniated Disk

Herniated intervertebral disks are more common in younger patients, with the average age being 35. The patients usually present complaining of back pain that radiates down one leg. The radiation associated with herniated disks is usually below the knee and into the foot. In some patients, the initial presentation may not include radiation but if a herniated disk is present, radiation of the pain will usually appear. Other complaints may include numbness and/or weakness in the lower extremity and aggravation of the pain by sitting, coughing, sneezing, straining, and defecation. Difficulty voiding and involuntary loss of stool are indications of central disk herniation and the Cauda Equina syndrome. This is a surgical emergency (see page 192).

When you first observe these patients in the examination room, they are usually standing and not sitting because sitting causes increased intervertebral pressure compared with standing. If nerve compression is significant, the patient may demonstrate weakness of toe walking or heel walking. Forward flexion will be decreased but backward extension will usually be normal. The straight leg-raising test will be positive and reveal a burning pain that radiates below the knee. Hamstring tightness is also common and causes pain over the back of the thigh and should not be confused with a positive straight leg test. Weakness of foot dorsiflexion and plantar flexion may also be present. Table 10.2 describes the common physical findings for L4, L5, and S1 nerve root compression. L5 and S1 are the most common nerve roots involved in herniated intervertebral disks.

5.1. Imaging

Initially, no studies are needed. Most patients with herniated disk will respond to conservative treatment much like mechanical back pain and not require any imaging studies. Nerve root compression will eventually disappear in all patients. The challenge is not to allow permanent damage to occur. If the root compression signs do not begin to diminish within 1 week or they worsen, it is advisable to consider neurosurgical evaluation. Some clinicians may wish to obtain an MRI at this point and use the MRI to help make a decision about further care. My preference is to consult a neurosurgeon and maybe order an MRI at the same time. Magnetic resonance imagings are positive for disk herniation in many patients who are asymptomatic and may not be conclusive in face of obvious nerve root compression. Plain films are of minimal value unless you suspect other bone pathology.

5.2. Treatment

As in the case of mechanical LBP, exercises are the mainstay of treatment. Exercises that make the pain worse should be avoided until they can be performed without discomfort. A physical therapist should be consulted to help the patient gradually initiate the exercises and avoid maneuvers that make the pain worse. Oral medications, like NSAIDs, and narcotics to relieve the pain

TABLE 10.2. Common findings with root compression of L4, L5, S1.

	L4	L5	S1
Motor weakness	Quadriceps extension	Dorsiflexion, great toe and foot	Plantar flexion, great toe and foot
Screening examination	Squat and rise	Heel walking	Toe walking
Reflexes	Knee jerk decreased	None reliable	Ankle jerk decreased

are indicated. Muscle relaxants can be used in the short term. Valium for 3 to 4 days is an excellent choice for muscle relaxation and sedation when the patient is in acute pain. Patients should be advised not to drive while using any sedating medication.

6. Spinal Stenosis

Spinal stenosis is a common cause of chronic back pain in patients over 60. It is secondary to the following progressive degenerative disease of the lumbar spine that occurs with aging:

1. Vertebral height decreasing because of the shrinkage of the intervertebral disks.
2. Disks becoming weaker and beginning to bulge into the spinal canal.
3. Other osteoarthritic changes that produce osteophytes and spurs that further increase compromise of the spinal canal.

The accumulation of these degenerative changes produces gradual narrowing of the cervical canal, and eventually compression of the spinal cord and neurological symptoms. The patient will usually have a 4- or 5-year history of back pain that becomes progressively worse. The pain starts in the lower back and eventually begins to radiate because of nerve root compression. The pain is worse with walking and back extension and relieved by rest and flexion. Walking uphill is usually worse because of the associated hyperextension that narrows the spinal canal. The physical examination may reveal signs of nerve compression, such as those noted in Table 10.2. An MRI is helpful in confirming the diagnosis. Plain films will reveal osteoarthritic changes but are not diagnostic. Treatment is a challenge. Intrathecal steroid injection helps some but not all patients and is dependent on the skill of the person performing the procedure. Surgery is indicated if the neurological deficit is progressive but pain alone is not an indication for surgery. Exercises are helpful, including walking to increase conditioning. Caution should be exercised in prescribing NSAIDs. These patients are older and the side effects and potential for drug interactions are greater in this age group. Tylenol is an excellent choice for short-term relief. Ten days of 3000 to 4000 mg daily is safe if the patient has no known liver disease or other contraindications to using Tylenol.

7. Cauda Equina Syndrome

The cauda equina (CE) is a collection of nerve roots beginning at the end of the spinal cord. Cauda is Latin for tail, and equina is Latin for horse, i.e., the "horse's tail." The CE syndrome is a rare but significant complication of herniated disks, trauma, and/or back infection. The cause is severe compression of the nerve roots of the CE that produces problems with urinary and fecal retention, severe back pain, lower extremity weakness and sensory loss. Delays of greater than 24 h in making this diagnosis can lead to significant disability. Keys to not missing this diagnosis are as follows:

1. Ask every patient with back pain about difficulty with urination and defecation.
2. Remember that the problem with urination is retention of urine and the patient may not feel the urge to urinate. Defecation problems are not as likely and when present usually present with fecal soiling.
3. A post-voiding urine test for residual urine may be indicated. Greater than 100 cc indicates retention.
4. Test the perineum for sensation. Saddle anesthesia may be present with compression of the CE.
5. Perform a rectal examination to test for decreased tone.
6. Keep a high index of suspicion in any patient with severe pain and neurologic deficit.

An MRI is helpful in making the diagnosis of CE compression but the clinical evaluation is the most reliable way to assess the significance of the CE compression.

8. Red Flags

8.1. Nighttime Pain

Back pain due to the above problems almost always improves when the patient is lying in bed and/or sleeping. If the pain is worse at night or when the patient is reclining or lying in bed, a fracture, a malignancy, or an infection should be considered the cause. Reclining, sleeping, and nighttime pain are an indication for an X-ray and further evaluation.

8.2. Localized Tenderness over the Spine

Acute onset of pain that is moderately severe and located in a specific area over the spine is worrisome. It may be caused by a fracture that is either associated with osteoporosis or a pathological fracture associated with a malignancy. In some cases, the pathological fracture may be the first sign of the malignancy. An X-ray is indicated when the onset of the pain is acute, severe, and associated with pinpoint tenderness over bone.

8.3. Fever

If fever and/or other signs of an infectious disease are associated with back pain, osteomyelitis of the spine should be considered. Appropriate imaging should be performed to rule out an infectious cause of the back pain.

9. Ankylosing Spondylitis

Ankylosing spondylitis (AS) is a rare but important cause of back pain in younger men because early recognition and treatment may decease disability. Unfortunately, AS is not usually recognized early. Consider AS if the patient is a male under 40 and has pain in the lower back that involves the SI and gluteal regions, and the pain is progressive for more than 3 months and accompanied by stiffness and reduced mobility of the spine. The hallmark of this disease is sacroiliitis. X-rays will demonstrate unilateral or bilateral erosions and sclerosis of the SI joint. Some of these patients may also have cardiac, pulmonary, and eye symptoms. The sedimentation rate is usually elevated and HLA-B-27 antigen may be positive. If you suspect AS, early physical therapy is important and consultation with a rheumatologist or a physician with an expertise in rheumatologic disease is advisable.

10. Spondylolysis

Spondylolysis is the most worrisome cause of back pain in adolescents. If back pain is present more than 2 weeks in an adolescent further evaluation with an x-ray is indicated. Spondylolysis causes 50% of chronic back pain in adolescents. Spondylolysis is a fatigue fracture of the bony pars interarticularis caused by repetitive hyperextension of the back. In adolescents the pars is thinner and more susceptible to the shear stress of back hyperextension. Risk factors for spondylolysis include hyperlordosis and specific athletic activities like gymnastics, weight lifting, dance, and football. The physical examination should include all the specific examination maneuvers suggested above plus the "stork test" (Figure 10.10). This test is performed by asking adolescents to stand on one leg and hyperextend their back. Reproduction of the pain is suggestive of spondylolysis.

When obtaining X-rays in adolescents with back pain, oblique views are important because standard posteroanterior (PA) and lateral views may not show the fractured pars interarticularis. A complication of pars interarticularis fracture is forward displacement of the vertebral body. This can cause an increase in the pain and compression of the spinal cord. When there is forward displacement the problem is called spondylolisthesis. There are four grades of forward displacement depending on the amount of displacement. The radiologist can provide the measurements.

Treatment for spondylosis and spondylolisthesis is most often nonoperative. The most common treatment includes relative rest from hyperextension, a nonrigid brace, and oral pain medications. If the spondylolisthesis slips to grades III and IV, the pain does not respond to conservative measures, or neurological symptoms appear, obtain an orthopedic consultation.

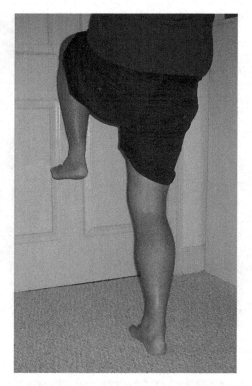

FIGURE 10.10. Stork test.

11. Back Exercises

Tell the patient to repeat each of the following exercises two times a day. Rotate from one exercise to the other. Do one set of exercises and then rotate to another exercise and do a set. Do not exercise past the point of pain. Pain means stop.

1. **Standing hamstring stretch (Figure 10.11)**: Place the heel of your leg on a stool or other object about 2 ft high. Keep your leg fully extended and lean forward. You will feel the back of your leg begin to stretch (your hamstring muscles). Remember to keep the leg straight and not bent and do not bend the back. Hold the stretch for 15 s. Hold the stretch for 15 s. Repeat five times alternating with each leg.

2. **Lying down hamstring stretch (Figure 10.12)**: Lie on your back and raise each leg straight (fully extended) until you feel the same stretch in the back of your leg. Bend your toes toward you to increase the stretch. Hold the stretch for 15 s. Repeat five times alternating with each leg.

3. **Pelvic tilt (Figure 10.13)**: Lie on your back with your knees bent about 45° and feet flat on the floor. Tighten your abdominal muscles and

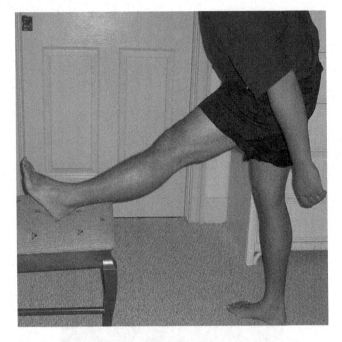

FIGURE 10.11. Standing hamstring stretch.

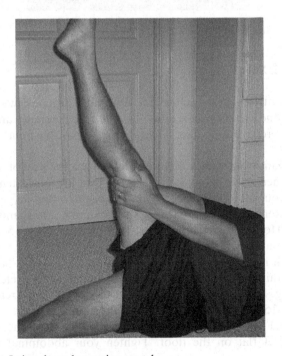

FIGURE 10.12. Lying down hamstring stretch.

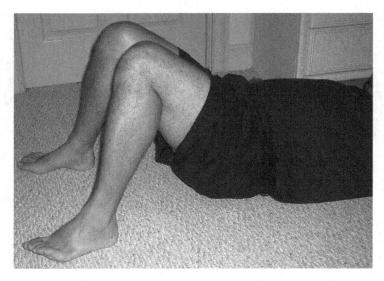

FIGURE 10.13. Pelvic tilt.

push your lower back into the floor. Hold this position for 5 s. Do three sets of 10.

4. **Partial curl (Figure 10.14)**: Lie on your back with your knees bent 45° and your feet on the floor. Tighten your stomach muscles and flatten your back against the floor. Place your chin onto your chest. Some individuals find that they need to support their neck with their hands clasped behind the neck to decrease discomfort. Start the curl by moving upper body toward your knees until your shoulders clear the floor. Hold this position for 5 s. Exhale with the curl and inhale as you return to the starting position. Initially repeat 25 times and then build up to 50 at each setting.

5. **Knee to chest stretch (Figure 10.15)**: Lie on your back with your legs straight out in front of you. Slowly bend one knee and bring it toward you. Clasp both hands around the knee and pull it toward your chest. Hold this position for 15 s and return to the starting position. Repeat the process on the other knee, then do both knees together, Repeat each one three times.

6. **Sacroiliac joint stretch (Figure 10.16)**: Lie on your back with your knees bent to 45° and feet on the floor. Place the ankle of one leg on the knee of the other and gradually externally rotate that leg until you feel the stretch in your back. Repeat with each leg and hold each external rotation for 15 s. Do each side 5 to 10 times.

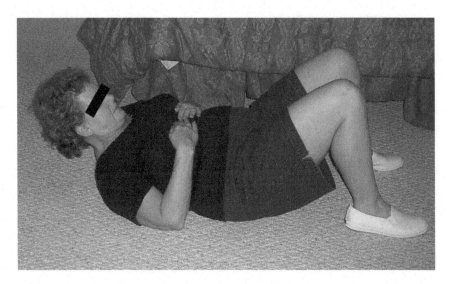

FIGURE 10.14. Partial curl exercise.

12. Back Hygiene

12.1. Sitting

- Head up not tilted forward or back.
- Thighs parallel to the floor. Knees bent to 90° and never higher than the hips.

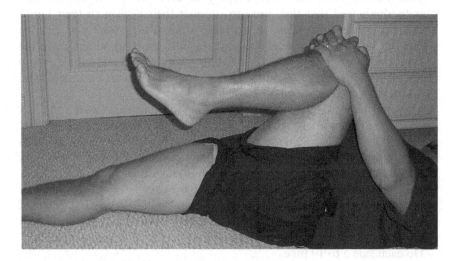

FIGURE 10.15. Knee-to-chest stretch.

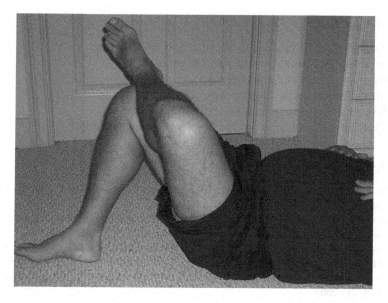

FIGURE 10.16. Sacroiliac joint stretch.

- Your feet should be flat on the floor.
- Make sure the chair has good lumbar (lower back) support. For additional support, use a small pillow or a rolled-up towel.
- Keep about 3 in. of space between the back of your knee and the edge of your seat.

12.2. When Using a Computer

- Keep the keyboard and monitor directly in front of you and the monitor should be at eye level.
- Bend elbows at a 90° angle and place wrists in a neutral position, not tilted up or down when using the keyboard.
- Use wrist rests for extra support.
- Avoid sitting for more than 1 h at a time. Get up and walk or stand for 1 or 2 min. Stretch your back and neck during the break.

12.3. Standing

- Have a place to rest your foot that is 6 in. high. Alternate each foot periodically.
- If working while standing, keep the work surface near waist level.

12.4. Lifting

- Stand as close as possible to the item you will be lifting.
- Place one foot slightly in front of the other.
- Bend your knees and squat down.
- Lift the object by pushing up with your legs and buttocks.
- Push or slide heavy objects rather than lift them.
- When retuning an object to the floor reverse the procedure.

Selected Readings

Rives PA, Douglass AB. Evaluation and treatment of low back pain in family practice. *J Am Board Fam Pract*. 2004;17:S23–S31.

Burton AK, Tillotson M, Main CJ, Hollis S. Psychosocial predictors of outcome in acute and subchronic low back trouble. *Spine*. 1995;20:722–728.

Thorson DC, Campbell R, Kuko O, et al. Health care guideline: adult low back pain. 9th ed. [monograph on the Internet]. Bloomington, MN: Institute Clinical Systems Improvement (ICSI); 2003, available from: http://www.icsi.org/, accessed June 26, 2005.

Part IV

Lower Extremity

11

Hip and Thigh Problems

Edward J. Shahady

Some common hip and thigh problems are encountered by the primary care practitioner. The problems will range from osteoarthritis (OA) of the hips in older patients to femoral stress fractures and muscle tears in younger athletic patients. As with all musculoskeletal problems, a good working knowledge of the epidemiology, anatomy, associated symptoms and examination reduce confusion and enhance the diagnostic and therapeutic process.

Caring for hip and thigh problems is enhanced with a few simple organizational steps:

1. Step 1 is to realize that 95% of patients seen in the office with hip and thigh complaints can be classified into the three categories of problems noted in Table 11.1.
2. Step 2 is to take a focused history that segments the categories into acute trauma, overuse trauma, medical disease and pediatric problems. You now have a manageable list to begin further investigation.
3. Step 3 is to perform a focused physical examination. With a focused history and examination you most likely now have the diagnosis or have decreased the possibilities to two or three diagnoses. Your knowledge of the usual history and examination associated with the most common problems has facilitated the diagnostic process.
4. Step 4 is ordering confirmatory studies if needed (many times they are not).
5. Step 5 is to start treatment. (This may include appropriate consultation.) Five percent of the time the diagnosis will not be so obvious. But not being one of the 95% is usually obvious. That is when additional confirmatory studies and/or a consultation will be required.

Rare or not so frequent problems are usually the ones that receive the most press. How often do you hear the words "I got burned once" mentioned about a rare problem that was missed in the primary care setting. Having a good working knowledge of the characteristics of common problems provides an excellent background to help recognize the uncommon. The uncommon is easy to recognize once you know the common. Be driven by the search for the common rather than the expensive intimidating search for the rare birds.

TABLE 11.1. Hip problems.

Overuse trauma
- Femoral neck stress fractures
- Avascular necrosis
- meralgia parasthetica
- Trochanteric bursitis

Acute trauma
- Hamstring muscle tears
- Quadriceps muscle tears
- Adductor muscle tears
- Myositis ossificans
- Hip pointer

Medical problem
- Osteoarthritis of the hip

Pediatric hip problems
- Avulsion fractures/apophysis injury
- Legg –Calvé–Perthes
- Slipped capital femoral epiphysis

1. Focused History

The first question relates to the acuteness of the problem. Did it just start or has it been present for a long period of time. The next question would depend on the answer to the first. If the onset is acute then ask patients what they were doing when the pain occurred and the location of the pain. Pain in the back of the leg that occurred immediately after the patient started running is probably a hamstring muscle tear. Age also helps with the diagnosis. Hip pain in older patients is most likely OA but in a 13-year-old, slipped femoral capital epiphysis is more likely. The sport the patient is involved in also helps. Runners are more likely to have stress fractures of the hip and soccer players are more likely to contuse and tear their hamstring and quadriceps muscles. The motion that aggravates the pain helps pinpoint location. Pain made worse by abduction of the hip may indicate trochanteric bursitis. Burning pain is commonly associated with nerve compression.

2. Focused Physical Examination

Six basic motions should be included in the examination of every patient with hip pain. Thigh pain examination includes the additional evaluation of knee extension and flexion. Perform these examinations when possible with the patient non-weight-bearing on the exam table.

- Hip extension, normal 15° (Figure 11.1)
- Hip flexion, normal 120° (Figure 11.2)
- Hip adduction, normal 30° (Figure 11.3)

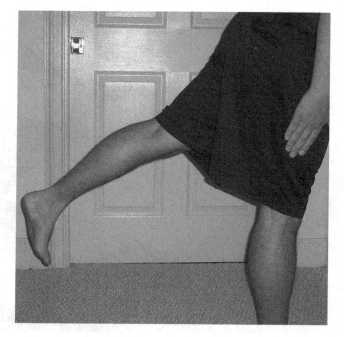

FIGURE 11.1. Hip extension.

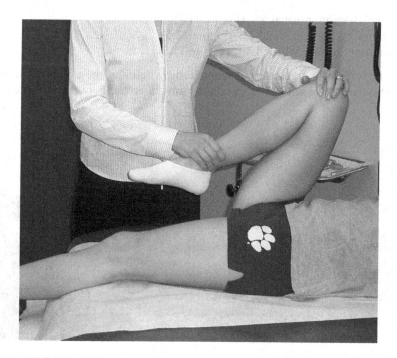

FIGURE 11.2. Hip flexion.

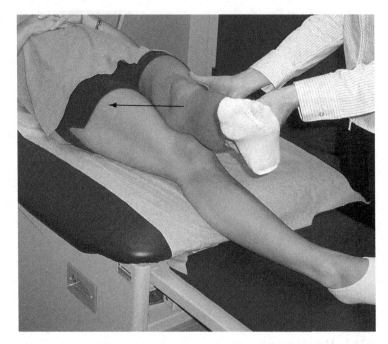

FIGURE 11.3. Hip adduction.

- Hip abduction, normal 50° (Figure 11.4)
- Internal rotation, normal 20° (Figure 11.5)
- External rotation, normal 40° (Figure 11.6)

It is important to start every examination by defining the range of motion (ROM) for each of the above and noting any difference between one side and

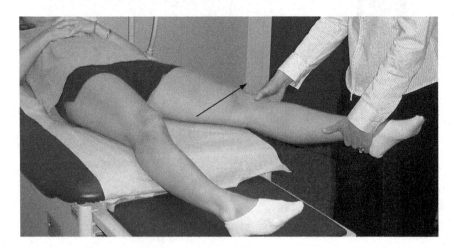

FIGURE 11.4. Hip abduction.

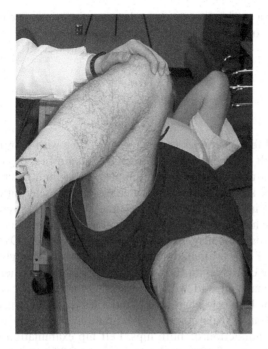

FIGURE 11.5. Internal rotation.

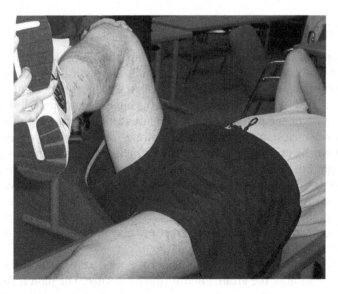

FIGURE 11.6. External rotation.

the other. Use a goniometer to assess degrees of motion. The focused history will guide the content of the remaining examination.

3. Case

3.1. History

A 22-year-old female runner comes to your office with complaints of right groin and thigh pain for the past 3 weeks. The pain first began after 25 min of running but now it starts within minutes of beginning her run. The pain stops when she stops running and the pain is not present with walking or at rest. She has increased her running time recently in preparation for a marathon. She has no history of hip or thigh problems in the past. She denies taking any chronic medicines or using alcohol excessively. Over the past few years, you have also evaluated her for inability to gain weight and amenorrhea. You have discussed an eating disorder diagnosis with her. Examination reveals a normal gait and with no excessive pronation or supination (see Chapter 15) of her feet. There is no tenderness over the greater trochanter. Hip examination reveals no pain or limitation of motion with extension, abduction, or adduction of both hips. Left hip examination elicits no pain and normal flexion of 120°, internal rotation of 20°, and external rotation of 50°. Right hip examination reveals pain and limitation of motion with flexion at 100°, internal rotation at 10°, and external rotation at 35°. Examination of her shoes reveals no excessive wear. A plain film X-ray of the hip is negative.

3.2. Thinking Process

Complaints of thigh and groin pain make hip pathology likely. Finding limitation of both internal and external rotation on physical examination confirms the suspicion of a hip problem. The first and most important diagnosis to think of in a runner with pain around the hip is a femoral neck stress fracture. Because of the potential negative consequences of missing this diagnosis it is reasonable to treat her like a stress fracture until you can prove yourself wrong or right. Other possibilities include avascular necrosis (AVN) of the right hip. Absence of chronic use of steroids and/or alcohol makes this diagnosis less likely. Hip OA is unlikely in a woman this age unless she had some type of prior problem with her hip like Legg–Calvé–Perthes or slipped capital epiphysis. A negative X-ray makes the AVN less likely but not the stress fracture. Femoral neck stress fractures may not be evident by plain film X-ray for 6 to 8 weeks.

The presenting symptoms of a femoral neck stress fracture include an aching sensation in the groin, anterior thigh, or knee. The pain is frequently associated with weight-bearing activity and stops shortly after cessation of activity. Physical findings include a limp and limitation of hip motion, particularly internal rotation. Tenderness by palpation is often minimal owing to the depth of soft tissue overlying the femoral neck. The above factors of (1) increased risk for osteoporosis (eating disorder), (2) history of recent increase in running mileage, (3) pain in the groin and thigh, (4) pain and limitation of motion with hip flexion and internal and external rotation are suggestive of a femoral neck stress fracture.

The negative X-ray is not surprising in the early stages of stress fractures. Obtain a bone scan or magnetic resonance image (MRI) when the history is suggestive and the plain film is negative. Magnetic resonance imaging has the advantage of grading the injury severity and differentiating other conditions like AVN and soft tissue injury. This patient's MRI revealed a fracture on the inferomedial aspect or the compression side of the femoral neck with no displacement.

3.3. Treatment

Because of the disability that can arise from femoral neck fractures, early diagnosis and aggressive treatment are necessary to prevent fracture displacement. Maintain a high index of suspicion in any patient, especially a runner, who presents with a story and examination suggestive of femoral neck stress fracture. If the initial radiographs are negative, recommend non-weight-bearing ambulation for 7 days, at which time repeat imaging or an MRI or bone scan is obtained.

Stress fractures occur with repetitive stress because bone resorption occurs at a greater rate than bone deposition. Simply stated, the bone does not have the time to heal and rebuild after the stress of exercise. Pace, intensity, and other factors like training routines, proper footwear, and running surfaces all play a part in the risk for stress fractures. Prevention and treatment of stress fractures need to include a discussion of these factors. It is also important to remember that femoral neck stress fractures are three times more common in females, probably related to amenorrhea, bone density, and diet. So in female patients, like the one above, counseling about appropriate diet and calcium supplementation are important. Screen all females with stress fractures for eating disorders.

Fractures of the femoral neck are of three categories. Compression fractures occur on the inferomedial side (close to the lesser trochanter) of the femoral neck. These are usually the most stable and are treated nonsurgically if they are not displaced. Tension fractures occur on the superolateral (close to the greater trochanter) aspect of the femoral neck. These fractures have a higher risk of displacement and usually require internal fixation. Displaced fractures are an orthopedic emergency that require immediate reduction and fixation. Avascular necrosis is more common with displaced fractures.

This patient was treated with crutches and remained non-weight-bearing until her plain X-ray indicated signs of healing. It took 4 weeks before sufficient healing was present. She gradually increased her ambulation and within 3 months she was back to running. A more sensible training routine was discussed and she has decided not to train for a marathon again.

4. Avascular Necrosis of the Femoral Head

Avascular necrosis of the femoral head is the result of interruption of the vascular supply to a segment of the femoral head. This leads to necrosis, collapse, and progressive arthritis of the hip joint. The causes can be traumatic or nontraumatic. Hip fractures and dislocations can disrupt blood supply and lead to necrosis. Use of systemic corticosteroids and alcohol abuse are nontraumatic causes. The dose and length of time of steroid administration has not been defined. The usual case is associated with patients like asthmatics who chronically take steroids but in one series the shortest period of steroid therapy associated with AVN of the femoral head was 30 days at 16 mg prednisone per day [1].

Patients with AVN usually present with groin or hip pain that is nonspecific. Patients with predisposing factors of alcohol abuse, steroid use, or past trauma should be suspected of AVN if they have hip pain. Predisposing factors are associated with most cases of AVN. On examination, hip ROM and gait may be normal early in the process but with time, limitation of internal rotation and flexion will appear.

Imaging is critical to making the diagnosis. Order X-rays of both hips. Changes do not usually occur during the first 3 months. The earliest finding is a mottled appearance of the anterosuperior aspect of the femoral head. As collapse progresses, the crescent sign appears. Secondary degenerative changes then follow as collapse progresses and arthritis of the joint evolves. If the X-ray is negative and AVN is suspected, obtain an MRI. Magnetic resonance imaging is a very specific and sensitive means of detecting AVN.

Treatment depends on the stage of the disease. For early disease, when no collapse is present, symptomatic treatment and restricted weight bearing may be used. Some authors feel this is worthwhile and others do not. Multiple surgical procedures including decompression, bone grafting, and arthroplasty are utilized depending on the stage of the disease. The key is initiating treatment before collapse of the femoral head has occurred. Without treatment, the disease will progress and most patients will require arthroplasty. The goal is to diagnose and treat the condition in its earliest stages. If you suspect AVN by history or X-ray, an orthopedic consultation is recommended.

5. Meralgia Parasthetica (Lateral Femoral Cutaneous Nerve Entrapment)

Entrapment of the lateral femoral cutaneous nerve is also called meralgia parasthetica. This nerve exits the pelvis under the inguinal ligament and passes medial to the anterior superior iliac spine (ASIS). It is solely a cutaneous nerve, supplying the skin of the anterolateral thigh down to the knee (Figure 11.7).

Primary care clinicians will see this problem in diabetics or obese patients who wear constricting garments around their waist like belts and girdles. The problem may also be seen in patients who have had surgical procedures of the abdomen and iliac crest like appendectomy, hysterectomy, and iliac bone grafting. Recent weight gain is a predisposing factor.

The common symptom is pain and/or numbness in the anterolateral thigh in the distribution of the lateral femoral cutaneous nerve (Figure 11.7). Hyperextending the hip and bending backwards at the back may make the symptoms worse. Tinel's sign (tapping on the area and reproducing the pain) is usually present 1 cm medial and inferior to the anterior superior iliac crest.

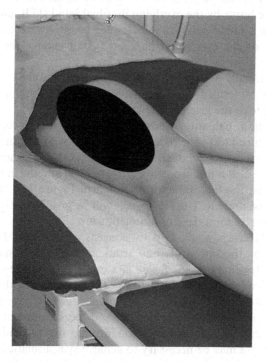

FIGURE 11.7. The lateral femoral cutaneous nerve sensory distribution.

Further testing is not indicated if the symptoms are classical and the patient responds to conservative measures listed below. If the patient does not respond to conservative measures, nerve conduction studies of the lateral femoral cutaneous nerve can be performed to access for nerve compression. Magnetic resonance imaging of the hip and pelvis are useful to rule out intra-articular derangement or intrapelvic causes of compression on the nerve.

The mainstay of treatment for entrapped lateral femoral cutaneous nerve is nonoperative. Weight reduction, decreased use of constrictive clothing, nonsteroidal anti-inflammatory drugs (NSAIDs), and local steroid injections succeed 90% of the time. If symptoms are persistent and disabling, surgical intervention is warranted. Local nerve block is a useful diagnostic tool and predictor of benefit from surgical decompression. If injection completely relieves the patients' complaints, surgery will usually help.

6. Trochanteric Bursitis

The trochanteric bursa lies over the greater trochanter of femur. Overuse is the usual cause of the bursitis. It is commonly associated with OA of the hip. Other factors that contribute to the etiology of trochanteric bursitis include irritation of the bursa by the overlying iliotibial band (ITB) and biomechanical factors like a broad pelvis in females, leg length discrepancy, and excessive pronation of the foot (see Chapter 15) that change the mechanics of the ITB.

The patient usually presents with an aching pain over the lateral hip that is made worse by prolonged standing, lying on the side, or stair climbing. The pain may radiate to the groin or the lateral thigh.

On examination, palpation along the posterior greater trochanter reveals tenderness (Figure 11.8). The pain is accentuated with external rotation and abduction and by resisted abduction. Patrick's (flexion, abduction and external rotation (FABER)) test is positive (Figure 11.9) and the hip abductors are often weak. Test the hip abductor as noted in Figure 11.4. Iliotibial band tightness may be present. The Ober's test will be positive if tightness is present. See Chapter 12 for a description of this test.

Treatment of trochanteric bursitis consists of rest, ice, ITB stretching, strengthening of the hip girdle and trunk musculature (especially gluteus medius), and stretching of the fascia lata and the ITB. The exercises at the end of this chapter describe how to do this. Leg length discrepancy and pronation need to be addressed. Inflammation generally responds to nonsteroidal anti-inflammatory medications and local treatment modalities. In some cases, local corticosteroid injection into the area of tenderness over the trochanteric bursa may be necessary to achieve symptomatic relief. Rarely, if the condition is refractory to conservative measures, operative release of the ITB may be required.

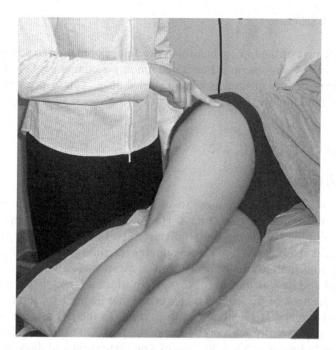

FIGURE 11.8. Point of tenderness in trochanteric bursitis.

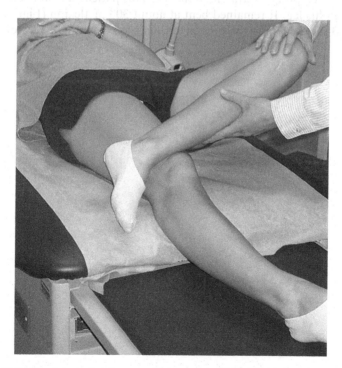

FIGURE 11.9. Flexion, abduction, external rotation (FABER) test.

Plain X-rays of the hip are helpful in the older population to access for the presence of OA. Trochanteric bursitis commonly accompanies OA of the hip. Magnetic resonance imaging is seldom needed unless you suspect tears of the abductor musculature.

7. Acute Trauma (Case)

7.1. History

A 38-year-old accountant comes to your office complaining of pain in the back of his leg for the past 3 days. He hurt the leg while playing softball with his family. He hit the ball and started to run to first base and felt a catch in the back of his leg. He was unable to continue playing because of the pain and inability to walk without assistance. The next day the pain increased and he was unable to work. He noticed a large "black and blue" area on the back of his leg. He is concerned that he has torn something and may need surgery. His general health is good. In the last few years, he has not been as physically active as he was in the past. On examination he walks with a slight limp and has a 30° loss of knee extension and discomfort with passive knee extension past 30°. Assess knee extension with the patient sitting and attempting to straighten the leg. This patient was not able to fully straighten his leg. It remained bent at about 30° of flexion (Figure 11.10). A 2-by 3-in. ecchymosis is present on his posterior thigh. Flexion of the

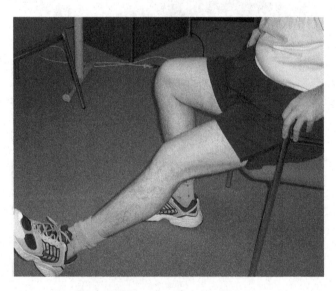

FIGURE 11.10. Knee extension limited to 30° while seated.

knee is painful. Palpation of the posterior thigh with the knee partially flexed against resistance (Figure 11.11) reveals mild tenderness and a palpable knot at the midthigh.

7.2. Thinking Process

This patient's history of acute onset of pain after starting to run, difficulty in walking, and the appearance of an ecchymosis is suggestive of a tear of one of his muscle groups. Being in the posterior thigh makes a hamstring tear likely, although adductor tears may produce posterior lateral pain. His physical examination supports the possibility of hamstring injury. Extension of the knee stretches the hamstring muscle and hamstring tears produce a spasm that limits extension. This patient has significant limitation of his knee extension and ecchymosis of the posterior thigh, so a hamstring muscle tear is most likely. Judge the severity or extent of injury by the degree of extension limitation and not by the size of the ecchymosis.

Palpation over the hamstring muscle group with resisted knee flexion may elicit tenderness, defects, and/or a mass when the hamstring is injured. Both tenderness and a mass are demonstrated in this patient with resisted flexion (Figure 11.11). More extensive tears are associated with palpable masses and

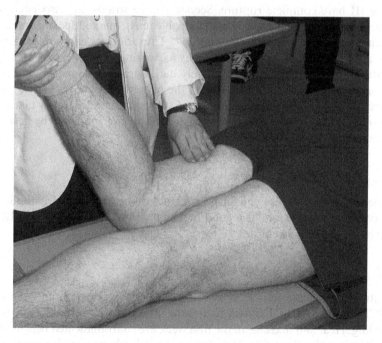

FIGURE 11.11. Knee partially flexed against resistance with muscle belly being palpated (patient on abdomen).

defects. Other factors responsible for hamstring injuries include inadequate warm-up, inflexibility, poor conditioning, and muscle strength imbalances between the hamstring and quadriceps muscles. This patient has decreased his physical activity in the last few years, is probably not well-conditioned, and did not stretch or warm up before he started playing.

Hamstring strains are the most common strain-related injuries seen by the primary care provider. They can be quiet disabling and lead to a loss of work and recreational time. The site of the tear in patients over age 25 is usually at the junction of the muscle and the tendon (musculotendinous junction). In patients under 25 the tear most likely occurs where the tendon attaches to the pelvis. The apophysis is the ossification center where the tendon attaches to the bones of the pelvis. These injuries will be discussed in Section 11 (Pediatric Hip Problems) (page 220).

The injury occurs during the stretching or eccentric phase of muscle contraction. The force generated during eccentric contraction is greater than the force generated during the concentric or contracting phase of muscle contraction. There are three muscles in the hamstring group: the biceps femoris, semimembranosus, and semitendinosus. The biceps femoris is the most commonly injured of the three.

Hamstring strains may be classified into three groups: mild (grade I), moderate (grade II), and severe (grade III). Grade I strains represent a small disruption of the musculotendinous unit. Grade II strains are partial tears and grade III have complete rupture. Second-degree strains are associated with immediate functional loss, a painful palpable mass, marked spasm, and a loss of knee extension between 20° and 25°. Third-degree tears are associated with a defect in the muscle, marked spasm, swelling, and an extension loss of greater than 45°. This patient probably had a grade II hamstring tear. It is important to classify the injury to give the patient a prognosis. Grade I tears take days to heal, grade II may take 4 to 6 weeks, and grade III may take up to 6 months. These times are approximations and are modified by response to treatment.

7.3. Diagnostic Studies

None are needed unless you suspect a fracture or an unusual pathological entity. Plain X-ray would be a good first step to look at bone and an MRI to rule out other muscle entities.

7.4. Treatment

Treatment for acute muscle strains is rest, ice, compression, and elevation (RICE) and NSAIDs. This will reduce the inflammatory process and control bleeding. Heat and massage in the first week are contraindicated because they will increase bleeding. After 3 to 5 days, a gradually progressive program of stretching is started. Range of motion is the key to judging progress. Once full extension is achieved and the pain has subsided, resistance exercises can be started. This is easier to reach in second-degree tears than in third-degree tears. For most patients the hamstrings are only 40% to 45% as strong as the quadriceps and this imbalance increases the risk of hamstring injury. Many hamstring injuries can be prevented if the hamstring strength in both legs is 60% of the quadriceps strength. The strength can be increased and measured at any gym that has leg flexion and extension machines. Remember to exercise one leg at a time to assure individual leg strength. A physical therapist can also be helpful in accessing muscle strength and recommending appropriate exercises.

8. Quadriceps Contusion

Direct blows to the quadriceps muscle can occur with certain sports like football and soccer or any activity that predisposes to contact with another person or object. The degree of disability depends on the amount of muscular hemorrhage that occurs. Slow bleeding may occur in the tissues surrounding the area of impact and the patient may not experience significant symptoms until the day after the injury. Symptoms include pain over the quadriceps and difficulty extending the lower leg.

Treatment is similar to that of the injured hamstring muscle. Start with RICE and NSAIDs. This will reduce the inflammatory process and control bleeding. Delay heat, massage, and vigorous physical therapy for 48 h or longer because they may increase bleeding. After 3 to 5 days a gradually progressive program of stretching is started. Range of motion is the key to judging progress. Once full extension is reached and the pain has subsided, start resistance exercises. The disability depends on the amount of muscle involved in the injury. One measure of severity is the ability to flex the knee. More severe injuries will have limited flexion. Some authors advise attempting to aspirate the hematoma but this has met with limited success and increases the risk of infection. Another popular treatment in the first 24 hours is to keep the knee flexed at 120 to 140 degrees with an Ace wrap. This treatment may decrease the flexion loss and enhance recovery. No randomized studies exist to support this treatment modality and it is difficult for the patient to tolerate the flexed position for the full 24 hours.

A major complication of quadriceps contusions is organization of the contusion hematoma into a calcified mass (myositis ossificans). This is a late occurring phenomena that is felt as a hard mass in the belly of the muscle. Patients may have forgotten that they had a contusion and may now feel a mass and become scared. Many of these patients are young so muscle and bone malignancies are possibilities that come to the mind of the clinician. Plain films usually reveal a calcified mass but the lateral film demonstrates that the mass is separate from bone. If the X-ray does not clearly show separation from bone, obtain an MRI.

9. Hip Pointer

This diagnosis includes any contusion or stretch that causes a tear or bleeding in the muscles that attach to the iliac crest (top of the hipbone). A subperiosteal hematoma and/or a separation of the muscle from the crest can be quiet disabling. The onset is acute and the degree of disability is determined by the degree of injury. The symptoms are pain over the iliac crest, point tenderness, and pain with stretching of the abdominal muscles. Treat by initiating RICE and NSAIDs. As the pain decreases start a stretching program. Ability to exercise and stretch without pain indicates it is okay to return to competitive activity. For adult athletes suffering from a hip pointer due to a contusion, judicious use of a local corticosteroid injection may help alleviate the pain and the disability from this condition and hasten the return to activity.

10. Case

10.1. History

A 60-year-old man presents to your office with increasing pain in his left hip. He has had some hip discomfort off and on for the past 3 years. He is in good health and takes no chronic medications. He denies smoking and heavy alcohol use. He has noted some periodic knee and back pain that responds to ibuprofen. Previously, the hip pain responded to heat and ibuprofen so he did not seek medical attention. The pain no longer responds to these measures, radiates down the lateral part of his leg, and causes a limp. He also notes a burning type of pain at night in his hip and lower leg. His work demands that he be on his feet most of the day and he is less able to do that. His past history is significant for periodic knee and back pain. He is also being treated for hypertension and type 2 diabetes. His main concern today is his ability to continue working. He wants to know if he should apply for disability. Examination of his hands reveals nonpainful Heberden's nodules of the distal interphalangeal (DIP) joints (see Chapter 8) in most fingers. Hip examination reveals some limitation of ROM. Internal rotation is 20° on the right but limited to 10° on the left with marked discomfort. Abduction is normal to 50° right but painful and limited to 20° on the left. Flexion is normal to 120° right but limited by discomfort to 80° left. External rotation, extension, and adduction are normal in both hips. He has tenderness over the greater trochanter and his Ober's test is positive on the left side.

10.2. Thinking Process

Osteoarthritis of the hip is the first thing that comes to mind given the patient's age and chronicity of the problem. There is no doubt the problem is in the hip given the history and the examination but is it OA or another disease process like AVN or a malignancy with bone metastasis. As noted previously, AVN is associated with excessive alcohol use and steroid use. He denies both, so AVN is unlikely. Prostate cancer is one of the cancers that can metastasize to bone so a rectal examination is in order. An X-ray will help rule out malignance and AVN and confirm OA.

OA is usually present in more than one joint. His history of knee and back pain and the presence of Heberden's nodules favors this diagnosis. Tenderness over the greater trochanter and a positive Ober's test now raise the suspicion of trochanteric bursitis and tightness of his ITB. Both of these entities commonly accompany OA of the hip. Iliotibial band tightness and OA of the hip can produce a burning pain at night in his hip and lower leg. Diabetic neuropathy may also cause the burning pain.

10.3. Diagnostic Studies

Unlike in the case of rheumatoid arthritis, blood tests are seldom used to diagnose OA. Rheumatoid arthritis is not usually a disease of the hip but a sedimentation rate of less than 20 usually confirms the absence of an inflammatory arthritis. Plain film X-rays will help confirm your suspicions. Joint space narrowing, osteophytes, sclerosis, and cyst formation are common. Radiographic changes of OA are common with aging and mean nothing unless the patient is symptomatic. The diagnosis and judgment of severity are made from the clinical picture and not the X-rays. This patient's films revealed loss of joint space and early osteophyte formation.

10.4. Treatment

The first line of treatment is to stretch and strengthen all of the hip musculature and the ITB. Exercises as described at the end of the chapter help accomplish this task. If trochanteric bursitis is present, treatment as outlined previously should be initiated. After the patient clearly understands how important the stretching and strengthening exercises are and you have demonstrated the exercises, discussion of oral medications can begin. Tylenol is very effective if used in a dose of 4000 mg a day for a minimum of 10 days. Patients may not understand the need to take the medication four times a day for 10 days continuously. Most patients think the medication is only for pain and will not take it if they do not have pain. Take a few extra seconds to help them understand and you will find that Tylenol is an effective drug. NSAIDs can be used as an adjunct to the exercises and Tylenol but not as first-line therapy. Try COX-1 agents first before going to the more expensive COX-2 agents. Also remember that many patients like the one above are older and have other chronic diseases like hypertension and diabetes that may be worsened by the use of NSAIDs. Some evidence suggests that glucosamine is an option but watch the patient's blood sugar as this medication may causes it to rise. Referral to a physical therapist is helpful to reinforce exercise therapy and for the use of other modalities like ultrasound. Some but not all patients may go on to require complete replacement of the hip but this is not the fate of all patients with hip OA. If all of your conservative measures fail, a consultation with an orthopedist will help answer this question.

This patient was taught stretching and strengthening of his hip musculature and ITB and prescribed 4000 mg of Tylenol a day. He did well and is being followed closely.

11. Pediatric Hip Problems

11.1. Avulsion Fractures of the Pelvis

These injuries account for 10% to 13% of pelvic fractures and are seen exclusively in children and young adults between 14 and 25 years of age. They occur at the apophysis or ossification center where the tendon attaches to bone. These ossification centers, as noted in Table 11.2, appear at age 11 or 12 and do not all fuse until age 25. The mechanism of injury is usually a sudden excessive muscle contraction that causes separation of the cartilaginous area between the apophysis and the bone. Splits done by young girls or sprints done by track athletes are two common activities that are associated with avulsion fractures at the apophysis. These injuries are referred to as an apophysitis.

Once the ossification center fuses, the same excessive muscle contraction produces injury in the musculotendinous junction of the muscle. Prior to ossification, the apophysis is the weakest link but after ossification, the musculotendinous junction is the weakest link, so injury will occur there.

Sprinters, jumpers, soccer, and football players have the most apophyseal injuries. There is usually no history of direct trauma but a sudden muscle contraction followed by immediate symptoms is the usual story. The same mechanism that results in a muscle or tendon strain in an adult will cause avulsion of an apophysis in an adolescent athlete. A good example is hamstring injury.

TABLE 11.2. Age of appearance and fusion of ossification centers in the hip and pelvis.

Location of ossification centers	Appearance (years)	Fusion (years)	Muscle(s) attachments
Anterior inferior iliac spine	13–15	16–18	Quadriceps
Anterior superior iliac spine	13–15	21–25	Sartorious
Lesser trochanter	11–12	16–17	Iliopsoas
Greater trochanter	2–3	16–17	Gluteal
Ischial tuberosity	13–15	20–25	Hamstrings
Iliac crest	13–15	21–25	Abdominal obliques, latissimus dorsi

Avulsion injuries associated with the hamstring, adductor, and sartorious muscle are the ones most commonly seen by the primary care practitioner. Knowing where these muscles attach to the pelvis and understanding which muscles are strained with certain sports or activities helps pinpoint the diagnosis. Ischial apophysis avulsion occurs with hamstring and adductor injury and ASIS avulsion occurs with sartorius injury.

Patients, usually young girls doing splits, sustain anterior ischial apophysis avulsion from adductor avulsion injuries. They usually feel an immediate pull or pain in the groin. They will present with a limp and groin pain on the involved side. Examination will reveal tenderness in the groin and pain with hip abduction and resisted adduction.

Posterior ischial apophysis avulsion is caused by maximum hamstring eccentric contraction. Hurdlers are most susceptible as they stretch the leg over the hurdling bar. Pain is immediate and in the posterior buttocks and groin. Lower leg extension with and without resistance produces symptoms.

X-rays may reveal avulsions of the ischium. Obtaining a comparison view of the uninjured side helps evaluate the degree of skeletal maturity and the status of the normal apophysis. Normal pelvic radiographs in this age group may look abnormal when they are not. The ischial apophysis appears at the age of 15 years and is one of the last to unite at about age 25.

Avulsion of the ASIS occurs with maximum pull of the sartorious muscle. This injury usually happens at the beginning of a race as the runner crouches with the back and hip extended and knee flexed. Coming up from the crouching position produces a sudden sartorious pull and avulsion at the ASIS. Examination will reveal tenderness over the rim of the pelvis at the ASIS and flexion and abduction of the hip will reproduce the pin. Radiographs comparing sides demonstrate displacement of the ASIS on the injured side. Avulsion of the anterior inferior iliac spine (AIIS) is less common. It ossifies earlier and has less stress placed on it. Contraction of rectus femoris muscle causes this avulsion. Kicking sports like football and soccer are usually the mechanism of injury. Examination reveals pain over the lower pelvic rim close to the groin. Asking the patient to go through the kicking motion reproduces the pain. Radiographs show distal displacement of a fragment of the AIIS. Full pelvis radiographs to include the acetabulum and head of the femur are important for side-to-side comparison to rule out acetabulum and femoral head injury. Slipped femoral capital epiphysis occurs in athletes of the same age group and needs to be ruled out. This is discussed later.

Treatment for avulsion fractures of the pelvis includes activity modification, NSAIDs, ice, and appropriate resting of the joint. Crutches to limit weight bearing may be needed to limit pain. Bed rest may be ideal but difficult to accomplish in this age group. Once the pain has diminished, gentle ROM exercises should begin. Once the ROM is accomplished with no pain, stretching and strengthening exercises for all the muscles of the hip should follow. Surgical intervention has been described in isolated cases but in most cases is not indicated and has no advantages over conservative care. Patients treated with positioning, protected weight bearing, and progressive rehabilitation can be expected to return successfully to full activity after 5 to 6 weeks.

12. Case

12.1. History and Exam

A 6-year-old boy presents to your office with a limp on his right side. He was playing soccer with his friends and kicking a ball when the limp became noticeable. The parents think the limp has been there for about 3 weeks. Initially the limp was present only after he played with his friends. Now the limp is there all the time and the parents are concerned. He also periodically complains of right knee and groin pain but no other symptoms. There is no change in his weight or eating behavior and he is "a normal active boy" according to the parents. His vital signs are normal and he is in no pain as he sits on the examination table. Right knee examination reveals no tenderness or instability. Examination of his hips is normal on the left with abduction to 65° but abduction on the right is limited to 25°.

12.2. Thinking Process

Limping in a child this age that lingers for 3 weeks must be taken seriously. Children in this age group seldom if ever take this route to gain attention. Possibilities include transient and bacterial synovitis, inflammatory arthritis, and Legg–Calvé–Perthes disease (LCPD).

Transient or toxic synovitis, a self-limited condition, is the most common cause of hip pain in children under 10 years of age. The onset is acute and may follow a recent upper respiratory infection or a traumatic event. There may also be a low-grade temperature elevation. The onset of symptoms in this boy was not acute and he is afebrile, making this diagnosis less likely. Bacterial or septic synovitis has a rapid onset and the patient is acutely ill, febrile, and refuses to bear weight. This is not the picture in this boy. Inflammatory arthritis is usually present in more than one joint but this may be the first manifestation of the disease so further evaluation and time will be needed to rule out this cause. Legg–Calvé–Perthes disease is characterized by gradual onset of a mild painful limp. The discomfort is relieved by rest and aggravated by weight bearing. This picture is certainly compatible with the story in this boy.

A radiograph of the hip is mandatory in any child with a limp. The X-ray in this boy revealed widening of the joint space and denseness of the femoral head suggesting early LCPD. Legg–Calvé–Perthes disease is an idiopathic osteonecrosis of the femoral head of unknown etiology. It is four times more common in boys and occurs between 4 and 10 years of age. Fifteen percent of cases are bilateral. The condition is self-limited but takes about 2 years to run its course. The most important part of treatment is early recognition and protecting the joint from further damage. Consultation with an orthopedic surgeon is recommended. Bracing and, occasionally, surgery is advisable.

13. Slipped Capital Femoral Epiphysis

Slipped capital femoral epiphysis is another problem that must be considered in an older child who is limping. Weakening of the epiphyseal plate of the head of the femur occurs and results in upward displacement or slippage of the femoral neck. It is seen most commonly in boys during their rapid growth spurt between 11 and 16 years of age. The boys are usually tall and thin or obese with underdeveloped sexual characteristics. The onset of symptoms is gradual. The symptoms are groin pain with radiation to the knee and a limp after activity in boys between 11 and 16. The examination reveals limitation of abduction and internal rotation. X-ray confirms the diagnosis. It is important to have the patient in a frog leg position to demonstrate the slippage of the upper segment. If diagnosis is suspected, give the patient crutches and obtain an orthopedic consultation. The treatment is usually surgical.

14. Hip Exercises

Repeat each of the following exercises two times a day. Rotate from one exercise to the other. Do one set of one exercise and then rotate to another exercise and do a set. Do not exercise past the point of pain. Pain means stop.

1. **Abduction (Figure 11.12)**: Stand facing a wall with both feet together and support yourself with both hands on the wall. Swing the fully extended leg away from the midline as far as it will go and hold for 10 s. Use ankle weights to increase the resistance. Bring the leg back to its prior position and repeat the process 10 times in each leg.
2. **Adduction (Figure 11.13)**: Stand facing a wall with both feet together and support yourself with both hands on the wall. Swing the fully extended leg across the opposite leg as far as it will go and hold for 10 s. Use ankle weights to increase the resistance. (Ankle weights can be purchased in most sports stores. They have inserts that allow you to increase the weights by 1/2 to 1 lb up to 5 lb total on each side.) Bring the leg back to its prior position and repeat the process 10 times in each leg.
3. **Backward extension (Figure 11.14)**: Stand facing a wall with both feet together and support yourself with both hands on the wall. Swing the fully extended leg back as far as it will go and hold for 10 s. Use ankle weights to increase the resistance. Bring the leg back to its prior position and repeat the process 10 times in each leg.
4. **Flexion (Figure 11.15)**: Stand facing an object like a counter top and grasp it for support and balance. Bend the knee up into your abdomen and hold it for 10 s. Use ankle weights to increase the resistance. Bring the leg back to its prior position and repeat the process 10 times in each leg.

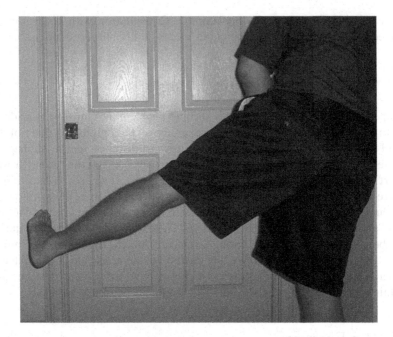

FIGURE 11.12. Abduction exercise.

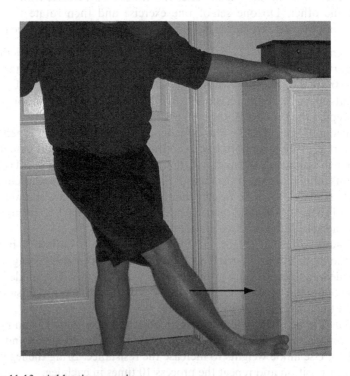

FIGURE 11.13. Adduction exercise.

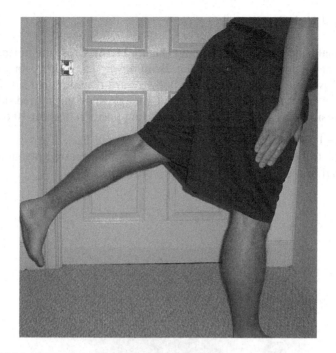

FIGURE 11.14. Backward extension exercise.

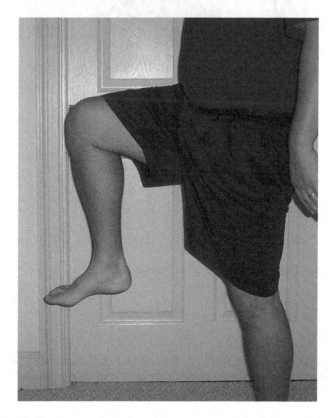

FIGURE 11.15. Flexion exercise.

5. **Iliotibial band stretching (standing) (Figure 11.16)**: Cross the normal leg in front of the injured or painful leg. Bend down, and touch your toes. You can move your hands across your body toward the uninjured side and you will feel more stretch on the outside of your thigh on the injured side. Hold this position for 10 s. Return to the starting position. Repeat 10 times.

Exercises 1, 2, and 4 can be performed lying on your back. Turn over on your abdomen to perform exercise 3. This may be the preferred position for an individual who is weaker or has balance problems.

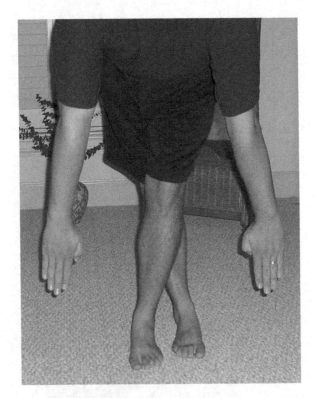

FIGURE 11.16. Iliotibial band stretching (standing).

Reference

1. McKee MD, Waddell JP, Kudo PA, Schemitsch EH, Richards RR. Osteonecrosis of the femoral head in men following short-course corticosteroid therapy: a report of 15 cases. *CMAJ*. 2001;164:205–206.

Suggested Readings

Boyd KT, Peirce NS, Batt ME. Common hip injuries in sport. *Sports Med.* 1997;24: 273–288.

Browning KH. Hip and pelvis injuries in runners, careful evaluation and tailored management, *Physician Sportsmed.* 2001;29:23–34.

12

Knee Problems

Jocelyn R. Gravlee and Edward J. Shahady

The primary care practitioner will encounter many common knee problems. The problems range from osteoarthritis (OA) in older patients to overuse injuries like iliotibial band syndrome (ITBS) and acute tears of the collateral or cruciate ligaments in the younger, more active patients. As with all musculoskeletal problems, a good working knowledge of the epidemiology, anatomy, associated symptoms, and examination reduce confusion and enhance the diagnostic and therapeutic process.

Caring for problems is easier if a few simple organizational steps are followed:

1. Step 1 is to realize that 95% of patients seen in the office with knee complaints can be classified into the categories of problems noted in Table 12.1.
2. Step 2 is to take a focused history that segments the categories into acute trauma, overuse trauma, medical disease, and pediatric problems. This process reduces the number to a manageable list to initiate further investigation.
3. Step 3 is to perform a focused physical examination. With a focused history and examination, you now most likely have a diagnosis. Your knowledge of the usual history and examination associated with the most common problems has facilitated this process.
4. Step 4 is ordering confirmatory studies if needed (many times they are not).
5. Step 5 is to start treatment. (This may include appropriate consultation.) Five percent of the time the diagnosis will not be so obvious. But not being one of the 95% is usually obvious. That is when additional confirmatory studies and/or a consultation will be required.

Rare or not so frequent problems are usually the ones that receive the most press. How often do you hear, "I got burned once," in reference to a rare problem that was missed in the primary care setting. Having a good working knowledge of the characteristics of common problems provides an excellent background to help recognize the uncommon. The uncommon is easy to recognize once you know the common. Be driven by the search for the common rather than the expensive intimidating search for the rare birds.

TABLE 12.1. Common knee problems.

Acute trauma
Anterior cruciate ligament rupture
Medial collateral ligament sprain
Meniscal tear
Patellar subluxation and dislocation
Loose bodies

Overuse
Patellofemoral pain syndrome (chondromalacia patellae)
Iliotibial band syndrome
Infrapatellar tendonitis (jumper's knee)
Prepatellar bursitis
Pes anserine bursitis

Medical problems
Degenerative joint disease (osteoarthritis)

Pediatric problems
Osgood–Schlatter disease
Physeal fractures

Bone does not provide stability for the knee. Ligaments, cartilage, muscle, and the capsule provide the support for the joint. The medial and lateral collateral ligaments, the posterior capsule, and the anterior and posterior cruciate (PC) ligaments are the most important structures for stability. Table 12.2 and Figure 12.1 show the anatomic location of ligaments, muscle, and their function.

TABLE 12.2. Anatomy and function of key structures of the knee.

Structure	Anatomy	Function
Medial collateral ligament	Originates below the adductor tubercle of the femur and attaches attaches to the upper medial tibia	It protects against medial collapse and assists with controlling rotation
Lateral collateral ligament	Originates on the lateral femoral epicondyle and attaches to the head of the fibula	It protects against lateral collapse
Anterior cruciate ligament	Intra-articular portions of the femur and tibia	Prevents anterior displacement of the tibia and helps control rotation of the tibia
Posterior cruciate ligament	Intra-articular portions of the femur and tibia	Prevents backward displacement of the tibia on the femur
Quadriceps muscles	Anterior thigh	Controls lower leg extension and prevents patellar dislocation
Hamstring muscles	Posterior thigh	Controls flexion and provides posterior support for the knee

1. Focused History

Establish whether the problem is acute or chronic or if other chronic diseases are present. This will get you started down the right path. The mechanism of injury will many times pinpoint the anatomy involved in the injury. Questions like the following help put the pieces of the puzzle together. Was there a direct blow to the knee? Was the foot planted? Was the patient trying to stop or slow down? Was there any twisting movement? Was the patient landing from a jump?

Medial collateral ligament injuries occur after a valgus load (stress going from the outside to the inside or lateral to medial) to the knee usually from a blow to the lateral aspect of the knee like clipping in football, or a fall while snow skiing or falling into an embankment that traps the leg. Quick stops or sharp cuts cause deceleration forces that can rupture the anterior cruciate ligament (ACL). Planting the foot and pivoting or twisting movements create shearing forces in the joint, causing meniscal cartilage tears. The twisting can be as benign as that associated with stepping off a curb and losing your balance. Overuse injuries are associated with discomfort that has developed over time. Certain characteristics like intensifying one's exercise routine, changing the terrain to hills or the beach, or different shoes are all areas that may be causative in the overuse syndrome. A good working knowledge of knee anatomy (Figure 12.1 and Table 12.1) will help you understand what structures were involved when the acute or overuse injury occurred.

Do not forget to ask about other medical problems. Diabetics have a greater incidence of OA. Patients with knee OA usually have evidence of other signs of OA in the hands (Heberden's nodes) and the hip or back. Gout can cause knee problems so a past history of gout would be an important piece of history. Other types of arthritis are possible but rarely involve the knee.

2. Focused Physical Examination

Begin by comparing the injured knee with the uninjured one. Look for erythema, swelling, and atrophy of the musculature. The quadriceps muscle will atrophy when the knee is injured because pain decreases use of the quadriceps muscles. The medial part of the quadriceps, specifically the vastus medialis obliquus (VMO), is the first portion of the muscle to atrophy. This atrophy can be appreciated by observation and palpation. Ask the patient to tighten this muscle by extending the knee and starting to lift the leg as noted in Figure 12.2. Palpate the muscle and compare one side with the other. Palpation should include all the major landmarks: patella, patellar tendon, tibial tubercle, quadriceps tendon, and medial and lateral joint lines (Figure 12.3). It is easier to find the joint lines with the knee flexed and the foot resting on the

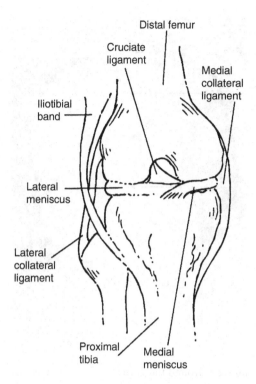

FIGURE 12.1. Anatomy of the knee. (Reproduced from Richmond J, Shahady E, eds. *Sports Medicine for Primary Care*. Cambridge, MA: Blackwell Science; 1996:392, with permission.)

examination table. Next, evaluate the range of motion (ROM) by flexing and extending the knee. Normal ROM is 0° to 10° of extension to 135° to 160° of flexion (Figure 12.4A and 12.4B). In one author's experience (ES), female and black patients are usually more flexible.

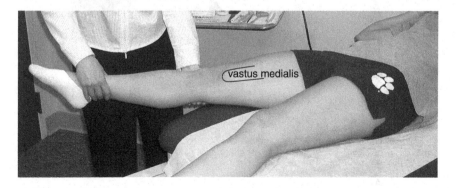

FIGURE 12.2. Partial leg lift to demonstrate vastus medialis muscle location.

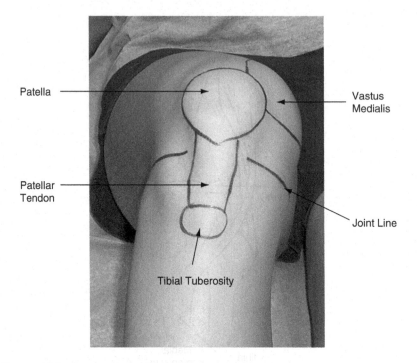

FIGURE 12.3. Landmarks around the knee.

Other knee evaluation tests include the following:

- Patellar compression test (Figure 12.5)
- Medial collateral ligament test (Figure 12.6A)
- Full extension test for capsular integrity (Figure 12.6B)

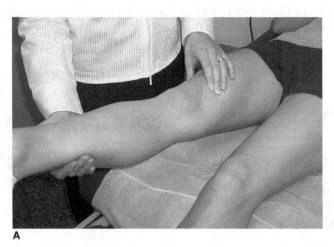

A

FIGURE 12.4. (A) Knee extension.

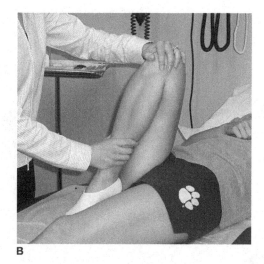

FIGURE 12.4. (B) Knee flexion.

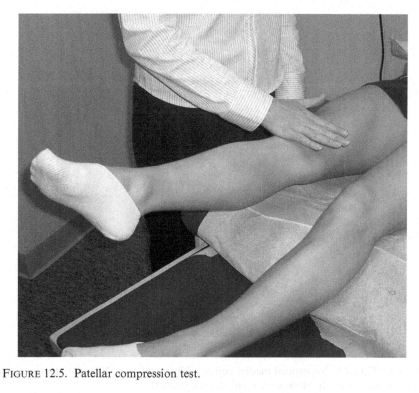

FIGURE 12.5. Patellar compression test.

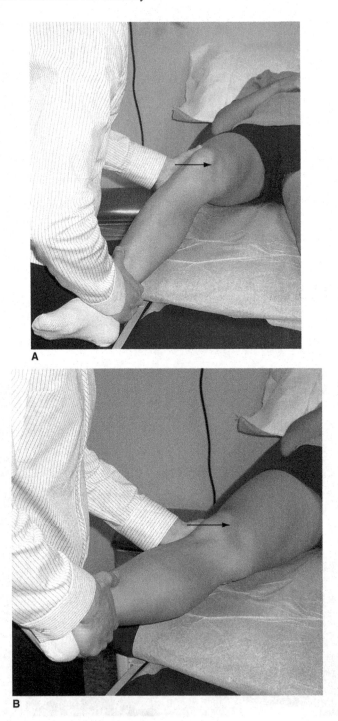

FIGURE 12.6. (A) Superficial medial collateral ligament test. (B) Full extension test for capsular integrity (deep medial collateral ligament).

- Lateral collateral ligament test (Figure 12.7)
- Anterior drawer (Figure 12.8)
- Lachman test (Figure 12.9)

3. Case

3.1. History and Exam

A 38-year-old recreational soccer player comes to see you in your office after hurting her right knee at last night's match. She complains of a swollen, painful right knee. She denies being hit, but remembers trying to stop suddenly to kick the ball and her knee giving away. She did not hear or feel a "pop" in her knee. The knee started to swell immediately and she could not bear weight because of the pain. She was unable to continue playing. She was very uncomfortable through the night and the knee is more swollen today. She has had no previous injuries to her knee and does not have any medical problems. She works as a legal secretary and wants to go back to work as soon as possible. Examination reveals a swollen knee held in 15° of flexion as the patient is lying flat on the examination table. Flexion is only possible

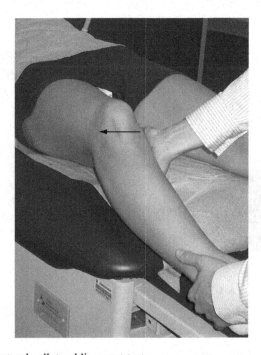

FIGURE 12.7. Lateral collateral ligament test.

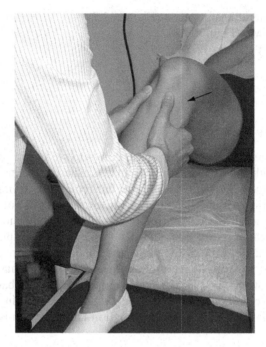

FIGURE 12.8. Anterior drawer test.

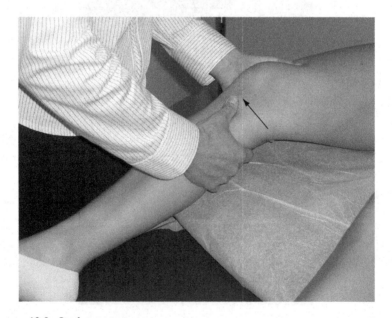

FIGURE 12.9. Lachman test.

to 80° and there is a 10° extension lag (unable to fully extend the knee through the last 10°). On the left, extension is full to −5° and flexion is possible to 145°. The rest of the knee examination is difficult to perform because of the swelling and discomfort.

3.2. Thinking Process

This is an acute injury in a person with no history of prior knee problems. Overuse injury and chronic arthritis are not likely. The history and mechanism of injury do not suggest collateral ligament injury because no direct blow to the knee occurred. A sudden stop and the knee giving away are suggestive of meniscus (cartilage) or ACL injury. Immediate swelling and inability to bear weight are suggestive of an anterior cruciate tear. Meniscal injuries do not usually swell for 12 to 24 h. Feeling or hearing a "pop" suggests an anterior cruciate tear but it is not always present. The examination is nondiagnostic because of the discomfort when trying other diagnostic maneuvers. The Lachman test is the more sensitive than the anterior drawer test but neither is very helpful at this stage of the injury. Examination immediately after injury is diagnostic but the swelling and pain will need to diminish before either test is of value. Imaging studies specifically magnetic resonance imaging (MRI) will help make the diagnosis at this stage and the MRI did indeed show a tear of the ACL.

There are several different mechanisms that can cause a tear of the ACL: hyperextension or valgus stress to the knee, a sudden deceleration and rotation of the lower leg, or any force causing the tibia to move anteriorly or forward relative to the femur when the knee is flexed. Injuries involving significant torsional or twisting rotation can also cause tearing of the meniscus, more commonly medial meniscus in addition to tearing of the ACL. Anterior cruciate ligament injuries occur more commonly in women than in men. The reason for this discrepancy is not clearly understood. Factors like joint laxity, differences in anatomy of the femur, hormonal influence, muscle strength, and skill development are thought to play a role in the risk of ACL rupture.

The majority of acute ACL tears will result in an acute swelling secondary to a bloody effusion. Range of motion of the knee will be decreased secondary to the effusion and pain. The Lachman test (Figure 12.9) assesses anterior or forward laxity of the knee. Lack of a firm end point to forward movement suggests a tear of the ACL. The Lachman test is more reliable than the anterior drawer test in assessing the integrity of the ACL ligament. When the knee is flexed 90° for the anterior drawer test the hamstrings will help stabilize the forward movement of the tibia and produce a false negative test. The Lachman is more difficult to perform on patients with a large leg circumference and physicians with smaller hands. Figure 12.10 demonstrates a Lachman when faced with patients who have thighs too large for the examiner. An assistant stabilizes the femur and the clinician tests the ACL for

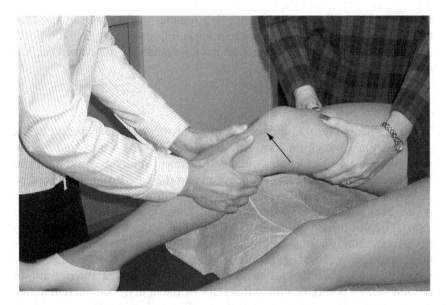

FIGURE 12.10. Alternative method for performing the Lachman test.

integrity. Diagnosis of ACL tears by physical examination is not possible after the first few hours of the injury because hamstring tightness and knee effusion limit the reliability of the Lachman and anterior drawer. When the effusion decreases and the pain is diminished the test will again be reliable. This usually takes 7 to 10 days.

Integrity of the PC ligament is tested the same way as the anterior drawer is tested (Figure 12.8) except the pressure is placed posterior rather than forward. Posterior cruciate ligament deficiency is also evaluated by placing both knees in 90° of flexion and observing the knees from the side. If one of the knees is PC-deficient it will sag further back than the other. Laxity testing for medial and lateral collateral injury (Figures 12.6A, 12.6B, and 12.7) and joint line tenderness (Figure 12.3) for meniscal injury should be done to rule out injury to these structures. Because of the anatomic proximity of the medial collateral ligament (MCL) and medial meniscus to the ACL, valgus stress (hit from the lateral side, Figure 12.11) can sometimes injure all three of the structures (terrible triad).

3.3. Imaging

Plain films are usually obtained to rule out fractures. Tibial plateau fractures can mimic ACL tears because of the acute swelling, inability to bear weight, and difficult initial examination. Magnetic resonance imaging is the gold standard for imaging ligamentous structures in the knee.

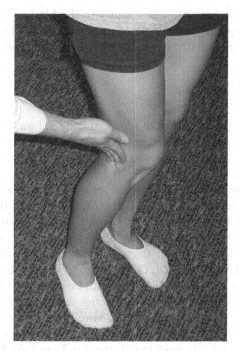

FIGURE 12.11. Valgus stress to lateral side.

3.4. Treatment of Anterior Cruciate Ligament Tears

The need for surgery depends in part on age, activity level, degree of knee laxity, and associated injuries. Certainly, any patient who wishes to remain active and participate in sports that require jumping, cutting, and pivoting would be recommended for surgery. However, this surgery is not emergent, and the outcome is usually better if the patient has full knee extension and minimal swelling prior to surgery. Most patients wait at least 1 month before considering surgery. Some patients complete a short course of physical therapy to achieve full extension and regain strength in the quadriceps prior to surgery. Inactive patients do not necessarily need to undergo ACL reconstruction but would need to be involved in a physical therapy program for quadriceps strengthening.

4. Medial Collateral Ligament Tear

This ligament is the most commonly injured ligament in the knee. The mechanism of injury is usually a forceful stress to the lateral side (Figure 12.11) while the foot is planted and the extremity is bearing weight. Any lateral or valgus stress to the knee can cause injury to the MCL. This can occur in a noncontact setting such as in skiing or swimming (whip kick in breaststroke) or in a contact situation involving a blow to the lower thigh while the foot is planted.

4.1. History and Examination

The patient usually cannot bear weight on the leg and may complain of the knee feeling "loose." Partial tears are usually more painful than complete tears. The severity of the pain does not always correlate with the degree of injury. Examination may reveal some mild effusion over the medial joint line if there is a more severe sprain. Pain localizes over the MCL on palpation. Complete tears usually occur in the middle of the ligament so the tenderness is in the joint line and partial tears occur at the insertion sites on the femur or tibia (Figure 12.1), so the tenderness will be there. Perform a valgus stress to the knee at 30° of knee flexion to assess the integrity of the MCL (Figure 12.6A). Also stress the knee in full extension (Figure 12.6B). The MCL cannot be accurately assessed with the knee in full extension, because the posterior capsule and the cruciate ligaments contribute to the stability of the knee in full extension. So if weakness exists in full extension, posterior capsule and cruciate damage is suspected. As previously mentioned, the MCL and ACL can be injured simultaneously.

Sprains to the MCL are classified as mild, moderate, and severe. Mild sprains cause some tearing of the individual ligament fibers, but no laxity is present on examination with valgus stress of the knee. Moderate sprains are partial tears but with minimal ligamentous laxity on examination. Severe sprains cause a complete disruption of the ligament, causing laxity and significant swelling. Another way to classify MCL sprains is by the degree of laxity or joint opening. Grade I shows very little laxity (up to 4 mm) with valgus testing. With grade II sprains, the joint opens no more than 9 mm, but there is a definite end point. Grade III sprains show significant laxity on valgus testing (10 to 15 mm) with no end point appreciated.

4.2. Imaging

The diagnosis is from history and physical examination. X-rays are not always indicated. If there is an effusion or the patient is unable to bear weight, obtain plain films to rule out a fracture or loose bodies; magnetic resonance imaging is indicated if associated injuries such as a meniscal tear or an ACL tear are suspected. Severe MCL sprains warrant an MRI for this reason. The MRI should be ordered to confirm what is already suspected and not to make the diagnosis.

4.3. Treatment of Medial Collateral Ligament Injuries

Almost all isolated MCL injuries are managed nonoperatively. Ice, nonsteroidal anti-inflammatory mediations, and rest are the first-line treatment. If the patient cannot walk without a limp, crutches should be used for protective weight bearing as tolerated. Early mobilization focusing on ROM should be initiated as soon as tolerated. The MCL heals by scarring down on itself. Usually, patients are back to their usual activities within 10 to 21 days, depending on the grade of sprain. Grade III sprains should be referred, as this injury may require surgery, depending on the degree of laxity.

5. Meniscal/Cartilage Injuries

The menisci or semilunar cartilage act as cushions or shock absorbers between the femur and tibia and assist with control of knee motion. Tears in the meniscus are the most common of knee injuries. Injuries to the medial meniscus are 10 times more common because it is less mobile and attached more firmly than the lateral meniscus, There are two types of tears: degenerative and activity-related (requiring pivoting movements).

5.1. History and Examination

Obtaining a good history can make the diagnosis the majority of the time. Most meniscal injuries result from a pivoting movement with the foot planted. Patients usually feel acute pain at the time of the tear. Delayed swelling usually occurs up to 12 to 24 h after the event in contrast to ligament tears that swell immediately because of the bleeding. Motion may be limited because of effusion or hamstring spasm. Once the acute symptoms subside, the patient may experience catching, buckling, or locking of the knee. They also will have difficulty walking up and down the stairs and squatting is avoided because of the pain. Patients with a long history of meniscal tear will report recurrent effusions and a lack of "confidence" in the knee. They are usually very hesitant with such movements as getting out of a car or making sudden changes in direction while walking.

Start the examination by comparing the injured knee to the uninjured side. Atrophy of the medial quadriceps may be present in chronic knee problems. Large effusions are obvious but smaller ones are more subtle. Effusion may cause the patella to be ballotable and produce a pouch over the joint lines, with milking down the suprapatellar pouch. Place the cupped hand above the patella and slowly push downward to see if any fluid can be "milked" out into the indented pouches below the patella. The patient may also sit with the knee slightly flexed because of effusion or a portion of cartilage blocking full extension. Palpation of the medial and lateral joint spaces will usually be tender. Tenderness in the joint space usually indicates a tear. The "squat" test is helpful in differentiating patellofemoral pain from a meniscal tear. The patient with a meniscal tear will report pain at the bottom of the squat, which localizes to either joint line. By contrast, the patient with patellofemoral pain will have pain anteriorly while descending and ascending from the squat. The McMurray test and Apley test are two provocative tests that may elicit symptoms from a torn meniscus. The McMurray test (Figure 12.12) is performed by first placing the knee in full flexion. The lower leg is then internally rotated with varus stress and externally rotated with valgus stress while passively bringing the leg into extension. One hand is placed over the joint line during this maneuver to feel for clicking. Suspect a meniscal tear if either pain or clicking is elicited. The Apley grind test (Figure 12.13) is similar to the McMurray test in that you are attempting to catch the torn cartilage with internal and external rotation of the lower leg. With the patient in the prone position, flex the knee to 90°, pull up on the tibia, and internally and externally rotate the tibia. This test is of most value if it is negative. If the McMurray or any other part of the examination is positive the Apley adds little but if all other tests are negative it will help rule out meniscal tears. As with any other potential injury to the knee, perform a complete evaluation of all ligamentous structures.

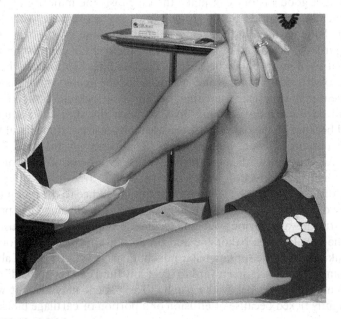

FIGURE 12.12. McMurray test.

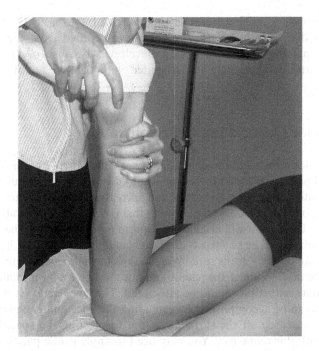

FIGURE 12.13. Apley grind test.

5.2. Imaging

Plain radiographs are helpful to rule out to rule out degenerative changes, loose bodies, and fractures. Magnetic resonance imaging is very effective at identifying meniscal tears. Use MRI to confirm a diagnosis formulated from a good history and physical examination.

5.3. Treatment of Meniscal Injuries

The initial treatment is conservative except in those cases where the knee is locked. Many tears especially peripheral ones can heal in a few weeks. Rest, ice, compression, and elevation should be started immediately. Use crutches as long as it is painful to bear weight. Quadriceps exercises should start early to help decrease the effusion and prevent atrophy. A physical therapist can help with effective strengthening and stretching exercises. As the pain decreases and motion returns, weight-bearing activity is gradually resumed. The key to treatment is the strengthening and stretching exercises of the quadriceps and hamstring muscles that are described at the end of the chapter. If the patient is unable to fully extend and flex the knee or the knee is locking, an orthopedic referral is in order.

Be sure that a meniscal tear is the source of the patient's symptoms. Vastus medialis obliquus atrophy may have resulted from the meniscus tear and patellar femoral tracking developed because of the atrophy. Buckling and catching can be associated with patellar femoral tracking problems

6. Patellar Dislocation and Subluxation

Patellar dislocation is not too common. It is usually caused by a direct blow to the lateral portion of the knee (valgus strain) or it can spontaneously occur in patients with patellar abnormalities and increased flexibility. They will have immediate pain and an obvious deformity that produces a considerable amount of anxiety. The patient will usually not want to move the leg and the deformity is usually obvious. The patellar is displaced laterally and the knee held in flexion. Swelling of the knee is usually rapid. The medial patellar retinaculum is torn on the medial side of the patella and knee will be tender medially.

Immediate reduction should be attempted. The key is relaxing the quadriceps. This can be accomplished by extending the knee and grasping the heel to lift the lower leg off the surface where it was resting. The patella usually reduces with this maneuver. You may need to apply gentle patellar pressure and ice to facilitate the reduction. On rare occasions, the patient will require further sedation for reduction to occur.

After the reduction, a knee immobilizer is used for 2 to 3 weeks and crutches are used until weight bearing can be performed without pain. This immobilization will enhance healing of the medial retinaculum and supporting structures of the patella. The immobilizer will cause quadriceps atrophy so quadriceps strengthening exercises should begin once the quadriceps can be stretched without pain. After the first 5 or 6 days, have the patient contract the quadriceps while in the immobilizer. After the second week a more extensive exercise program should begin. Some suggested quadriceps exercises are included at the end of the chapter. Consultation with a physical therapist will help train the patient to do appropriate quadriceps exercises. Recurrent subluxation is a complication of acute dislocation and quadriceps exercises help decrease their occurrence. An X-ray is indicated to rule out a patellar fracture and/or the formation of a loose body from a patellar fracture.

Recurrent patella subluxation is a common and often undiagnosed disorder because the symptoms are similar to other knee derangements. The usually story is one of recurrent pain, swelling, and leg giving out. Examination will reveal tenderness on medial side of the patella. A classic finding with this injury is a positive apprehension test. Perform this test by placing your thumb on the medial aspect of the patella and gently displacing it laterally while the knee is flexed 15° to 20°. The test is positive if significant discomfort and apprehension occurs with lateral movement. There may also be hypermobility compared with the other side. It is important to not confuse the apprehension test with the patellar compression test (Figure 12.5) that is used to help diagnose patellar femoral pain syndrome (PFPS).

Anteroposterior, lateral, merchant, and notch knee radiographs are indicated to look for osteochondral or avulsion fractures and the position of the patella. These fractures may produce a loose fragment that will eventually become a loose body. Lateral subluxation of the patella may be noted on the merchant view and/or a high-riding patella (patella alta) observed on the lateral view. Patella alta is thought to be associated with an increased risk of subluxation/dislocation.

7. Loose Bodies

Loose bodies also known as a *joint mouse* can be found in the knee joint. They may be present because of a prior osteochondral fracture or osteochondritis. The patients are usually young and complain of pain and intermittent swelling and locking or catching. Sometimes the patient feels the lump or loose body. The loose body can be felt anywhere in the joint or the suprapatellar pouch. Radiographs may demonstrate the loose body. The treatment is surgical if the loose body can be palpated and easily removed.

The symptoms of a loose body can be similar to recurrent subluxation and PFPS and these entities can coexist with each other. The patient may have dislocated the patella and sustained an osteochondral fracture that formed a loose body. The catching and discomfort from the loose body can lead to atrophy of the VMO. This atrophy predisposes the patient to PFPS (discussed next). The loose bodies are not always easy to find clinically or by imaging. If a patient is not responding to the quadriceps muscle strengthening program, consider a loose body. It may take a little time for it to show up but they usually do.

Loose bodies may have arisen from osteochondritis dissecans (OD). The knee is the most common site for OD. It also occurs at the capitellum of the elbow and the talar dome of the ankle. Osteochondritis dissecans results from a piece of bone undergoing avascular necrosis. The segment of bone separates and become a loose body. If a loose body is noted on a traditional X-ray, obtain a tunnel view to look for the donor site (where the bone was previously located). The lateral surface of the medial femoral condyle is the most common donor site. If OD is suspected, an orthopedic consultation is appropriate.

8. Case

8.1. History and Exam

A 22-year-old student presents to your office with complaints of right anterior knee pain. The pain started about 3 months after she began a walking/running program to help her loose weight. The pain now makes it difficult for her to do much exercise and she experiences periodic giving away and locking of her knee. Walking up and down the stairs and sitting for long periods at her desk increases the pain. She has no medical problems and no previous injuries to the knee. The examination reveals some atrophy of her right VMO by observation and palpation. Palpation also reveals tenderness around the anterior patella and no lumps are found in the joint spaces. There is no joint line tenderness and the McMurray and apprehension tests are negative. The patella compression test (Figure 12.5) produces retropatellar pain and palpable crepitus below the patella. No ligamentous instability is noted and neither foot has excessive pronation.

8.2. Thinking Process

Since there was no acute trauma, the list is narrowed to include overuse syndromes or medical problems. Her history is negative for medical problems and her age does not favor degenerative joint disease. The history of pain aggravated by going up and down the stairs and prolonged sitting is classic for PFPS. Locking and giving away can be present with PFPS but it also can be indicative of several other entities that include meniscal tears, recurrent patellar subluxation, and loose bodies. The examination helps rule out these entities. No lumps are felt so a loose body is less likely, the apprehension test is negative ruling out patellar subluxation and the lack of joint line tenderness, and a negative McMurray make meniscal damage unlikely. The patellar compression test is positive, further indicating that the PFPS is the diagnosis in this patient. The patellar compression test is performed with the knee slightly flexed, one hand compresses the patella, and the leg is extended (Figure 12.5). Atrophy of the VMO is associated with any of the above entities. The VMO keeps the patella centered in the patellar sulcus of the femur so a decrease in VMO strength creates patellar displacement. This displacement places increased pressure on the lateral portions of the patellar sulcus and degenerative changes occur. This helps explain why the compression test produces pain and crepitus. Pronation of one or both feet is associated with multiple leg and foot problems including PFPS. It is not always present but if it is, it needs to be recognized and treated.

This patient most likely has PFPS. It is one of the most common disorders of the knee and is seen frequently in the primary care setting. Women are affected more than men, and it is thought to occur because of abnormal tracking of the patella causing microtrauma. Factors responsible for the syndrome may include weakness of the hip girdle, increased quadriceps (Q) angle, high-riding patella, imbalance between the vastus lateralis and the weaker VMO, and misalignment of the lower extremity. The Q angle is measured by drawing a line from the anterior superior iliac crest through the midpoint of the patella. Draw another line from the tibial tuberosity through the midpoint of the patella. The angle formed at the intersection of the two lines is the Q angle (Figure 12.14).

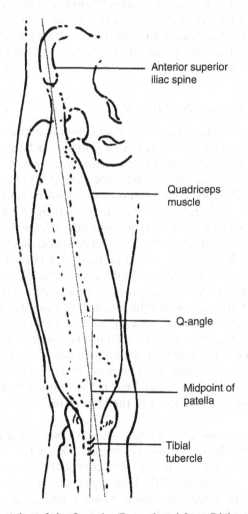

Anterior superior iliac spine

Quadriceps muscle

Q-angle

Midpoint of patella

Tibial tubercle

FIGURE 12.14. Drawing of the Q angle. (Reproduced from Richmond J, Shahady E, eds. *Sports Medicine for Primary Care*. Cambridge, MA: Blackwell Science; 1996: 398, with permission.)

8.3. Imaging

Imaging is only needed to rule out other entities. The PFPS diagnosis is clinical.

8.4. Treatment of Patellar Femoral Pain Syndrome

Quadriceps strengthening especially the VMO is the cornerstone of treatment to help improve the tracking of the patella. Quadriceps exercises are described at the end of the chapter. Exercise 3, straight leg raising, is very helpful for PFPS. Ice, nonsteroidal anti-inflammatory drugs (NSAIDs), and arch supports to correct ankle pronation are also suggested interventions. Patella bracing and bands are commonly used with varying effectiveness. The great majority of the time, conservative measures are effective. Surgery is a rare option for resistance cases.

8.5. Iliotibial Band Syndrome

Iliotibial band syndrome (ITBS) is another common overuse syndrome associated with running and other knee flexion activities such as cycling, skiing, or weightlifting. It is the most common overuse syndrome in distance runners and the most common cause of lateral knee pain. It is more common in men than in women. Iliotibial band syndrome is caused by faulty training techniques (running on hilly terrain) and anatomic malalignment.

The usual presentation is a sharp burning lateral knee pain that may radiate up into the lateral thigh or down to Gerdy's tubercle of the tibia (is easily palpated on the tibia just lateral to the distal portion of the patellar tendon, Figure 12.15). Runners often describe a specific, reproducible time when their symptoms start. They also note more pain with downhill running because of the increased time spent in the impingement or friction zone. This zone is the area between 20° and 30° of flexion that the iliotibial band (ITB) crosses over the lateral femoral condyle. Friction from excessive flexion and extension produces inflammation of the ITB. Fast running and sprinting does not cause pain because the athletes' knee spends more time in angles greater than 30° and not in the impingement zone. Riding a bike can increase the time spent in the impingement zone and produce or aggravate ITBS.

Physical examination should begin with an observation for swelling and atrophy especially the vastus medialis muscle. The vastus medialis will atrophy with many knee injuries. Range of motion of the hip and knee should be evaluated and any limitation of the injured side when compared with the normal side should be noted and used to follow treatment progress. Be on the lookout for hip abductor weakness as it is common with ITBS. Physical examination in ITBS usually reveals tenderness over the lateral femoral epicondyle when the knee is flexed greater than 30° (Figure 12.16). A Noble

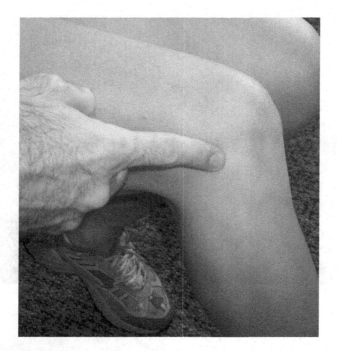

FIGURE 12.15.   Gerdy's tubercle.

compression test is performed by applying pressure to the lateral femoral epicondyle while the knee is fully extended (Figure 12.17A). The knee is slowly flexed. The compression test is positive if the patient reports pain at 30° of knee flexion (Figure 12.17B) and/or the examiner palpates a rubbing or snapping sensation as the ITB passes over the lateral femoral epicondyle. Ober's

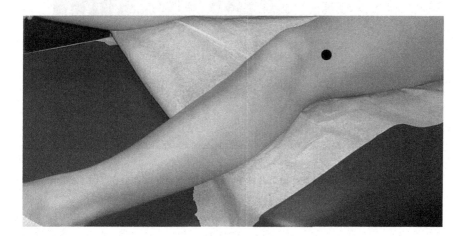

FIGURE 12.16.   Lateral femoral condyle of ITB.

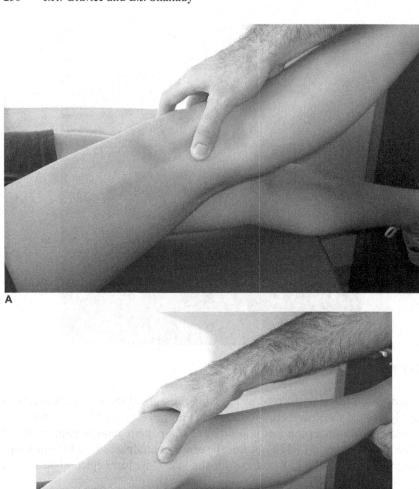

FIGURE 12.17. (A) Noble test at full extension. (B) Noble test at 30° of flexion.

test (Figure 12.18) assesses ITB tightness that is associated with ITBS. The patient lies on the unaffected side. The unaffected hip and knee are both flexed to 120°. The involved knee is flexed to 90°, and the hip is abducted and hyperextended. After helping the patient do the maneuvers let the leg drop. A tight ITB will prevent the extremity from dropping below the imaginary horizontal noted in Figure 12.18.

8.6. Imaging

X-rays are not needed to make the diagnosis of ITBS. Magnetic resonance imaging is done to rule out other causes. If the patient is not responding to conservative measures after 3 months an MRI is helpful to rule out other causes of the pain.

8.7. Treatment of Iliotibial Band Syndrome

Most patients with ITBS respond to nonoperative measures. Activity modification, exercises to strengthen hip abductor weakness, and hamstring and ITB stretching should be instituted. The exercises at the end of Chapter 11 and this chapter contain those exercises. Prescribe a short course (7 to 10 days) of NSAIDs. If excessive foot pronation is present suggest that the

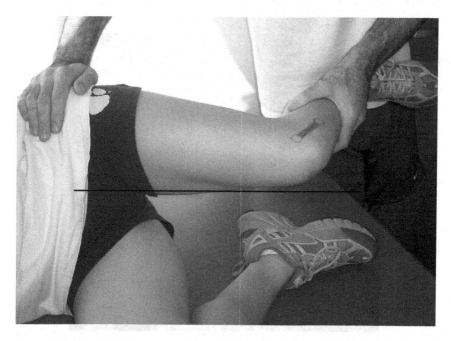

FIGURE 12.18. Ober test.

patient use orthotics. Chapter 15 has a more extensive discussion of the use of orthotics. After a short period of avoiding running or cycling for 7 to 10 days (okay to walk) patients slowly start back with their running and biking. Symptoms and conditioning guide this process. Stretching of the ITB and strengthening of the medial abductors should start with the diagnosis and should be continued after return to activity. Most patients' symptoms improve by 3 to 6 weeks. A corticosteroid injection (Figure 12.19) into the underlying bursa can be considered in refractory cases. Treatment and prevention of future injury can be accomplished by looking for training errors. This may involve decreasing mileage, altering stride length, avoiding hills, or periodically changing direction when running on a sloped surface. In cyclists, the seat height or the foot position may need to be changed.

Surgery may be considered after at least 6 months of nonoperative management. After arthroscopy to exclude intra-articular pathology, surgical excision of a portion of the ITB is performed.

9. Infrapatellar Tendonitis (Jumper's Knee)

Anatomically this is not a tendon but a ligament because it goes from bone to bone. Tradition refers to it as a tendon so for the sake of communication between health professionals it will be referred to as a tendon. This overuse injury is seen more commonly in patients who participate in activities that

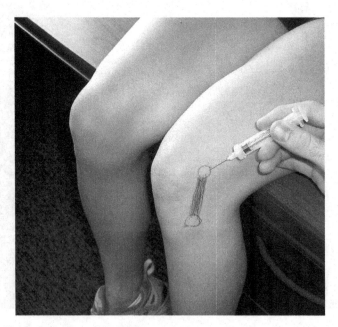

FIGURE 12.19. Injection of the ITB.

require a lot of jumping or squatting like basketball, volleyball, and weight lifting. The patellar tendon originates on the inferior pole of the patella and attaches to the tibial tubercle. Look at Figure 12.3 for all of these landmarks. Repeated forces at the inferior pole of the patella or the tibial tubercle cause microtrauma that results in microscopic tearing of the fibers and tendonitis. Direct palpation of the inferior pole of the patella, the patellar tendon, or less commonly over the tibial tubercle will cause pain, as will resisted knee extension. Be sure the tendon is intact and not ruptured by having the patient perform a straight leg raise with the knee in extension. A patient with a torn tendon would not be able to extend the knee and lift the leg. The rest of the examination for meniscal tears and ligamentous instability should be normal.

X-rays are usually normal, but may demonstrate calcification within the patellar tendon or a small avulsion fracture from the inferior pole of the patella. In a younger patient the tibial tubercle may be tender and look unusual because of an entity known as Osgood–Schlatter disease. This will be discussed in the pediatric section.

9.1. Treatment of Patellar Tendonitis

Activity modification along with ice and NSAIDs are the mainstays of treatment. The patient should avoid leg extension exercises, as this puts an unnecessary load on the patellar tendon. Physical therapy for long-term treatment focuses on hamstring and quadriceps muscle strength, Achilles tendon stretching and ankle dorsiflexion flexibility. Steroid injection is not recommended due to the increased risk of tendon rupture.

10. Bursitis

There are several bursas around the knee. Two of them, the pes anserine and the prepatellar, can become inflamed and present to the primary care clinician. Being able to differentiate these two problems from other knee problems is an important skill. Figure 12.20 depicts the location of the bursa.

10.1. Pes Anserine Bursitis

This bursitis can be confused with a MCL sprain, medial meniscus tear, and OA because it causes medial knee pain. The bursa overlies the tibial attachment site of the sartorious, gracilis, and semitendinosus muscles and is located about 2 in. below the medial joint line. It is most common in middle-aged to older patients who are overweight. It can become inflamed from overuse or a direct contusion. The symptoms usually include sense of fullness in the area of the bursa and pain that can worsen with repetitive flexion and extension. Valgus stress testing in the supine position or resisted knee flexion in the prone position may reproduce the pain.

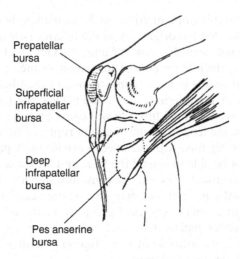

Prepatellar
bursa

Superficial
infrapatellar
bursa

Deep
infrapatellar
bursa

Pes anserine
bursa

FIGURE 12.20. Drawing of the knee bursa. (Reproduced from Richmond J, Shahady E, eds. *Sports Medicine for Primary Care*. Cambridge, MA: Blackwell Science; 1996: 431, with permission.)

Treatment is directed at decreasing the inflammation of the pes bursa area. Limitation of or change in any aggravating activity, use of moist heat, ultrasound, iontophoresis, and a stretching and strengthening program are usually successful. Use the hamstring and calf stretching and strengthening exercises described at the end of the chapter. Physical therapy consultation for iontophoresis and ultrasound with progression to resistance exercises can be helpful. Cortisone injections into the bursa are usually successful (Figure 12.21). Return to recreational activities and work is dependent on regaining muscle strength and flexibility in addition to decreasing inflammation. Some of the patients with this bursitis may also have OA so be alert for the dual diagnosis. Imaging plays no role in making this diagnosis but may be helpful to rule out other entities.

10.2. Prepatellar Bursitis

The prepatellar bursa is located directly above the patella (Figure 12.20). Its superficial location makes it susceptible to acute and chronic trauma. Acute injury is not as common as chronic microtrauma. In both acute and chronic bursitis the examination is similar but the history is different. An acute fall will produce bleeding, immediate swelling, and the appearance of a baseball-sized mass directly over the knee cap. The appearance can sometimes be quiet frightening to the patient and the novice practitioner. The chronic microtrauma is usually occupational. Any occupation that requires patients to be working on their knees can cause this bursitis. The chronic microtrauma usually appears

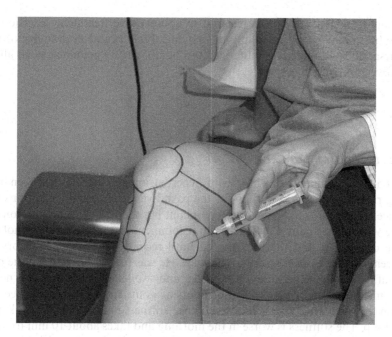

FIGURE 12.21. Injection of the pes anserine bursa.

the day after patients have spent a long time on their knees with their occupation. This is why this entity is sometimes called housemaid's knee.

The examination reveals a tight tender baseball-sized mass over the patella. Flexion and extension of the knee may be limited because of the mass. Be sure no other cystic structures like a Baker's cyst (bulge behind the knee) or a meniscal cyst (bulge lateral to joint line) are present. Another rare entity to rule out is septic prepatellar bursitis. Septic patients complain of sudden onset of redness, warmth and swelling, fever, and/or chills. Examination reveals erythema and swelling over the patella with surrounding soft tissue edema. All patients with prepatellar bursitis will have some degree of tenderness and warmth but not the extensive amount that is associated with septic bursitis.

Aspirating the bursa is the key to diagnosis and treatment. The fluid in acute trauma is bloody and may clot. In chronic microtrauma the fluid is dark red but does not clot. The fluid in septic bursitis is usually turbid but can also be blood-tinged. Obtain cultures and smears for bacteria if sepsis is suspected. Most of the time the diagnosis is chronic microtrauma.

Treatment consists of draining the fluid and injecting a steroid and lidocaine. A large-bore needle (18 gauge) is used because the fluid is thick and may be difficult to drain. Advise the patient to avoid kneeling and if that is not possible protect the knee with some type of padding.

Occasional surgery may be required for recurrent prepatellar bursitis. This is usually because of the synovial thickening similar to olecrenon bursitis (see

Chapter 6) that will not to respond to conservative treatment. Excision of the bursa may be indicated in these patients. Pigtail catheter drainage of the bursa, inserted under computerized tomography (CT) guidance, is an alternative approach to surgery.

11. Case

11.1. History and Exam

A 65-year-old man with a history of hypertension and diabetes has been having right knee pain off and on for the past 3 years. He usually mentions the knee pain as an "oh, by the way" complaint but today the primary reason for the visit is knee pain. Previously you recommended that he take Tylenol for the discomfort and that has helped until recently. There is no history of recent trauma or past injury to the knee. He was told 1 year ago that he had gout in his big toe because it was tender and swollen. His uric acid has never been elevated and he had no prior bouts of gout. He is not on any medication for gout. He also has had some knee stiffness and pain in his back and left hip. The stiffness is worse in the morning and takes about 10 min to wear off. The pain is now impacting his life as it keeps him from exercising and his blood sugar is running over 200 in the morning. He has no complaints of buckling or catching of his right knee but he does note periodic swelling especially after he tries to walk.

When walking he has a significant limp and does not want to bear weight on the right leg. He is afebrile. When reclining on the examination table you note that the right knee is mildly swollen and he is holding the knee in about 15° of flexion. The knee joint seems warmer than the rest of the leg but no redness is present. Milking down the suprapatellar pouch is positive for fluid, his VMO is weaker on the right by palpation, flexion is limited to 90° by pain, and he is not able to fully extend his knee without pain. Examination does not suggest ligamentous laxity but all maneuvers for ligamentous and meniscal damage are difficult because of the pain. The rest of the examination is negative. He does have Heberden's nodes on the distal interphalangeal (DIP) joints of multiple fingers. Aspiration of the knee joint fluid reveals a light straw-colored fluid. When the fluid-filled tube is placed next to newsprint you can read newsprint. The white cell count of the fluid is 500 mm^3 and no crystals are noted. An X-ray of his right knee compared with that of the left knee reveals narrowing of the medial joint space and osteophytes.

11.2. Thinking Process

The patient's age, morning stiffness that rapidly clears, and Heberden's nodes of the DIP suggest OA but other diagnoses should be ruled out. No history of injury, buckling, or catching, and a stable knee on examination helps rule out ligamentous and meniscal damage. Septic joint should always be ruled out because the joint can be destroyed if a bacterial infection is not treated quickly. Warm joints are common in OA. The septic joint is usually hot, tender, and red. Septic joint fluid is a turbid yellow and the cell count is greater than 60,000. One quick way of deciding on the turbidity of the fluid is to place the fluid-filled tube in front of some newsprint. In OA you should be able to read the print. With other inflammatory arthritis and sepsis, the print is not visible. This patient has a low cell count, the color is light straw-colored, and you can read newsprint through it. Gout is ruled out by the absence of crystals in the fluid. The history of gout is probably a red herring. The classical "big toe" gout usually occurs for the first time in 35- to 40-year-old men and not at age 64. Osteoarthritis is the most common cause of big toe arthritis in this age group. Gout of the big toe usually causes a much greater degree of swelling and redness than OA. The X-ray with narrowing of the joint space is highly suggestive of OA.

This patient was diagnosed with OA and treated with Tylenol and quadriceps strengthening exercises. He now uses the Tylenol prn and does his strengthening exercises faithfully and he is doing well.

11.3. Imaging

When OA is suspected, recommended radiographs include weight-bearing and non-weight-bearing views. Some of the classical findings include joint space narrowing, subchondral bony sclerosis, cystic changes, and hypertrophic osteophyte formation. The X-ray should never be used to make a diagnosis or judge degree of severity of OA. Many individuals over the age of 50 will have radiographic evidence of OA but do not seek or require medical attention. Some patients may be symptomatic and have minimal radiographic changes. Osteoarthritis is a clinical and not a radiographic diagnosis.

11.4. Treatment of Osteoarthritis

Quadriceps strengthening is the mainstay of treatment for knee OA. Many patients and clinicians do not understand this important concept and start treatment with medication. Quadriceps strengthening exercises, many times, are all that is needed to reduce the pain and return the patient to an acceptable level of function. Unfortunately, most patients with knee OA are like the patient above. They have other medical problems that bring them to the clinician and the knee complaints are mentioned casually at the end of the visit ("oh, by the way"). The clinician is about out of the door and takes the quickest strategy for treatment: a "pill." The authors are also human and have done the same thing but only to regret it later because the patient does not value exercises like medication. Taking the extra minute and give the patient a list of exercises like the ones at the end of this chapter and reserve medication as a second line of treatment. This strategy pays dividends for future care. The above patient may have avoided much of his disability if he had been taught exercises when he initially complained of the knee pain.

The first medication used after exercises are started is Tylenol, 4 grams a day. Tylenol treatment will fail if the dose is not correct or the patient just uses it as needed. At least a 10-day course of Tylenol at 4 g a day is recommended. Other effective medications are NSAIDs, topical capsaicin cream, and glucosamine sulfate. Caution should be exercised with long-term use of NSAIDs because of bleeding, renal dysfunction, and hypertension. Glucosamine can elevate blood sugar and if used in combination with NSAIDs can increase bleeding tendencies. Monitor for these problems when NSAIDs are used long term.

A regular exercise program can reduce the symptoms of pain by increasing ROM of the joint and reducing overall weight on the arthritic joint. Most patients will be able to perform low-impact activities such as biking and swimming without pain.

Injections with lidocaine and a steroid like Depo-Medrol can provide effective short-term relief. This short-term relief (4 to 6 weeks) of pain and enhanced ability to flex and extend the knee permits the initiation of a program of quadriceps strengthening. Once the quadriceps strength has increased the patient usually does well. For the injection the lateral approach is most commonly used. For this approach, lines are drawn along the lateral and proximal borders of the patella. The needle is inserted into the soft tissue between the patella and the femur near the intersection point of the lines (Figure 12.22) and directed at a 45° angle toward the middle of the medial side of the joint.

In the anterior approach, the knee is flexed 90°, and the needle is inserted just medial or lateral to the patellar tendon and parallel to the tibial plateau (Figure 12.23). This technique is preferred by some physicians. It is more difficult to enter the joint space if significant OA is present and may produce more pain. But this approach is more likely to deposit the steroid and lidocaine in the joint. Injections with exogenous hyaluronic acid (viscosupplementation) may improve pain and function. These solutions are not long term, but may delay the need for surgery up to 6 months.

Surgical options are reserved for those patients who fail conservative measures. Debridement of the articular cartilage has no proven benefit. Significant improvement can be seen in patients undergoing partial and total knee replacements.

12. Case

12.1. History

A 11-year-old boy who is in good health complains of a "bump below his kneecap" that hurts to touch and when he jumps. The pain has been present for 1 month and is increasing in intensity. The patient plays basketball every

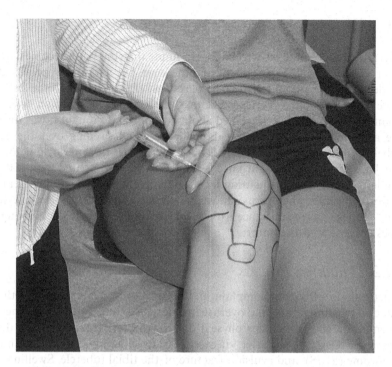

FIGURE 12.22. Lateral injection of the knee.

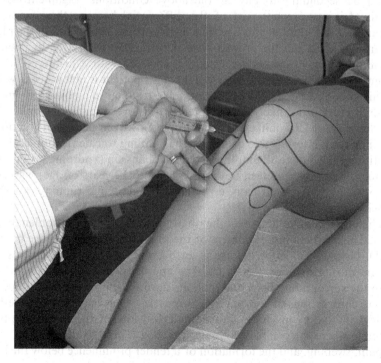

FIGURE 12.23. Anterior approach injection of the knee.

day after school and on weekends. He notes that the pain becomes worse after a lot of jumping or if he falls on the knee, but it always improves after he decreases the amount of time he plays basketball. He fell on the anterior knee yesterday and experienced a marked increase in the pain over the "bump." The mother is concerned about a tumor and thought it was time to see a doctor. Examination reveals tenderness and swelling over the tibial tubercle on the right knee. There is no tenderness at the inferior pole of the patella. Flexion of the right knee is limited to 120° compared with 150° on the left. Kneeling and squatting increase the pain. There is no ligamentous laxity of the knee when varus and valgus stress is applied. He is able to extend the right leg against resistance with equal strength to the left side although it does induce some discomfort.

12.2. Thinking Process

Knee pain is a frequent complaint in this age group. Trauma, from either a fall or a twisting injury, and overuse injuries need to be considered. The differential diagnosis includes physeal or growth plate fracture of the distal humerus, Osgood–Schlatter disease (OSD), Sinding–Larsen–Johansson syndrome (SLJS), and avulsion fracture of the tibial tubercle. Swelling and tenderness in one knee, which is exacerbated by activity and relieved by rest, could be secondary to any of the above conditions. Ligamentous and meniscal injury are not part of the differential because they are a rare occurrence in a child of this age. The ligaments are stronger than the physis or growth plate and the growth plate will fracture before the ligament or meniscus tears. Fractures are usually associated with a history of recent trauma and the inability to bear weight. This patient is able to bear weight on his knee and there is no history of acute trauma, so a physeal or growth plate fracture is not likely. Lack of tenderness over the inferior pole of the patella makes SLJS unlikely. This entity results from persistent traction at the immature inferior pole of the patella, leading to calcification and ossification at this junction. Sinding–Larsen–Johansson syndrome occurs most frequently in active preteen boys (usually 10 to 12 years of age) who complain of activity-related pain, especially with jumping, running, kneeling, or with stairs.

The presence of a lump over the tibial tubercle suggests a problem in that area. The most common problem of the tibial turbercle in this age group is OSD. Osgood–Schlatter disease is an overuse injury of adolescents that occurs during their growth spurt. The apophysis in this region is weaker than the surrounding bone and tendons during the growth spurt. Repeated strong contractions of the quadriceps muscle—such as occur in basketball, volleyball, and gymnastics—cause small avulsions of the developing tibial tubercle where the patellar tendon is attached. These small avulsions result in pain, swelling, and the formation of a tender prominence below the knee, as in this boy. The condition, once seen exclusively in boys, is now seen in girls who are involved in jumping sports. The age of appearance ranges between 11 and 17 years.

Acute avulsion fracture of the tibial tubercle is a rare complication in an adolescent with OSD. If it occurs, it is dramatic and precipitated by a sudden acceleration or deceleration of the extensor mechanism of the knee. An immediate disability is noted and the patient cannot fully extend the knee. This patient is able to fully extend his knee against resistance, indicating that the extensor mechanism is intact and no avulsion fracture is present. The remaining parts of the history and physical in this patient are consistent with OSD.

12.3. Imaging

The lateral radiograph of the knee outlines the tibial tubercle. In an adolescent between 9 and 17 years of age, the normal tubercle has varying degrees of fragmentation and apparent separation. Normal will look abnormal so compare one knee with the other. The diagnosis is made on clinical criteria. Be cautious with making a diagnosis based on radiographic findings. Clinically significant separation indicating avulsion fracture is made by limitation of quadriceps function and the X-ray only serves to confirm and not make the diagnosis.

12.4. Treatment

Osgood–Schlatter disease is a self-limited condition that is treated conservatively. Three out of four patients will have no limitation of activity and their only complaint is tenderness over the tibial tuberosity and inability to kneel. They may or may not need a knee pad. The great majority of the remaining 25% do well with knee pads and common sense. Limiting the adolescent from participation is usually unnecessary. Protection through the use of knee pads, periodic use of NSAIDs, and postexercise icing for 4 to 6 months is all that is needed most of the time. It may take 9 to 18 months for complete resolution of symptoms and the "bump" may persist into adulthood. Immobilization or surgery is reserved for those adolescents who fail all other measures or have avulsed the tendon.

13. Physeal Fractures

In the adolescent, the vulnerability of the physis or growth plate makes it the site of injury rather than ligaments or cartilage when there is trauma to the knee. So the same mechanism of injury that produces tears of the knee ligaments and their insertions in an adult will injure the physis in a young person who has open growth plates. This is sometimes forgotten in skeletally immature adolescents who sustain injuries to their knees.

Of the growth plates, the distal femoral physis is most frequently injured. In this injury the adolescent may report being hit on the lateral side of the knee and experiences immediate medial knee pain and inability to bear weight. Examination reveals point tenderness in the vicinity of the attachment of the MCL. A valgus stress produces discomfort similar to a medical collateral ligament tear and there may be some laxity. If the clinician's thinking is oriented toward adults a diagnosis of MCL tear will be made. The treatment for a fracture is different from the treatment for a ligamentous sprain.

A high index of suspicion for physeal fractures should lead to a low threshold for obtaining X-rays in skeletally immature children and adolescents compared with adults. Physeal fractures are classified as Salter–Harris types I, II, and III. Types II and III are usually seen on the X-rays but type I physeal fractures are difficult to diagnose radiographically unless they are displaced. Armed with this knowledge the clinician should make a tentative diagnosis of physeal fracture in any skeletally immature patient with significant pain, inability to bear weight, and a negative X-ray. If you suspect a physeal fracture of the distal humerus an orthopedic consultation is recommended. Treatment usually consists of a closed reduction and a long leg cast for 6 to 8 weeks.

14. Knee Exercises

Repeat each of the following exercises two times a day. Rotate from one exercise to the other. Do one set of one exercise and then rotate to another exercise and do a set. Do not exercise past the point of pain. Pain means stop.

1. **Quadriceps stretch (Figure 12.24)**: Stand in front of a wall. Brace yourself by keeping the hand on side of the uninjured leg against the wall. Grasp the ankle of the injured leg with your other hand and pull your heel toward your buttocks. Do not arch or twist your back and keep your knees together. Hold this stretch for 10 s. Repeat five times on the injured leg and three times on the noninjured leg.
2. **Wall slide (Figure 12.25)**: While standing with your back, shoulders, and head against a wall, slide down the wall, lowering your buttocks toward the floor. Place your feet about 1 to 2 ft away from the wall. Initially only lower the buttocks for a few degrees and then gradually increase until your buttocks are almost at the same level as your knees. It is not advisable to have your buttocks go past the knees. Make sure that you have sufficient strength to push yourself back to the starting position, Tighten the thigh muscles as you slowly slide back up to the starting position. Gradually increase the amount of time you are in the lower position from 5 to 20 s. Repeat this exercise 10 times and do it twice a day.
3. **Straight leg raise (Figure 12.26)**: Lie down on your back with your legs straight in front of you. While keeping the leg straight, tighten up the thigh

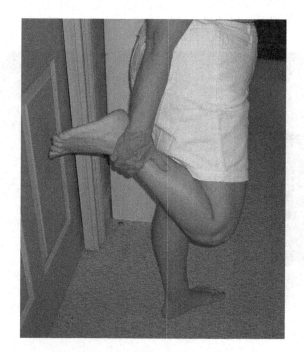

FIGURE 12.24. Quadriceps stretch.

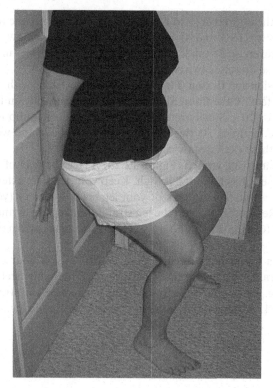

FIGURE 12.25. Wall slide.

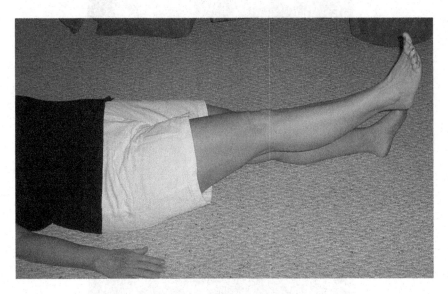

FIGURE 12.26. Straight leg raise.

muscle on the injured leg and lift that leg about 8 in. off the floor. Hold leg raise for 10 to 15 s and slowly lower your leg back down to the floor. Repeat the exercise 25 times in the injured leg and 10 times in the uninjured leg. Do these exercises twice a day.

4. **Knee extension and flexion (Figure 12.27)**: Sit in a chair with the knees bent to 90° and feet on the floor. Slowly extend the knee fully and hold it in full extension for 10 s. Slowly return the knee to its original position. Repeat the exercise 25 times. As this becomes easier, you can add weights to your ankle. Do these exercises twice a day.

5. **Standing hamstring stretch (Figure 12.28)**: Place the heel of your leg on a stool or other object about 2 ft high. Keep your leg fully extended and lean forward. You will feel the back of your leg begin to stretch (your hamstring muscles). Remember to keep the leg straight and not bent and do not bend the back. Hold the stretch for 15 s. Repeat five times alternating with each leg.

6. **Lying down hamstring stretch (Figure 12.29)**: Lie on your back and raise each leg straight (fully extended) until you feel the same stretch in the back of your leg. Bend your toes toward you to increase the stretch. Hold the stretch for 15 s. Repeat five times alternating with each leg.

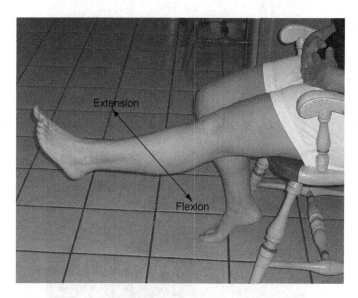

FIGURE 12.27. Knee extension and flexion.

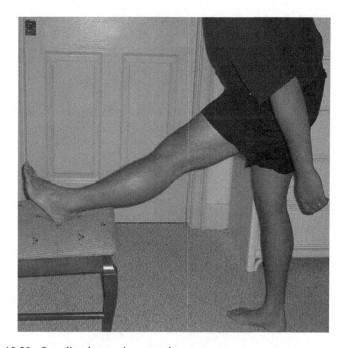

FIGURE 12.28. Standing hamstring stretch.

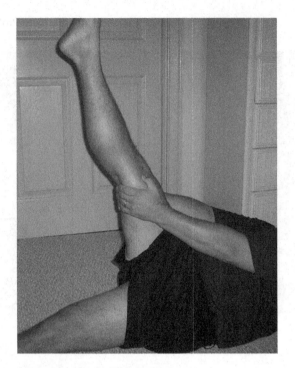

FIGURE 12.29. Lying down hamstring stretch.

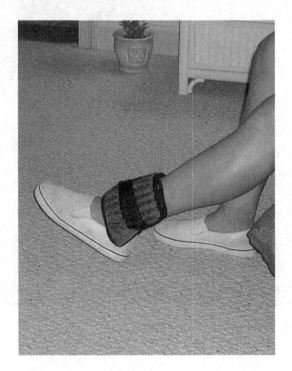

FIGURE 12.30. Ankle weights.

Ankle weights (Figure 12.30) can be purchased in most sports stores. They have inserts that allow you to increase the weights by 1/2 to 1 lb up to 5 lb total on each side.

Suggested Readings

Calmbach W, Hutchens M. Evaluation of patients presenting with knee pain: Part II. Differential Diagnosis. *Am Fam Physician*. 2003;68:917–922 (available at www.aafp.org).

Siva C, et al. Diagnosing acute monoarthritis in adults: a practical approach for the family physician. *Am Fam Physician*. 2003;68:83–90 (available at www.aafp.org).

13

Lower Leg Problems

EDWARD J. SHAHADY

This chapter covers primary care problems that occur between the ankles and the knees. Many common lower leg problems will be encountered by the primary care practitioner. Most patients seen with lower leg pain are physically active and their pain is related to exercise. Direct trauma and neurovascular disease can be associated with lower leg pain. Overuse is the cause of most of the problems in active patients, with shin splints topping the list. Shin splints are a waste-basket term and a more specific diagnosis like medial tibial stress syndrome (MTSS) or tibial stress fracture should be sought. Direct trauma may lead to a fracture or significant contusion. Spinal stenosis (see Chapter 10), osteoarthritis of the hip (see Chapter 11), and iliotibial band syndrome (see Chapter 12) can all refer pain to the lower leg and exercise can make the pain in all these entities worse.

As with all musculoskeletal problems, a good working knowledge of the epidemiology, anatomy, associated symptoms, and examination reduce confusion and enhance the diagnostic and therapeutic process.

Caring for problems is easier if a few simple organizational steps are followed:

1. Step 1 is to realize that the majority (95%) of patients seen in the office with lower leg complaints can be classified into the categories of problems noted in Table 13.1.
2. Step 2 is to take a focused history that segments the categories into acute trauma, overuse trauma, and medical disease. This process reduces the possibilities to a manageable list that helps initiate further investigation.
3. Step 3, performing a focused physical examination, builds on the detective work of the first two steps. With a focused history and examination, you now most likely have a potential diagnosis. Your knowledge of the usual history and examination associated with the most common problems has facilitated this process.
4. Step 4 is ordering confirmatory studies if needed (many times they are not).
5. Step 5 is to start treatment. (This may include appropriate consultation.) Five percent of the time, the diagnosis will not be so obvious. However, not being one of the 95% is usually obvious. That is when additional confirmatory studies and/or a consultation will be required.

TABLE 13.1. Classification of lower leg problems.

Overuse
Medial tibial stress syndrome
Stress fractures
Compartment syndromes
Gastrocnemius tears
Popliteus tendonitis
Retrocalcaneal bursitis
Achilles tendonitis and rupture

Acute trauma
Fracture of the tibia
Fracture of the fibula

Medical problems
Spinal stenosis

Rare or not so frequent problems are usually the ones that receive the most press. How often do you hear the words "I got burned once" mentioned about a rare problem that was missed in the primary care setting. Having a good working knowledge of the characteristics of common problems provides an excellent background to help recognize the uncommon. The uncommon is easy to recognize once you know the common. Be driven by the search for the common rather than the expensive intimidating search for the rare birds.

1. Anatomy

The two major bones of the lower leg are the tibia and fibula. They are connected by a superior and inferior tibiofibular joint and an interosseous membrane. The interosseous membrane is most important at its distal portion because it keeps the two bones together and helps provide for a stable ankle mortise. Disruption of the membrane distally leads to ankle joint dysfunction. This is discussed in Chapter 14.

The lower leg is divided into anterior, lateral, superficial posterior, and deep posterior compartments. Figures 13.1 and 13.2 describe the compartments and the contents of the compartments. Knowledge of the structures in these compartments aids in the diagnosis and treatment of lower leg problems. The anterior compartment contains the tibialis anterior, the long toe extensor muscles, the deep peroneal nerve, and the anterior tibial artery. The nerve supplies sensation to the first web space of the foot and the muscles are responsible for dorsiflexion of the foot. The lateral compartment contains the peroneus longus and brevis and the superficial peroneal nerve. These two muscles evert the foot and the nerve supplies sensation to the dorsum of the foot. The posterior compartment of the leg is divided into superficial and deep compartments. The superficial compartment contains the gastrocnemius, plantaris, and soleus muscles and the sural nerve. The muscles aid in

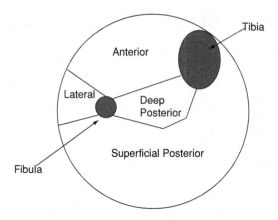

FIGURE 13.1. Compartments of the lower leg.

plantar flexion and the nerve supplies the lateral side of the foot and the distal calf. The deep posterior compartment contains the tibialis posterior muscle, the long toe flexor muscles, the posterior tibial and peroneal arteries, and the tibial nerve. The muscles aid in plantar flexion and eversion and the nerve supplies sensory function to the plantar aspect of the foot. The popliteal artery provides the vascular supply to the lower leg. The artery divides to form three branches: the anterior tibial artery, the posterior tibial artery, and

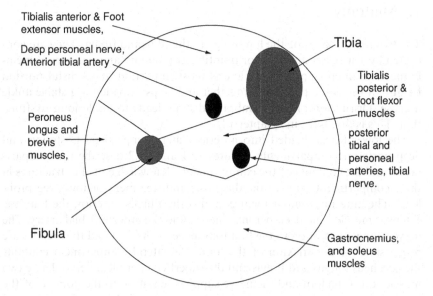

FIGURE 13.2. Anatomical structures in lower leg.

the peroneal artery. Palpating the dorsalis pedis artery over the dorsum of the foot assesses the anterior tibial artery. The posterior tibial artery is palpated posterior to the medial malleolus.

2. Focused History

Establish whether the problem is acute or chronic or if other chronic diseases that have musculoskeletal components are present. This will get you started down the right path. The mechanism of injury will many times pinpoint the anatomy involved in the injury. Questions like the following help put the pieces of the puzzle together: Was there a direct blow to the leg like being kicked in soccer or football? If the problem is chronic and getting worse ask how it is related to exercise. Is it only present with exercise? Does it stop or continue after exercise is over? Certain characteristics like intensifying one's exercise routine, changing the terrain like hills or the beach, or a change of shoes are all areas that may be causative in the overuse syndrome. Be alert for symptoms of neurological or vascular compromise. Compartment syndromes can produce neurological symptoms like numbness and/or a foot drop. Spinal stenosis can produce a burning pain and weakness of foot movement secondary to nerve root compression. A good working knowledge of lower leg anatomy as outlined above will help you understand what structures were involved when the injury occurred.

Do not forget to ask about other medical problems. Patients with osteoarthritis usually have evidence of other signs of osteoarthritis in the hands (Heberden's nodes). Rheumatoid arthritis commonly involves the ankle and foot and the first signs of rheumatoid may be in the foot and ankle.

3. Focused Physical Examination

Begin by comparing the injured leg with the uninjured one. Look for erythema, swelling, and atrophy of the musculature. Have the patient walk without shoes and socks and observe from behind for pronation. Pronation is excessive eversion (Figure 13.3). Ask the patient to point with one finger to the site of the pain. Pinpoint pain is more characteristic of fractures and more diffuse pain suggests MTSS. Location of the pain is also diagnostic, as will be pointed out when specific problems are discussed. Use a tuning fork above the area of pain to see if the vibrations reproduce the patient's pain. The tuning fork test helps diagnose stress fractures. Hopping up and down on the foot of the involved leg is usually painful in tibial stress fractures. Plantar flexion aggravates the pain of the MTSS and posterior tibial tendonitis. Dorsiflexion aggravates the pain of anterior tibial tendonitis. Anterior and posterior tibial tendonitis cause pain to the foot, so they will be discussed in Chapter 15.

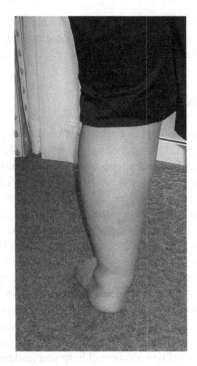

FIGURE 13.3. Eversion–pronation.

4. Case

4.1. History

A 17-year-old boy presents to your office with left lower leg pain of 3-week duration. He began football practice 3 weeks ago. The pain initially was present at the end of practice and quickly disappeared. It now is present as soon as he starts practice and it increases in intensity to the point he cannot continue to practice after 1 h. The pain persists for 1 to 2 h after practice. He does not note any numbness or loss of ability to move his foot. He did not stay in shape over the summer, so he was not well-conditioned at the start of practice. Examination reveals no gross difference in the appearance of the lower extremity. He does pronate when he walks. He points to a general area on his posterior medial tibia that is painful (Figure 13.4). The tuning fork test is negative. Resisted plantar flexion and standing on his tiptoes on the left reproduces the pain. He has no neurological deficit. His shoes are 2 years old and were used by his brother for a full season. They provide minimal support medially and the cleats are worn out on the medial side.

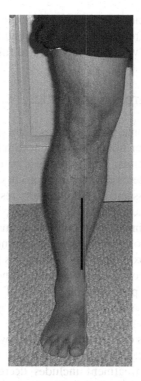

FIGURE 13.4. Location of pain in medial tibial stress syndrome.

4.2. Thinking Process

This is most likely an overuse injury given the patient's age, lack of acute trauma, gradual onset of symptoms, and recent onset of intense physical activity. The location of the pain over the posterior medial tibia area is characteristic of stress fractures and the MTSS. The negative tuning fork test and the lack of pinpoint tenderness make a stress fracture less likely. The lack of neurological symptoms like numbness and foot drop make compartment syndrome less likely. Compartment syndrome pain is usually located on the anterior lateral portions of the lower leg (see Figure 13.6). Compartment syndrome is discussed later in this section. Pronation predisposes the patient to excessive pull of the posterior musculature on the tibia. This pull or stretch causes a periosteal reaction on the tibia at its posterior medial border. His shoes provide minimal medial support and aggravate the medial tibial stress. This points to a diagnosis of MTSS and increase of the pain with resisted plantar flexion and standing on his tiptoes help confirm the diagnosis.

The patient was informed of the most likely diagnosis and was asked not to run for 1 week. He was treated with nonsteroidal anti-inflammatory drugs (NSAIDs), cross training on a stationary exercise bike, and exercises to stretch his posterior muscles. He obtained a new set of cleats with an orthotic to decrease pronation. After 1 week, he was encouraged to gradually increase his running and within 3 weeks, he was back to full participation.

5. Medial Tibial Stress Syndrome

Medial tibial stress syndrome, also known as "shin splints syndrome," is caused by traction of the posterior tibial, flexor digitorum longus, and soleus muscles on the periosteum of the tibia. This anatomy is noted in Figure 13.2. The individual muscles and the interosseous membrane attach to the tibia. The traction produces an overload stress and an inflammatory response on the periosteum of the tibia (periostitis). Some authors feel this syndrome may represent a continuum from an initial inflammatory response to a unique type of stress fracture.

The pain of MTSS is located over the posteromedial tibia from just above the medial malleolus proximally for 4 to 5 in., as noted in Figure 13.4. It is activity-related, and neurologic symptoms are generally absent. Diffuse pain and tenderness along the posteromedial border of the tibia that is aggravated by plantar flexion are characteristic findings on examination. Pronation of the foot of the symptomatic leg may be present.

Treatment for MTSS is conservative. Running will need to stop for a short period but alternative activities like a stationary bike or swimming can be substituted. Additional treatment includes decreasing inflammation with anti-inflammatory drugs (NSAIDs), orthotics for pronation, and exercises to strengthen the calf muscles (exercises described at the end of this chapter).

Medial tibial stress syndrome is an overuse syndrome caused by a mismatch between overload and recovery. The repetitive overload on tissues that are not able to adapt to new or increased demands leads to tissue breakdown and the clinical syndrome. Multiple factors contribute or increase the risk of overload. Prior injury and/or lack of conditioning leads to muscle imbalance, inflexibility, weakness, and instability. Other factors include poor technique, improper equipment, and changes in the duration or frequency of activity (training errors). Some individuals seem to be more vulnerable to the overload syndrome. The individual discussed in the case above was not conditioned when he began to practice. His equipment was faulty (shoes) and he pronated. His anatomy predisposed him to overload his posterior musculature and his lack of conditioning contributed muscle weakness and lack of flexibility. He was an MTSS waiting to happen.

6. Tibial Stress Fractures

Stress fractures of the tibia are one of the most common of activity-related stress fractures. It is also called a fatigue fracture because of its cause. Like MTSS, stress fractures are a result of overload without adequate recovery.

Bone is constantly remodeling itself. Bone responds to overload or additional stress by increasing its rate of turnover and repairing itself. A balance between bone resorption and bone formation keeps the bone intact. A stress fracture occurs when the repetitive load disrupts the balance, resulting in a spectrum of injury that results in a fracture through the cortex.

The balance between normal repair and bone breakdown can be compromised for several reasons. The majority of the time excessive training and/or training errors like a change in footwear, training on different surfaces (hard surfaces or the sand on the beach), or failure to modify activities at the onset of symptoms compromises the balance. The clinician should also be alert to the possibility of a stress fracture with normal stress applied to abnormal bone. The abnormal bone is usually osteoporotic secondary to an underlying metabolic or endocrine disorder. If overuse or training error is not obvious, these possibilities should be in the back of the clinician's mind when caring for stress fractures. Underlying conditions that predispose bone to stress fractures include amenorrhea, female athletic triad, hyperparathyroidism, hypothyroidism, osteoporosis, Paget's disease, rheumatoid arthritis, and steroid use or abuse.

Screen for the female athletic triad in all women who are less than ideal body weight and have recurrent or difficult to heal stress fractures. The triad consists of amenorrhea, an underlying eating disorder, and osteoporosis. Patients are often reluctant to discuss disordered eating behaviors until a reasonable degree of trust exists with their clinician.

The history is similar to the MTSS but the examination helps differentiate the two issues. The pain is usually exertional and located on the posteromedial aspect of the tibia. The pain and tenderness may be alleviated by rest initially, but with time continues in the resting state. If the exertional activity is not modified the pain will occur earlier in the activity. Occasionally, a history of trauma preceded by an aching discomfort in the leg may exist. On examination, the tenderness is localized to a specific area (Figure 13.5) rather than the diffuse tenderness of MTSS (Figure 13.4). Other helpful signs include pain with a one-leg hop, and reproduction of the pain with percussion or use of a tuning fork at sight on the tibia distant to the area where the patient complains of the pain.

6.1. Imaging

Plain film radiographs may not show signs of a fracture for up to 12 weeks. Bone scans are helpful but magnetic resonance imaging (MRI) is more precise. If the history and examination are suggestive, a negative plain film or bone scan does not rule out the diagnosis. Most clinicians would treat the patient as if they have a stress fracture and follow up with plain films or a bone scan. The cost of an MRI is significant and unless it will change the way you may treat the patient, is it really needed? There are some indirect clues that indicate periosteal new bone formation or cortical breaks.

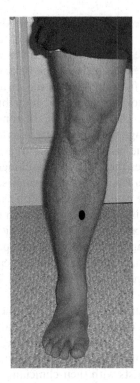

FIGURE 13.5. Location of pain in a tibial stress fracture.

Radiologists often report these signs when clinicians share their suspicion of a stress fracture.

6.2. Treatment

Relative rest and restricted weight bearing combined with short-term NSAIDs are the foundation of treatment. Crutches should be used until there is no pain with walking. Non-weight-bearing activities for 4 to 6 weeks like riding a bike, pool exercises, and upper body strengthening should be encouraged. Stretching and strengthening the anterior and posterior tibial muscle groups should be encouraged as soon as the patient can bear weight without pain. Exercises are listed at the end of the chapter. A cast is rarely required for proximal and distal tibial stress fractures. Symptoms usually resolve in 2 to 4 weeks if the diagnosis is not delayed and the patient is adherent to the treatment suggestions. After symptoms resolve, the patient is encouraged to gradually increase activities on soft surfaces. Walking and running combinations should be used with running time gradually increasing and walking time decreasing. Non-weight-bearing activities should still be employed on alternate days initially and gradually decreased over a 6-week period. Most patients are going to do what they feel comfortable doing so a flexible rehabilitation program that incorporates what the patients desire guarantees success. Avoidance of training errors, proper footwear, sensible diet, and correcting biomechanical problems should be stressed. Orthotics, if recommended, should gradually be adapted for use. More extensive discussion of orthotics will be found in Chapter 15.

Anterior tibial shaft stress fractures are less common but more problematic. They have an increased incidence of delayed union, nonunion, and progression to complete fracture. Casting is recommended for these types of fractures and close follow-up is indicated. When an anterior tibial shaft fracture is present, discussion with an orthopedist and potential referral is recommended.

7. Exertional Compartment Syndrome

Exertional compartment syndrome (ECS) must be distinguished from acute compartment syndrome (ACS) because of the urgent need for surgery in ACS. Acute compartment syndrome of the lower extremity is almost always preceded by some type of acute trauma like a tibial fracture. When the diagnosis of ACS is made, the compartments must be decompressed as soon as possible. Exertional compartment syndrome, on the other hand, is chronic and is the result of exercise causing increased intracompartmental pressure.

The muscles of the lower limb are divided into compartments enclosed by relatively noncompliant fascia. With exercise the intracompartmental pressure increases but the majority of the time this increase does not create problems. Patients with ECS have a more than usual increase in compartment pressure that produces pain and nerve compression. The anterior compartment is more commonly involved and accounts for approximately 70% to 80% of the cases. The anterior tibial musculature and the deep peroneal nerve are usually involved. This produces symptoms in the foot extensors and the patient will have problems with dorsiflexion. Posterior compartment involvement is less common and is usually associated with MTSS. The posterior tibial musculature is usually involved and this produces foot flexor symptoms and plantar flexor problems.

Exertional compartment syndrome in the anterior compartment produces a dull achy pain and swelling in the anterior lateral tibial area (Figure 13.6). The pain occurs with exercise and disappears with rest. Cramping, associated muscle tightness, and paresthesias will occur if exercise continues. The diagnosis of anterior ECS is one of exclusion. Anterior tibial stress fractures produce pain in the same location. Stress fracture pain is more localized and persists after exercise. Percussion and use of a tuning fork distal to the area of the pain will not reproduce the pain of ECS as it does in stress fractures. Stress fractures do not usually produce neurological symptoms like numbness or tingling. Posterior compartment

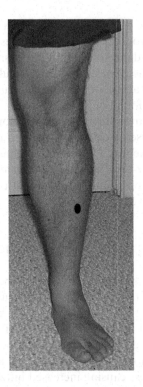

FIGURE 13.6. Location of pain in anterior compartment syndrome.

ECS can be confused with MTSS because of the location of the pain on the posterior medial tibial area.

7.1. Diagnostic Studies

The gold standard for making a diagnosis of compartment syndrome is measurement of compartmental pressure. Measurement can be accomplished with catheters or needles. One of the most popular devices is the Stryker stic. The stic is a portable handheld device that contains a scale for direct measurement and is easily operated in an outpatient setting. Resting pressure, immediate postexercise pressure, and continuous pressure measurements for 30 min after exercise help confirm the diagnosis. A study is considered positive if the immediate postexercise pressure is greater than or equal to 30 mmHg, or if the pressure at 15 min post exercise fails to return to normal or exceeds 15 mmHg.

Other diagnostic studies like plain films, MRI, or nerve conduction studies are of limited value. They help rule out other entities but do not help make the diagnosis of compartment syndrome. Measuring intracompartmental pressure is the gold standard for confirming the diagnosis.

7.2. Treatment Options

Conservative treatment is not too helpful unless there is a dramatic change in exercise intensity or the patient is willing to changing to another sport or form of physical activity. Operative treatment is indicated for patients who have appropriate clinical presentations with confirmatory pressure measurements and are unwilling to modify or give up their choice of exercise or sport. Although various techniques have been described, the two-incision fasciotomy of both the lateral and anterior compartments is indicated. If the symptoms are posterior, and elevated posterior compartment pressures are documented, a single incision is used to release the tibialis posterior and remainder of the deep compartment.

8. Case

8.1. History and Exam

A 29-year-old account executive comes to your office complaining that he felt a pop and immediate pain in the back of his calf of the left lower leg 1 day ago while playing basketball. You recently encouraged him to be more physically active in order to lose weight. He was dribbling the ball and came to an abrupt stop to shoot. The pain occurred before he was able to shoot. He had to stop playing and was unable to walk without severe pain. The pain and disability is not improving and he is seeking your advice about returning to work. Observation reveals that he walks with the foot held in plantar flexion and has swelling and ecchymosis in the popliteal fossae. He is unable to perform a single-leg toe raise with his left leg. Palpation reveals significant tenderness over the medial head of the gastrocnemius muscle in the popliteal fossae (Figure 13.7). There was no tenderness over the anterior tibial or posterior medial tibial area. No neurological deficit was present and both dorsalis pedis and posterior tibial pulses were normal. Knee flexion and extension did not change the strength of the pulses. There was no tenderness over the posterior lateral joint line of the knee and resisted external rotation produced no pain (Garrick test, see Section 10 (Popliteus Tendonitis)).

8.2. Thinking Process

The patient was deconditioned and started a strenuous exercise program abruptly. This lack of a gradually conditioning program made him more susceptible to muscle and ligament injury. The acute onset of pain accompanied by feeling a pop suggests a muscle or ligament tear. The mechanism of injury suggests that his calf muscles were maximally stretched as he stopped and was about to shoot. This is the usual position for tears of the gastrocnemius muscle. The location of the pain in the popliteal fossae and tenderness over

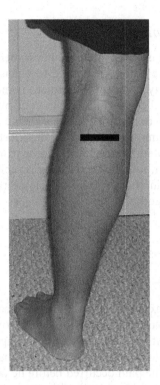

FIGURE 13.7. Location of pain in gastrocnemius tear.

the head of the gastrocnemius muscle suggests a tear of that muscle. A desire to keep the foot plantar-flexed and inability to perform a single toe raise with his left leg further indicates a problem with the gastrocnemius muscles. Lack of tenderness over the tibia is against an acute fracture. No decrease in pulses in the foot with knee flexion and extension suggests an intact popliteal artery. A ruptured popliteal cyst (Baker's cyst) is not likely as it usually occurs in patients over 55 and he has no history of degenerative arthritis or a prior history of an uncomfortable fullness in the popliteal fossae.

The patient was diagnosed with an acute tear of the gastrocnemius muscle "tennis leg." He was treated initially with the rest, ice, compression, and elevation (RICE) protocol and NSAIDs. He was able to return to work but required crutches for the first 5 days and was then able to walk with minimal pain. He was referred to physical therapy for a gradual program of stretching and eventual strengthening. After 3 months, he was able to return to his usual recreational activities. He was instructed to stretch all of his muscle groups before playing, do some laps around the gym before playing. He was also encouraged to start a walking–jogging program to enhance his conditioning before playing in the recreational league next season.

9. Gastrocnemius Tears

Gastrocnemius tears or strains (tennis leg) usually occur at the muscle–tendon junction of the medial head of the gastrocnemius muscle. It is most common in middle-aged tennis players, but may also be seen in other racket sports, basketball, running, and skiing. The patients are usually between 20 and 50 years of age, and are always engaged in physical activity at the time of the injury. Predisposing factors include increasing age, inadequate stretching, fatigue, and previous muscle injury. The injury usually occurs acutely and complaints include a sudden pain in the back of the leg over the medial head of the gastrocnemius muscle. The muscle is usually stretched and not contracted when the tear occurs. The patient prefers not to dorsiflex the foot because this movement aggravates the pain. The patient may walk with the foot plantar-flexed and on examination be unable to stand on the tiptoe of the affected leg.

If examined immediately after the injury a defect may be palpable over the area of the tear. Within 24 h, there will be significant swelling and ecchymosis. Again similar to hamstring tears the patient may become more alarmed about the ecchymosis than the original injury. Be sure to warn the patient that it is normal for an ecchymosis to appear and becoming more extensive is part of the normal course of events. The history and exam should contain elements that rule out other causes of posterior leg pain like a baker's cyst and popliteus tendonitis (PT). These entities are discussed later in this chapter.

Poor preparticipation stretching or conditioning is a common comorbid condition. Many times clinicians encourage patients to become more active to counteract recent weight gain, hypertension, and diabetes but do not give them an exercise prescription that takes into account their prior conditioning. See Chapter 2 for suggestions on exercise prescriptions.

9.1. Imaging

Plain films and/or MRI are not usually needed. The history and examination are sufficient to make the diagnosis. If the diagnosis is in question, imaging may be of help to rule out other entities.

9.2. Treatment

Treatment for muscle–tendon injuries depends on the severity of injury. NSAIDs and RICE usually work well for the initial stages. Crutches may be needed for the first week or so. Within 1 week, passive stretching should begin followed by strengthening exercises. Evaluation and treatment by a physical therapist may be helpful. Immobilization with a cast or splint to allow healing of the injured muscle–tendon unit may be needed for a more severe injury. It may take up to 3 months before the patient can return to full involvement in strenuous physical activity. Return to full activity should be accompanied by preparticipation conditioning and stretching exercises.

10. Popliteus Tendonitis

This is not a common problem but one that needs to be considered in patients with pain in the popliteal area (the back of the knee). The popliteus is the primary internal rotator of the tibia. Its origin is the posterior, medial border of the tibia. It inserts on the lateral femoral condyle anterior and inferior to the origin of the fibular collateral ligament. Popliteus tendonitis can be confused with lateral meniscus and lateral collateral ligament injury as well as gastrocnemius injury.

The patients usually complain of posterolateral knee pain that extends into the popliteal fossae. The onset of symptoms is gradual and it increases with activity. Examination reveals tenderness in the popliteal fossae and the posterior lateral area of the knee. Resisted external rotation (Figure 13.8) while palpating the popliteus produces pain. This test is performed with patients lying on their back with the painful leg placed in 90° of hip flexion

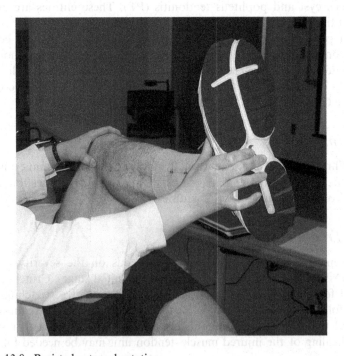

Figure 13.8. Resisted external rotation.

and 90° of knee flexion. The clinician stands on the lateral side of the knee with one hand supporting the knee and the other placed on the foot resisting external rotation.

10.1. Imaging

An MRI may be needed to make a definitive diagnosis.

10.2. Treatment

Excessive quadriceps fatigue strains the popliteus so a rehabilitation program emphasizing strengthening of the quadriceps muscle should be instituted. A 2-week course of NSAIDs should also be included in the treatment. Recalcitrant cases may require a local injection of a steroid. Maintaining good quadriceps strength is the key to preventing a recurrence.

11. Retrocalcaneal Bursitis

The retrocalcaneal bursa is located behind the calcaneus and in front of the Achilles tendon at its insertion site onto the calcaneus. The history is generally that of slow onset of dull aching pain in the retrocalcaneal area aggravated by activity and certain shoe wear. A common complaint is start-up pain after sitting or when arising in the morning. Examination reveals swelling in between the Achilles tendon and the calcaneus. There is generally a prominence in the area of the superior portion of the heel. Palpation may reveal the presence of fluid within the bursa. Dorsiflexion of the foot usually increases the pain in the area. Retrocalcaneal bursitis may be a manifestation of systemic arthritis or gout. Treatment is similar to that used for Achilles tenonitis.

12. Achilles Tendon Disorders

Commonly called "Achilles tendinitis" by many clinicians, posterior heel pain in the setting of exercise and overuse represents spectrum of problems caused by both inflammation and degeneration. Entities include tendonitis with and without partial rupture, retrocalcaneal bursitis, and complete tear caused by an acute injury. Achilles tendon disorders occur most often in patients involved in activities where running is an important part of the activity. Like other overuse injuries, training errors, improper footwear, and foot pronation predispose to Achilles injury. Long standing tendon degeneration may occur without symptoms or pain. But if a change in exercise intensity occurs the patient will develop symptoms.

A classic history is postexercise pain usually relieved by rest. The pain is located about 4 to 6 cm proximal to where the tendon inserts on the heel.

A change in activity levels or training techniques usually precedes the onset of symptoms. Patients usually take some NSAIDs, rest a little, and return to activity. If no change in training or correction of other predisposing factors occurs, the pain will return quickly. As the tendonitis continues, pain may occur during exercise and interfere with activities of daily living. Familial hypercholesterolemia, which is present in one of 500 patients, is associated with recurrent Achilles tendonitis. So inquiring about a family history of premature cardiovascular disease or lipid disorders is appropriate if recurrent Achilles tendonitis is present. A complete rupture of the tendon is usually an acute event accompanied by pain and inability to plantar-flex the foot. The patient usually complains of a sudden severe calf pain as if someone hit them with a rock. They will have difficulty bearing weight.

Clinical examination of the foot should be performed with the patient first standing and then prone. Inspection for pronation and palpation of the tendon for swelling, asymmetry, thickening, erythema, tenderness, crepitation and nodules should start the examination. Pain anterior to the tendon at its insertion is a sign of retrocalcaneal bursitis. If the tendon has ruptured acutely, the patient may have a defect in the tendon about 2 to 3 in. from its insertion. The Thompson test (Figure 13.9) should be performed to assess the integrity of the Achilles tendon. With the patient kneeling on a chair grasp the calf and note the ability of the foot to plantar-flex. Plantar flexion will not occur with a torn tendon. The test is best performed within 48 h of the rupture.

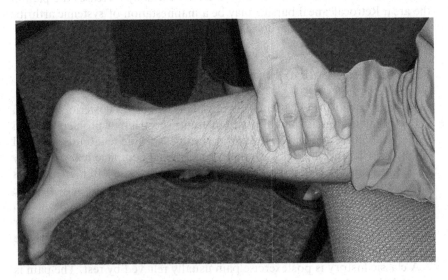

FIGURE 13.9. Thompson test.

12.1. Diagnostic Tests

Ultrasound and MRI are sometimes used if it is difficult to make the diagnosis. Although ultrasound is less expensive, both are costly and should be used with discretion. History and examination are usually sufficient to make the diagnosis and start treatment unless a complete tear is likely.

12.2. Treatment

Initial management should focus on symptom relief and correcting the training errors and mechanical problems. Cessation of running and cross training with a stationary bike or swimming plus the use of NSAIDs will help decrease the symptoms. There is no place for injection of steroids into the tendon but steroid injection may be considered for retrocalcaneal bursitis. Ice massage as described in Chapter 1 can also decrease symptoms and help with inflammation. Exercises to stretch and strengthen the tendon as described at the end of this chapter are important. Orthotics for pronation and a heel lift also help. The heel lift should be used for a short time to decrease the discomfort. Operative treatment may be needed in a small number of patients for excision of adhesions and degenerated nodules, or decompression of the tendon by longitudinal tenotomies. If the tendon is completely ruptured, surgery may be indicated depending on the age, level of activity, and medical status of the patient.

13. Fractures of the Tibia and Fibula

Fracture of the tibia secondary to trauma are not usually a diagnostic problem. Type 1 growth plate fractures in children may be a little more difficult to diagnose because the X-ray is usually negative. Any child or adolescent less than age 16 may have open growth plates. Any child in this age group with significant lower leg pain, inability to bear weight, and a negative X-ray should be considered to have a growth plate fracture until proven wrong. The key symptom is inability to bear weight. Because of the potential impact on bone growth, a consultation with an orthopedic surgeon is recommended.

Isolated fibula fractures, especially of the distal fibula, are not usually problematic because the fibula is not a weight-bearing bone. Proximally the fibula anchors the lateral supports of the knee and distally it is the lateral buttress for the talus and ankle joint. In patients with tibial fractures, stability of the fibula assumes more importance. Fixation of the fibula may be indicated in order to restore stability and alignment for the tibia. An intact fibula in association with a tibial shaft fracture is actually a marker for a less severe injury and an improved prognosis.

Most fibular fractures are distal and associated with an ankle inversion injury. If there is a fracture in the proximal fibula be alert for a Maisonneuve's fracture. This is a proximal fibula fracture with an associated ankle fracture or ankle deltoid ligament tear. This fracture is also associated with partial or complete disruption of the syndesmotic membrane between the tibia and fibula. An orthopedic surgeon should manage Maisonneuve's fracture.

Treatment of truly isolated fibular shaft fractures is symptomatic. A well-padded splint or cast may be useful briefly for comfort, but is not required. A lightly wrapped elastic bandage is applied over the padding. Elevation, ice, crutches (with weight bearing as tolerated), and NSAIDs as needed are helpful. Once the pain and swelling have largely resolved (usually in 1 to 2 weeks), progressive weight bearing is encouraged, and activities are encouraged. This fracture is treated as inversion ankle injury, which is discussed in Chapter 14.

14. Medical Problems

14.1. Baker's Cyst

A Baker's, or popliteal, cyst should be considered in a patient with a bulge or pain in the back of the knee, also known as the popliteal region. The cyst represents a herniation of the synovial membrane through the posterior aspect of the capsule of the knee. Fluid may escape through the normal communication of the bursa with the knee joint producing a budge. The herniation can sometimes also occur laterally. The underlying problem is always internal derangement of the knee (loose body, meniscal tear, and degenerative arthritis) that produces synovitis and fluid accumulation. As the severity of the synovitis increases more fluid is produced and the size of the cyst (bulge) will increase. This is an important piece of information in the history, as these patients may not have a prior history of posterior pain but one of a posterior knee mass that fluctuates in size.

The clinical challenge comes when there is rupture of the cyst and escape of fluid into the calf. This produces significant pain and a clinical picture similar to thrombophlebitis and gastrocnemius strain or tear. Baker's cyst are usually present in older not-too-active patients who have a history of osteoarthritis and a fluctuating posterior knee mass. Nevertheless, there are active patients in their middle ages that can have a baker's cyst and/or tear their gastrocnemius muscle. A meticulous history and physical using the suggestions listed in other parts of this chapter will usually help establish the diagnosis. If knee pathology is present, a focused knee history and examination, as discussed in Chapter 12, should help establish the diagnosis of the knee problem. The diagnosis of thrombophlebitis will be by exclusion of the other entities and presence of circumstances that predispose the patient to thrombophlebitis. If you suspect thrombophlebitis, please consult another source of information.

Treatment for Baker's cyst is primarily for the underlying cause of the cyst (usually osteoarthristis). Spontaneous disappearance is common but occasionally aspiration and or surgical excision may be required. Differentiation from other clinical entities may require aspiration, ultrasound, or an MRI scan. Once the underlying intra-articular pathology is understood, appropriate treatment and prevention measures can be instituted.

15. Spinal Stenosis

Spinal stenosis is mentioned in this chapter because it can cause exertional lower leg pain (neurogenic claudication). The patients are usually over age 60 and have had a 5- to 10-year history of back pain and other signs of osteoarthritis of large joints like the knees or the hips. The classical symptoms are back pain radiating into the calf and foot brought on by exercise. It is also classical that the symptoms are relieved by bending over and rest. Bending backward as demonstrated in Figure 10.3 (page 183) increases all the symptoms. Chapter 10 has a more extensive discussion of spinal stenosis. Vascular claudication must also be ruled out by accessing for loss or diminishing of dorsalis pedis and posterior tibial pulses with exercise in these patients. Both entities may be present in some patients.

16. Lower Leg Exercises

Figures for these exercises can be found in Chapter 14.

1. **Towel stretch (see Figure 14.10):** Sit with your injured leg stretched out in front of you. Loop a towel around the ball of your foot and pull the towel toward your body keeping your knee straight. Hold this position for 10 s then relax. Repeat five times.
2. **Standing calf stretch (see Figure 14.12):** Facing a wall, put your hands against the wall at about eye level. Keep the injured leg back, the uninjured leg forward, and the heel of your injured leg on the floor. Slowly lean into the wall until you feel a stretch in the back of your calf. Hold for 15 to 30 s. Repeat three times. Do this exercise several times each day.
3. **Anterior leg muscle stretch (see Figure 14.13):** Stand next to a chair or the kitchen counter and grasp one of them with your hand to maintain balance. Bend your knee and grab the front of your foot on your injured leg. Bend the front of the foot toward your heel. You should feel a stretch in the front of your shin. Hold for 10 to 15 s. Repeat five times.
4. **Heel raises A (see Figure 14.14):** Stand behind a chair or counter to balance yourself. With your feet internally rotated, raise your heels by standing on the tips of the toes for 5 s. Do this 20 times and repeat two times a day.

5. **Heel raises B (see Figure 14.15)**: Stand behind a chair or counter to balance yourself. With your feet straight, raise your heels by standing on the tips of the toes for 5 s. Do this 20 times and repeat two times a day.
6. **Heel raises C (see Figure 14.16)**: Stand behind a chair or counter to balance yourself. With your feet externally rotated, raise your heels by standing on the tips of the toes for 5 s. Do this 20 times and repeat two times a day.
7. **Heel raises on the stairs (see Figure 14.17)**: Stand on a stairs (grab a banister for support) and support your body weight on the tips of your toes. Rise up on your toes for 5 s and then lower the heel down below the toes to increase dorsiflexion for 5 s. Work up to achieving 10 repetitions three times a day. The ankle will be stiff and hard to dorsiflex (see Fig. 14.3 on page 293) initially but will become more flexible with increased repetitions. Once the degree of dorsiflexion in the injured ankle is the same as the uninjured ankle, activity-specific training can begin.
8. **Standing toe raises (see Figure 14.18)**: Stand with your feet flat on the floor, rock back onto your heels, and lift your toes off the floor. Hold this for 5 s. Repeat the exercise 10 times and do it two times a day.
9. **Activity-specific training**: If you will be involved in a recreational activity or competitive sport, gradually acclimatize your ankle to the routines and stress of this activity. Start with a combined walk–jog–run that is characteristic of this activity/sport. The running/jogging component should gradually increase and replace the walking. Gradually increase the distance and add figures of eight and backward walking/jogging to the routine. The last routine attempted should be sharp cutting movement after coming to a stop.

A trainer, physical therapist, or coach may be able to help you with all of the above exercises.

Suggested Readings

Hootman JM, Macera CA, Ainsworth BE, et al. Predictors of lower extremity injury among recreationally active adults. *Clin J Sport Med*. 2002;12(2):99–106.

Glorioso J, Wilckens J. Exertional leg pain. In: O'Connor F, Wilder R, eds. *The Textbook of Running Medicine*. New York: McGraw-Hill; 2001:181–198.

14

Ankle Problems

EDWARD J. SHAHADY

This chapter covers primary care problems that occur with the ankle. The most common problem seen by primary care clinicians is the common ankle sprain. Unfortunately, ankle sprains are not always treated appropriately. Often, a patient is evaluated in the emergency department where an X-ray is performed without much of a history and physical examination and the recommended treatment is "take it easy or use a set of crutches until you see your doctor" and no rehabilitation exercises are prescribed. Nonindicated X-rays raise the cost of initial care and lack of appropriate rehabilitation delays return to activity and increases the risk of recurrent ankle injury. Other ankle problems like fractures and osteoarthritis (OA), although less frequent, are discussed.

A focused history that includes the mechanism of injury will help categorize the problem so that a focused examination can be performed. Common ankle problems seen in primary care are listed in Table 14.1. The decision to obtain X-rays with acute trauma is facilitated by following the Ottawa ankle rules (Table 14.2). Following these rules helps decrease unneeded X-rays. An effective treatment plan should include some form of rehabilitation exercises. As with all musculoskeletal problems, a good working knowledge of the epidemiology, anatomy, associated symptoms, and examination reduce confusion and enhance the diagnostic and therapeutic process.

1. Anatomy

The talus articulates with the tibia and fibula to form the ankle joint. The talar dome is wider at its anterior margin than the posterior margin by an average of 2 to 3 mm. This difference in width imparts relative ankle instability in plantar flexion and increased stability during ankle dorsiflexion. This partially explains the reason why ankle injury is most common in the plantar-flexed position. Lateral ankle stability is enhanced by the lateral ankle ligaments. The lateral ankle ligaments include the anterior talofibular ligament (ATFL), the calcaneofibular ligament (CFL), and the posterior talofibular ligament (PTFL) (see Fig. 14.1). The ATFL and CFL are the most important clinically because they are the most commonly injured ankle ligaments.

TABLE 14.1. Common ankle problems.

Ankle sprains
- Lateral ankle sprains
- Medical ankle sprains
- High ankle sprains

Fractures
- Lateral and medial malleolus
- Talar dome
- Maisonneuve fracture

Arthritis
- Osteoarthritis
- Rheumatoid arthritis

TABLE 14.2. Ottawa ankle and foot rules.

An ankle radiographic series is indicated if a patient has
1. Inability to bear weight immediately in the emergency department or physician's office or
2. Pinpoint bone tenderness at the posterior portions of the lateral and medial malleolus

A foot radiographic series is indicated if a patient has pinpoint pain over the base of the fifth metatarsal or the navicular bones
Adapted from Stiell IG, McKnight RD, Greenberg GH, McDowell I, Nair RC, Wells GA, et al. Implementation of the Ottawa ankle rules. *JAMA*. 1994;271:827–832.

The ATFL originates from the anterior aspect of the distal fibula and inserts on the lateral aspect of the talar neck. The CFL originates from the distal tip of the fibula and inserts at the lateral wall of the calcaneus (Figure 14.1). When the ankle is in dorsiflexion, the ATFL is perpendicular to the axis of the tibia and the CFL is oriented parallel to the tibia. In neutral dorsiflexion, the CFL provides resistance to inversion stress or varus tilt of the talus. In plantar flexion, the most common position for lateral ankle inversion injuries, the ATFL is parallel and the CFL is perpendicular to the axis of the tibia. This position places the ATFL in the precarious situation of providing resistance to inversion stress.

Isolated testing of the individual ankle ligaments demonstrates that the ATFL is the first to fail and the ATFL is considered the weakest lateral ankle ligament. Sixty-five percent of ankle sprains are secondary to partial or complete rupture of the ATFL. (Figure 14.2). Another 30% are caused by a sprain or rupture of both the ATFL and the CFL. As previously mentioned, the PTFL is seldom, if ever, involved in ankle sprains seen in the primary care setting.

Medial ankle stability is provided by the strong deltoid ligament, the anterior tibiofibular ligament, and the bony mortise. The anterior tibiofibular ligament is located between the distal portions of the tibia and fibula. The deltoid ligament is composed of four strong ligaments: posterior and anterior tibiotalar ligament, tibiocalcaneal ligament, and the tibionavicular ligament. They are named for the bones where they originate and insert.

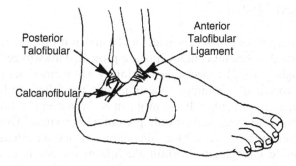

FIGURE 14.1. Lateral ankle ligaments. (Reproduced from Shahady E, Petrizzi M, eds. *Sports Medicine for Coaches and Trainers*. Chapel Hill, NC: University of North Carolina Press; 1991:119, with permission.)

Because of the support of the bony articulation between the medial malleolus and the talus, medial ankle sprains are less common than lateral sprains. In medial ankle sprains, the mechanism of injury is excessive eversion and dorsiflexion. Medial ankle sprains are more problematic and take more time to heal.

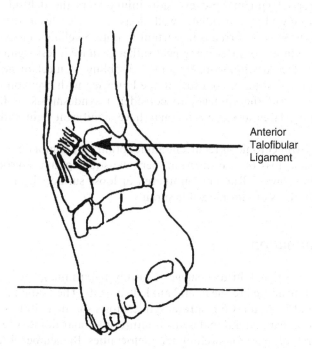

FIGURE 14.2. Anterior talofibular ligament tear. (Reproduced from Shahady E, Petrizzi M, eds. *Sports Medicine for Coaches and Trainers*. Chapel Hill, NC: University of North Carolina Press; 1991:120, with permission.)

2. Focused History

Establish whether the problem is acute or chronic or if other chronic diseases that have musculoskeletal components are present. This will get you started down the right path. The mechanism of injury will many times pinpoint the anatomy involved in the injury. Questions like the following help put the pieces of the puzzle together. If the problem is chronic and getting worse ask how it is related to exercise. Is it only present with exercise? Does it stop or continue when exercise is over? Certain characteristics like intensifying one's exercise routine, changing the terrain like hills or the beach, or a change of shoes are all areas that may be causative. Chronic problems like OA usually wax and wane with time. Patients with OA usually have evidence of other joint involvement like the hands (Heberden's nodes) and large joints like the knees and hips. Rheumatoid arthritis (RA) may involves the ankle and foot and the first signs of rheumatoid may be in the foot and ankle.

Ask about prior ankle injury. Old ankle sprains that were not properly rehabilitated lead to increased risk of new ankle sprains. Ability to bear weight after acute trauma is a critical piece of information. Third-degree ankle sprains and fractures are likely when the patient is unable to bear weight. How the injury occurred also helps. Inversion injury leads to tears of the lateral ligaments and eversion injury tears the deltoid ligaments. A "pop" followed by immediate swelling usually indicates a torn ligament. When the swelling occurred is important to note. Swelling that occurred the day after an injury or after using heat rather than ice is less significant than swelling that occurs immediately and is disabling. A mechanism of injury that leads to twisting or rotation of the lower leg with eversion and inversion should lead the clinician to consider a syndesmosis or high ankle sprain injury. High ankle sprains may have significant pain with minimal swelling.

Patients with chronic or recurrent ankle sprain may complain of weakness, apprehension, loss of coordination, periodic swelling, and episodes of the ankle "giving away." Running on uneven or loose surfaces brings out many of the symptoms of chronic ankle sprains.

3. Examination

Even if the patient's history suggests an inversion injury, the examination should not be limited to the lateral ankle ligaments. The examination should rule out ATFL sprain, CFL sprain, syndesmosis sprain, deltoid sprain, peroneal tendon tear, lateral malleolus fracture, and talar dome osteochondral injury. First, observe for swelling and deformities. Remember RA may first manifest itself in the ankle and foot. Palpation for tenderness over the ATFL and the CFL as well as the bones of the navicular, malleoli, and the fifth metatarsal should be performed. Feel for nodules of the

Achilles tendon and other extensor surfaces. These nodules may be associated with RA or familial hypercholesterolemia. Range of motion of the ankle is assessed with the patient seated and relaxed. Maximal dorsiflexion and plantar flexion are observed both passively and actively. Dorsiflexion (Figure 14.3) can normally be accomplished to 15° to 20° and plantar flexion up to 40° to 55° (Figure 14.4). Compare the injured to the uninjured side to access for differences. Initial measurements can be used as a baseline to evaluate progress.

Next, a series of tests to evaluate for ligamentous injury and stability are performed. The squeeze test identifies tibiofibular syndesmosis disruption (the interosseus membrane between the tibia and fibula). The test is performed by compression of the midleg from posterior lateral to anterior medial area, as noted in Figure 14.5. This test is positive when the compression produces pain secondary to separation of the fibula from the tibia in the lower ankle.

The talar tilt test is performed with the lower leg secured with one hand and the heel grasped from behind with the opposite hand. An inversion force is placed in an effort to produce a talar tilt. Perform the test against resistance in both ankle neutral and plantar-flexed positions (Figure 14.6). Inversion

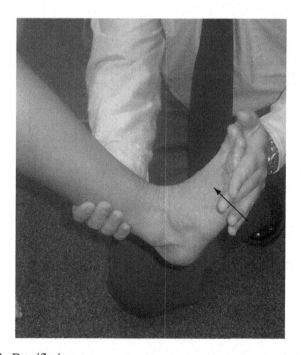

FIGURE 14.3. Dorsiflexion.

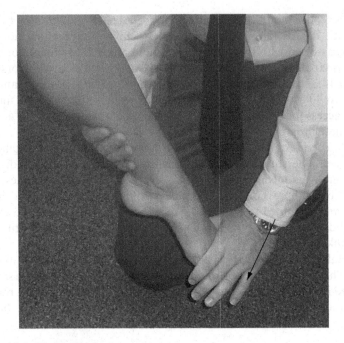

FIGURE 14.4. Plantar flexion.

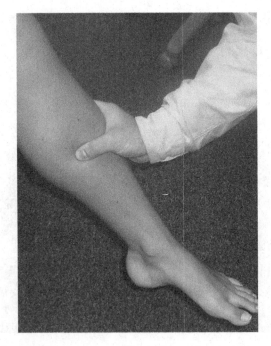

FIGURE 14.5. Squeeze test.

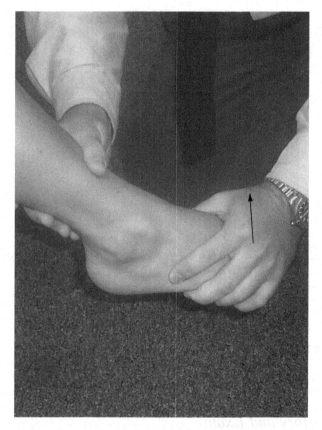

FIGURE 14.6. Talar tilt (inversion stress).

stress in the neutral position tests the stability of the CFL and inversion stress
in the plantar-flexed position tests the stability of the ATFL.

4. Test

The anterior drawer test tests the integrity of the ATFL. While the patient is
seated the lower leg is grasped with one hand and the foot with the other
(Figure 14.7). An anterior force (see arrow in Figure 14.7) is used in an effort
to produce forward translation. Perform the test in both ankle neutral and
plantar flexion positions. A few millimeters of translation is normal.
Compare one side with the other. The test is more reliable in chronic instability than in acute because of the negative inhibition of pain during an acute
sprain. Thus, a negative test is not always reliable with acute ankle sprain and
should be repeated when the pain subsides.

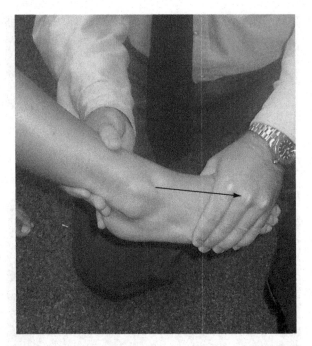

FIGURE 14.7. Anterior drawer.

5. Case

5.1. History and Exam

A healthy 23-year-old female student who regularly runs 3 miles three times per week comes to your office with ankle pain and swelling. She tripped on a tree root in the woods yesterday while running and twisted her right ankle. She did not hear or feel a pop, but noticed immediate pain on the lateral side of the ankle. She was able to bear weight and walk out of the woods. As she walked, the ankle became more painful and began to swell. She has no history of past ankle injuries and she has no known medical problems. Based on the advice of a friend she used a heating pad to help decrease the swelling and pain. The next morning she noted increased swelling and moderate discomfort while walking.

The examination revealed swelling, ecchymosis, and diffuse tenderness over the anterior portions of right lateral malleolus. Dorsiflexion is limited to 10° on the right foot compared with 20° on the left. Plantar flexion is equal bilaterally to 45°. The anterior and medial portions of the malleolus are tender but not the posterior portion of the lateral malleolus. The squeeze and anterior drawer tests are negative. The talar tilt test produces pain in the plantar flexed position but no instability. Palpation of the base of the fifth metatarsal reveals no tenderness.

The patient was prescribed a nonsteroidal anti-inflammatory drug (NSAID), and taught some initial exercises to stretch and strengthen her ankle ligaments. After 2 weeks, the patient returned to running but was unable to complete her runs without lateral ankle pain. She then was treated by a physical therapist and after 2 months has returned to her full routine of running.

5.2. Thinking Process

The history suggests that the patient has probably stretched or torn one of her lateral ankle ligaments. The anterior talar fibular and CFLs are the most common lateral ankle ligaments injured. The immediate swelling indicates bleeding and the use of a heating pad suggests increased bleeding secondary to the vasodilatation caused by the heat. The ability to walk and bear weight is a significant piece of history. Fractures and complete ligamentous tears are associated with an inability to bear weight. Therefore, the diagnosis is most likely a first- or second-degree sprain. Her lack of a history of ankle injury goes against this, being a chronic ankle sprain. Rheumatoid arthritis can present with ankle pain but it is not usually associated with an acute event. There is no pinpoint tenderness over the posterior portions of the lateral and medial malleolus tests, indicating fracture is unlikely. A negative squeeze test makes a syndesmosis tear unlikely and the negative anterior drawer suggests that the ATFL is intact. The talar tilt test produces pain in the plantar-flexed position but no instability, indicating complete stability of the ATFL and CFL. An avulsion fracture of the fifth metatarsal at the insertion of the peroneus brevis is not likely because no tenderness was demonstrated at the base of the fifth metatarsal. After reviewing the Ottawa Ankle Rules (Table 14.2) a decision was made not to perform an X-Ray of the ankle or foot. The patient was able to bear weight and had no pinpoint tenderness on the posterior portions of the lateral malleolus or the base of the fifth metatarsal.

6. Ankle Sprains

Ankle sprains are classified according to signs and symptoms. Grade I is characterized by a stretching of the ATFL and the CFL, producing mild tenderness and swelling. Usually no ecchymosis is present and no loss of function or motion. The patient is able to bear weight and walk with minimal pain. Examination reveals no instability with the talar tilt and anterior drawer test. The patient usually recovers with minimal treatment in 6 to 8 days.

Grade II is an incomplete tear of the ATFL and stretching of the CFL with moderate pain and swelling. There is ecchymosis, more swelling and tenderness, and some loss of function and motion. The patient has pain with weight bearing but is able to walk usually with a limp. Examination reveals mild to moderate instability with the tilt and anterior drawer tests. These patients may take 3 to 6 weeks to recover and chronic instability is more likely.

Grade III is a complete tear of the ATFL and CFL and partial tears of the posterior talofibular and the tibiofibular ligaments. There is immediate and significant swelling. The ecchymosis is more significant. The patient loses function and motion and is unable to bear weight or ambulate. The talar tilt test and anterior drawer tests are positive indicating significant instability. Many times the tests cannot be performed because of the marked discomfort with movement. These patients are probably best referred to an orthopedic surgeon. It is debatable whether they do better with surgery or casting.

7. Mechanism of Injury

Up to 90% of ankle sprains are caused by inversion of the plantar-flexed ankle. The ATFL and CFL ligaments are the most commonly injured when the ankle is inverted and the ATFL is the most easily injured. Significant instability can occur when both ligaments are injured. Both grade II and III sprains can lead to significant chronic instability if effective rehabilitation is not accomplished. Excessive eversion and dorsiflexion produces sprains of the strong deltoid ligament medially. Medial injury is not that common because of the stability provided by the bony articulation. Injury to the (syndesmosis) tibiofibular ligament and the interosseus membrane between the tibia and fibula (Figure 14.8) usually occurs with a combination of twisting and plantar flexion.

8. Evaluation

The evaluation includes an assessment of the grade of sprain and an application of the Ottawa ankle rules (Table 14.2). After this evelution the clinician can more readily make decisions about imaging, prognosis and treatment. The history should include a description of the mechanism of injury, past history of ankle problems, ability to bear weight after the injury, and what treatment the patient used prior to your evaluation. Examination should include inspection, palpation of the malleoli, weight-bearing status, and all the tests listed in the focused examination. If you suspect a syndesmosis injury, palpate the entire length of the tibia and fibula to detect a fracture of the proximal fibula (Maisonneuve fracture). Palpate the base of the fifth metatarsal to rule out an avulsion fracture.

Two unusual but significant scenarios should be kept in mind. One is a possible talar dome fracture. These patients will not be able to bear weight but the X-ray may not be positive for 2 to 4 weeks. The fracture may be between the talus and the fibula or the talus and the tibia. Persistent pain and limitation of dorsiflexion and plantar flexion should raise suspicion of this fracture. The other scenario is significant pain and disability, minimal swelling, and tenderness over the distal tibiofibular joint. This usually indicates a syndesmosis

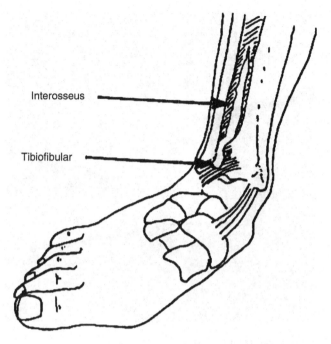

Interosseus

Tibiofibular

FIGURE 14.8. Injury to the tibiofibular ligament and the interosseus membrane between the tibia and fibula. (Reproduced from Shahady E, Petrizzi M, eds. *Sports Medicine for Coaches and Trainers*. Chapel Hill, NC: University of North Carolina Press; 1991:120, with permission.)

sprain or high ankle sprain. In addition to the "squeeze test" (Figure 14.5) for disruption of the syndesmosis, an additional test called the "external rotation test" will also help identify syndesmosis disruption. This test (Figure 14.9) is performed by externally rotating the foot with the ankle in dorsiflexion. Pain in the distal tibiofibular junction indicates syndesmosis injury.

9. Imaging

The Ottawa ankle rules (Table 14.2) can be used to determine when radiographic studies are needed. Location of the pain and inability to bear weight are the key indicators. Use of these rules has decreased costs, waiting time, and unneeded tests. The rules are highly sensitive for malleolar and midfoot fractures. If X-rays are obtained, they should include anteroposterior, lateral, and mortise views to rule out the most common types of fractures. In addition to looking for fractures, observe for an increase in the space between the tibia and fibula. This so-called "clear space" is increased in size with disruption of the syndesmosis. Talar dome fractures are not always seen initially on the X-ray. If after 6 weeks, the patient has persistent symptoms and the X-ray

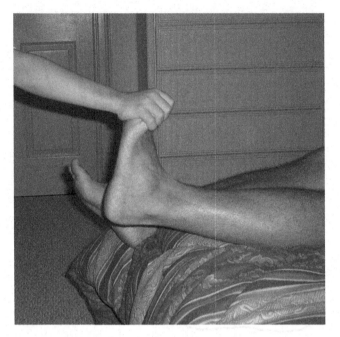

FIGURE 14.9. External rotation test.

remains negative, a magnetic resonance imaging (MRI) or computerized tomography (CT) scan may be helpful.

10. Treatment

Most ankle sprains can be managed conservatively. Disability from sprains is related to the loss of motion especially dorsiflexion. Initial goals are to prevent or decrease swelling and maintain motion. Rest, ice, compression, and elevation (RICE) are the keys to early management. Initially use crutches to decrease weight bearing and provide relative rest for 48 to 72 hours and ice to decrease pain and swelling. The ice can be placed in a plastic bag applied to the ankle over a thin cloth. Ice decreases metabolism and limits hypoxic injury. Immersion in a cold-water bath can also be used. Ice massage can be applied by filling paper cups with water and placing them in a freezer. The patient then removes the cup and peels a portion of the rim to expose the ice and use it to massage the ice into the area affected. The ankle should be cooled for 20 min every 3 to 4 h during the first 48 h. Heat should not be used for an acute ankle sprain because it increases swelling and inflammation. Compression with an ace wrap on the ankle helps limit the swelling. Elevation is the most poorly followed of all the components of RICE. The elevation should be above the level of the heart to not only decrease the swelling but also displace it. Effective elevation will cause the blood to pool away from the area of injury and go to a higher spot on the leg or into the lower foot. Blood is a proinflammatory agent. If the blood stays in the area of the torn ligaments, it aids in the promotion of the inflammation. Elevation causes the blood to go away from the area of the original ligamentous tear. Following these few simple steps will decrease recovery time.

Prolonged immobilization of ankle sprains is a common treatment error. Movement of the ankle stimulates the incorporation of stronger replacement collagen. Sprained ankles tend to stiffen in a plantar-flexed, slightly inverted position and preventing this stiffening is critical to more rapid recover. Rehabilitation begins on the day of injury and continues until pain-free gait and activity can be attained. Range-of-motion and muscle strengthening exercises and proprioceptive and activity-specific training are the key components of rehabilitation. Grade I and II rehabilitation can start immediately but grade III sprain rehabilitation will not begin until the ankle is judged stable. Rehabilitation begins with ROM and progresses to muscle strengthening followed by proprioceptive and activity-specific training.

Painless ROM exercises should begin within hours of the injury. Patients are asked to write the alphabet with their toes on the floor without bearing weight and pull a book on a towel toward them. After 48 h, instruct patients to pull their toes with a towel to stretch the Achilles tendon and prevent loss of dorsiflexion (Figure 14.10). Once they are able to bear weight without pain and a limp they can use an air-filled or gel-filled ankle brace. These braces restrict inversion–eversion and allow plantar and dorsiflexion. Casting is

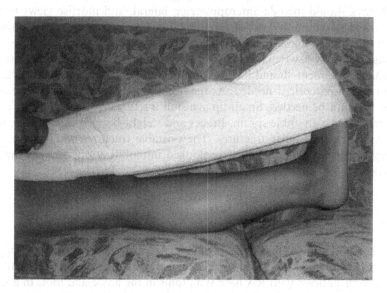

FIGURE 14.10. Towel stretch.

discouraged as it limits plantar flexion and dorsiflexion. Other exercises are now started to regain strength and balance. These exercises are described at the end of the chapter. A program for activity-specific training should also be recommended. A physical therapist can also be a big help if the patient needs more encouragement or is not responding as well as anticipated.

Occasionally it may be necessary for the clinician to recommend no weight bearing and use crutches or a cast for 10 to 14 days and then reevaluate for recovery or the presence of a talar dome or other fracture.

11. Fractures

Ankle fractures can occur at the lateral malleolus (distal fibula), medial malleolus, posterior portion of the medial malleolus, and the talar dome. Stable ankle fractures involve only one side of the ankle joint like the distal fibula fracture with no involvement of the medial bony or ligamentous structures. Unstable ones involve two or three sides of the ankle joint. Bimalleolar fractures include fractures of the lateral and medial malleoli or the lateral malleolus and a disrupted deltoid ligament. Trimalleolar fractures have the additional involvement of the posterior portion of the medial malleolus. Stable fractures are treated nonoperatively but the unstable ones require orthopedic evaluation and possible surgery. The history is usually one of acute twisting trauma and immediate onset of pain. The examination will reveal an immediate effusion and significant pinpoint tenderness. Palpation should always include the proximal fibula to rule out the Maisonneuve fracture and tenderness of the tibiofibular ligament and the syndesmosis.

X-rays should include anteroposterior, lateral, and mortise views to rule out the most common types of fractures. Talar dome fractures are not always seen initially on the X-ray. If after 6 weeks, the patient has persistent symptoms and the X-ray remains negative an MRI or CT scan may be helpful.

Initial treatment should include protection of the ankle, ice, and relief of pain with a narcotic if needed. As the fibula is a non-weight-bearing bone a cast may not be needed. Small tip avulsion fractures of the distal fibula can be treated like an ankle sprain. Braces and weight-bearing casts can be used for other distal fibular fractures. The unstable fractures will require non-weight-bearing casts and more prolonged immobilization. Surgery may be needed for some unstable fractures.

12. Arthritis

Rheumatoid arthritis may affect the ankle. Ankle swelling without trauma in a patient less than 50 should make the clinician suspicious of RA. Ten to fifteen percent of patients with RA have symptoms in the ankle and foot. In a small percentage, the first symptoms may be in the ankle and foot. The talonavicular joint is the most common one involved in RA. Swelling and decreased ROM (mostly dorsiflexion) are the most common presenting symptoms. Foot symptoms may also be present. The gait may be abnormal because of the pain with walking. Examination may reveal a warm tender joint that has decreased plantar flexion and dorsiflexion. Rheumatoid nodules (firm nontender movable masses) on the extensor surfaces may also be present. X-rays may show joint space changes early in the disease. If RA is suspected, be sure to obtain appropriate laboratory tests and consider referral for disease-modifying drug therapy. Many of these patient eventually become candidates for surgery.

Osteoarthritis is the most common nontraumatic cause of ankle pain. These patients are usually over 50 and may have had some type of trauma to the ankle in the past. The tibiotalar, talonavicular, and talocalcaneal joints are most commonly affected by OA. Other joints like the first metatarsal phalangeal, hip, knee, and distal interphalangeal are commonly involved at the same time as the ankle. Symptoms are pain, swelling, and difficulty walking. Examination may reveal decreased ROM and walking with the leg externally rotated. Treatment consists of using Tylenol and/or NSAIDs, orthotics, and firm but comfortable shoes. Ankle injection with lidocaine and a steroid may also help. The injection should be into the tibiotalar joint. Palpate for a soft area just medial to the anterior tibial tendon to identify the tibiotalar joint (Figure 14.11).

13. Ankle Exercises

Tell the patient to repeat each of the following exercises two times a day. Rotate from one exercise to the other. Do one set of one exercises and then rotate to another exercise and do a set. Do not exercise past the point of pain. Pain means stop.

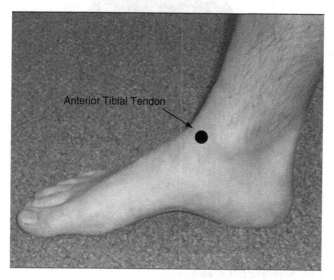

FIGURE 14.11. Area for injection of the tibiotalar joint.

1. **Towel stretch (Figure 14.10)**: Sit with your injured leg stretched out in front of you. Loop a towel around the ball of your foot and pull the towel toward your body keeping your knee straight. Hold this position for 10 s, then relax. Repeat five times.
2. **Standing calf stretch (Figures 14.12)**: Face a wall, and put your hands against the wall at about eye level. Keep the injured leg back, the uninjured leg forward, and the heel of your injured leg on the floor. Slowly lean into the wall until you feel a stretch in the back of your calf. Hold for 15 to 30 s. Repeat three times. Do this exercise several times each day.
3. **Anterior leg muscle stretch (Figure 14.13)**: Stand next to a chair or the kitchen counter and grasp one of them with your hand to maintain balance. Bend your knee and grab the front of your foot on your injured leg. Bend the front of the foot toward your heel. You should feel a stretch in the front of your shin. Hold for 10 to 15 s. Repeat five times.
4. **Heel raises A (Figure 14.14)**: Stand behind a chair or counter to balance yourself. With your feet internally rotated, raise your heels by standing on the tips of the toes for 5 s. Do this 20 times and repeat two times a day.
5. **Heel raises B (Figure 14.15)**: Stand behind a chair or counter to balance yourself. With your feet straight, raise your heels by standing on the tips of the toes for 5 s. Do this 20 times and repeat two times a day.

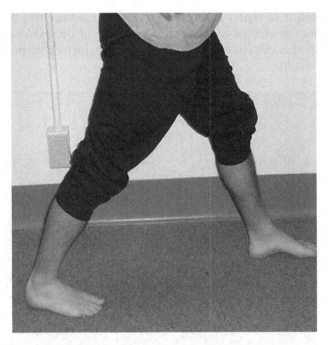

FIGURE 14.12. Standing calf stretch.

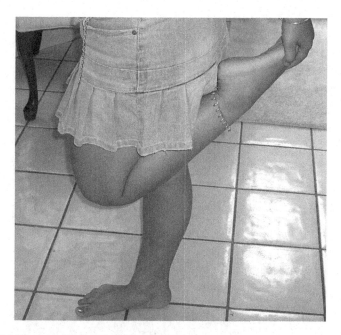

FIGURE 14.13. Anterior leg muscle stretch.

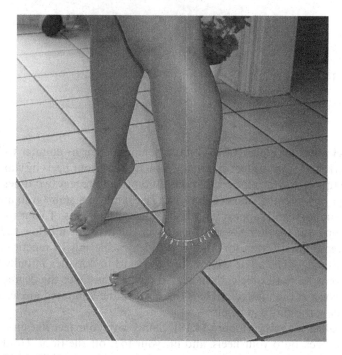

FIGURE 14.14. Heel raises A.

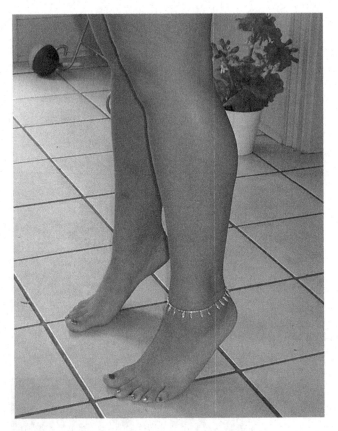

FIGURE 14.15. Heel raises B.

6. **Heel raises C (Figure 14.16)**: Stand behind a chair or counter to balance yourself. With your feet externally rotated, raise your heels by standing on the tips of the toes for 5 s. Do this 20 times and repeat two times a day.
7. **Heel raises on the stairs (Figure 14.17)**: Stand on a stair (grab a banister for support) and support your body weight on the tips of your toes. Raise up on your toes for 5 s and then lower the heel down below the toes to increase dorsiflexion for 5 s. Work up to achieving 10 repetitions three times a day. The ankle will be stiff and hard to dorsiflex initially but will become more flexible with increased repetitions. Once the degree of dorsiflexion in the injured ankle is the same as the uninjured ankle, activity-specific training can begin.
8. **Standing toe raises (Figure 14.18)**: Stand with your feet flat on the floor, rock back onto your heels, and lift your toes off the floor. Hold this for 5 s. Repeat the exercise 10 times and do it two times a day.

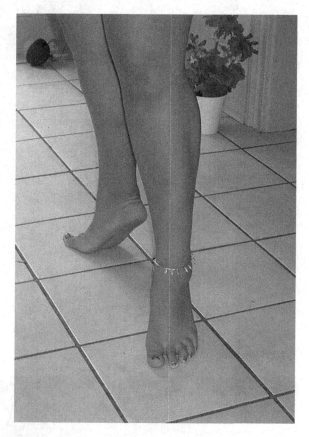

FIGURE 14.16. Heel raises C.

9. **Proprioceptive training**: Once all the above exercises are performed without pain, start this training. Walk on an uneven surface, heel to toe, for 50 ft slowly. Once you are able to do this with no difficulty close your eyes and repeat the process. Initially only close your eyes for few steps then gradually increase the time with your eyes closed. Have a partner with you when you walk with your eyes closed.

10. **Activity-specific training**: If you will be involved in a recreational activity or competitive sport, gradually acclimatize your ankle to the routines and stress of this activity. Start with a combined walk–jog–run that is characteristic of this activity/sport. The running/jogging component should gradually increase and replace the walking. Gradually increase the distance and add figures of eight and backward walking–jogging to the routine. The last routine attempted should be sharp cutting movement after coming to a stop.

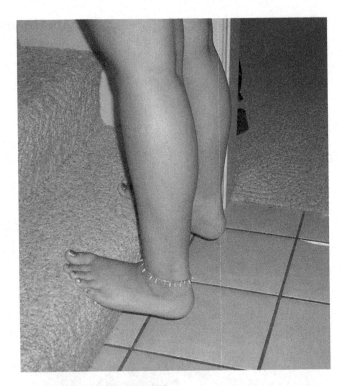

FIGURE 14.17. Heel lowering on the stairs.

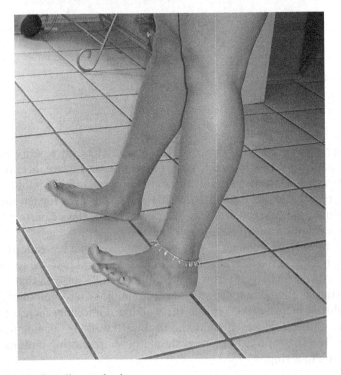

FIGURE 14.18. Standing on heels.

A trainer, physical therapist, or coach may be able to help you with all of the above exercises.

Suggested Readings

Stiell IG, McKnight RD, Greenberg GH, et al. Implementation of the Ottawa ankle rules. *JAMA*. 1994;271:827–832.

Wolfe MW, Uhl TL, Mattacola CG, et al. Management of ankle sprains. *Am Fam Physician*. 2001;63:93–104.

15

Foot Problems

MIKE PETRIZZI AND EDWARD J. SHAHADY

Foot pain is a common and troubling problem for primary care clinicians. It can be quite disabling because it can interfere with the ability to work, perform activities of daily living (ADL), and participate in recreational activities. Many patients with common chronic diseases like osteoporosis, diabetes, and obesity have foot problems that limit their ability to treat their disease with exercise. The foot is exposed to forces equal to two or four times the body weight with prolonged walking, running, and jumping. This exposure makes the foot the site of many problems seen in primary care. Table 15.1 lists some of these common problems.

Foot problems are categorized in a variety of ways. Overuse versus acute injury or division by anatomic areas like rearfoot, midfoot, and forefoot. Combining both categories helps the clinician think through the differential diagnosis. Diagnostic evaluation begins with a focused history that includes the mechanism of injury. The history focuses the problem so that a more efficient examination can be performed. The foot examination always includes an evaluation of gait and shoes. X-rays should be part of the diagnostic evaluation when fractures or arthritis is part of the differential diagnosis. Treatment options include strengthening and stretching exercises, change in training routine, use of corrective shoe wear, nonsteroidal anti-inflammatory drugs (NSAIDs), and orthotics and splinting. When conservative measures are not effective, surgery may be required. As with all musculoskeletal problems, a good working knowledge of the epidemiology, anatomy, a focused history, and examination reduce confusion and enhance the diagnostic and therapeutic process.

1. Anatomy

The foot is divided into three segments (Figure 15.1). Clinical problems will be presented as they occur in each of these segments. Knowledge of the bones, joints, and ligamentous structures in each of the segments facilitates the clinician's diagnostic and therapeutic process. The rearfoot (first segment) contains the talus and calcaneus; the midfoot (second segment) contains the navicular, cuboid, and three cuneiforms; and the forefoot (third segment)

TABLE 15.1. Classification of foot problems.

Rearfoot pain
- Plantar fasciitis
- Fat pad syndrome
- Tarsal tunnel syndrome
- Posterior tibial tendonitis
- Calcaneal stress fracture
- Sever's disease

Midfoot pain
- Lisfranc ligament sprains
- Navicular stress fracture
- Köhler's disease (avascular necrosis of the navicular)

Forefoot pain
- Fifth metatarsal fractures
- Metatarsal stress fractures
- Metatarsalgia
- Morton's neuroma
- Sesamoiditis
- Turf toe

contains the metatarsals, phalanges, and sesamoid bones. The main joints of the rearfoot are the talocrural (ankle joint), the talocalcaneal (subtalar joint) joints, the midfoot joints, the tarsometatarsal joints, and the forefoot metatarsophalangeal joints. The joints and their ligamentous interconnections contribute to the shape and function of the foot.

Multiple muscles from the lower leg attach to the various bones of the foot. The main foot flexors or plantar flexors are the posterior tibial, flexor hallucis longus, and flexor digitorum longus. The posterior tibial also maintains the arch of the foot and aids with eversion. Problems with these muscles, especially the posterior tibial, create problems with plantar flexion and inversion of the foot. The foot extensors or dorsiflexors are the anterior tibial, extensor hallucis longus, and the extensor digitorum longus. Problems with this group of muscles create problems and difficulties with dorsiflexion. The everters are the peroneus brevis and longus. Inflammation or tears of these two tendons can produce problems with eversion of the foot.

The shape and function of the foot is dependent on the longitudinal and the transverse arches. The longitudinal arch runs from the calcaneus to the metatarsal heads on the medial side of the foot. Loss of the longitudinal arch produces pes planus or flat foot. The prime dynamic stabilizer of the longitudinal arch is the posterior tibial muscle, secondarily supported by the anterior tibial and peroneus longus muscles. The transverse (metatarsal) arch is located in the frontal plane in the forefoot. It is apparent only when the foot is non-weight-bearing. The transverse arch is supported by the intermetatarsal ligaments and collapses with weight bearing to allow weight to be distributed to all metatarsal heads.

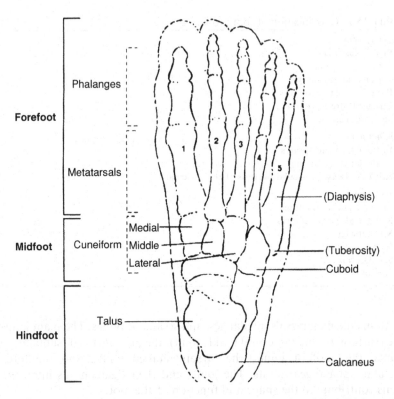

FIGURE 15.1. Three segments of the foot with bones. (Reproduced from Richmond J, Shahady E, eds. *Sports Medicine for Primary Care*. Cambridge, MA: Blackwell Science; 1996:502, with permission.)

2. Biomechanics

Understanding the biomechanics of the foot during running and walking helps the clinician understand and treat many foot problems. The gait cycle begins with the heel strike of one foot and ends with the heel strike of the same foot (Figure 15.2). The foot extensors maintain the foot in dorsiflexion and supination at heel strike. Next is the stance phase. During this phase the foot goes from supination to pronation and rigid to flexible. Both feet are on the ground during the stance phase of walking but there is only a single limb support during the stance phase of running. There is a float phase in running, where both feet are off the ground. The stress on the foot is greater with running because the total weight of the body is transferred to one foot during running. With heel strike the foot tends to supinate at the subtalar (talocalcaneal) joint. As the foot begins to flatten to bear weight in the stance phase and right before toe off, the foot now tends to pronate (everts, Figure 15.3) at the subtalar joint. If the pronation is

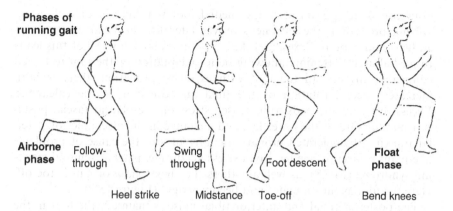

Phases of running gait

Airborne phase Follow-through   Swing through   Foot descent   **Float phase**

Heel strike   Midstance   Toe-off   Bend knees

FIGURE 15.2. Phases of running gait. (Reproduced from Richmond J, Shahady E, eds. *Sports Medicine for Primary Care.* Cambridge, MA: Blackwell Science; 1996:503, with permission.)

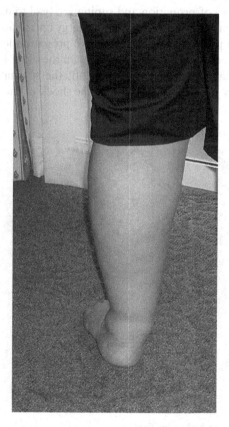

FIGURE 15.3. Eversion–pronation.

exaggerated, it appears as if the medial foot is rolling in or collapsing. During pronation, the calcaneus moves laterally, the head of the talus adducts and plantar–flexes, and the tibia rotates medially. All of this leads to medial arch flattening, allowing better adaptation of the foot to varied contacted surfaces. In the foot with excessive pronation, there is both increased medial rotation of the tibia and eversion of the calcaneus. Excessive pronation leads to increased stress on the plantar fascia, posterior musculature of the lower leg, and a change in the mechanics of patellar tracking. Exaggerated pronation contributes to the cause of problems like plantar fasciitis, medial tibial stress syndrome, patellar femoral tracking syndrome (PFTS), as well as others. The next phase of gait is toe off. Here the foot again supinates and becomes rigid (Figure 15.2).

The posterior tibial and anterior tibial muscles maintain the foot in the supinated position during the swing phase of gait. This dissipates some of the energy (three to four times body weight) that must be absorbed with each step. In the stiffer high-arched (cavus) foot (Figure 15.4), very little energy is dissipated, and excessive forces are transmitted up the leg, leading to leg, knee, or thigh injuries.

Excessive degrees of pronation and supination lead to injury. Even though the foot needs to pronate both to dissipate energy and to adapt to uneven surfaces, there is the trade-off because excessive pronation leads to an increase in torsional forces on the connective tissues. On the other hand, although the supinated foot may be great for pushing off, the supinated foot is a rigid structure that may not be able to dissipate the shock of the forces transmitted

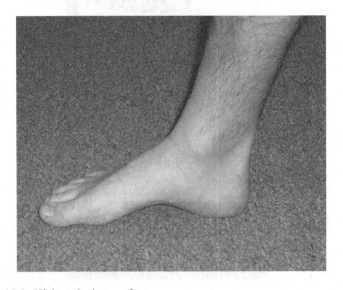

FIGURE 15.4. High-arched cavus foot.

to it. Appropriate balance of these forces is the key to injury prevention and treatment.

3. Shoes

There has been an explosion in the types of athletic footwear over the past 40 years. Beginning with running shoes in the late 1960s, the number and complexity of shoe types have increased. It is important to understand basic terminology and construction of these athletic shoes.

- The *last* is the basic shape of the shoe—it can be a board last (stiffer = more support) or a slip last (more flexible = more cushion).
- The *counter* is the heel cup configuration of the shoe. It should be firm, well-padded, and rigidly attached to the last. With alignment abnormalities of the foot, the counter and its attachment to the last are often the first part of the shoe to break down.
- The *toebox* is the portion of the shoe that accommodates the forefoot. It should have enough room to allow for easy motion of the toes. There should be 1/4 to 3/8 in. in front of the long toe. Excessive space, however, can cause trouble if the foot slides in the shoe.
- The shoe should have an adequate *arch support*. This is most often supplied as a separate insert in running or walking shoes and as a glued-in support in other athletic footwear. Typically, the arch support supplied will accommodate a foot with a normal arch. Athletes with either a flat foot or a high-arched foot will usually require a more substantial, often custom-made, orthotic for comfort and to reduce the risk of injury.
- The *sole* of athletic shoes these days is usually a composite of several layers. The outer sole typically is designed for either traction or abrasion resistance, while the main sole structure is for cushioning and flexibility. Shoes for distance running should be flexible in the forefoot; shoes for walking or racquet sports should have a stiffer forefoot. More expensive running shoes often have a gel or airbag system in the heel to help absorb energy. Most running shoe companies have a shoe designed for the pronated foot, which uses a stiffer material for the sole on the medial heel and arch.

4. Focused History

First, determine if the problem is acute and caused by trauma or chronic and related to overuse in a recreational or occupational activity. The mechanism of injury also helps. Was there a fall or unusual stress on the foot? Was there a history of chronic pain that preceded the acute pain? If the problem is more chronic, ask about risk factors such as a change in shoes, change in activity level or surface where the activity is conducted, change in intensity, or a change in jobs. A past history of lower extremity problems may trigger you to consider anatomic or biomechanical abnormalities. Diet and menstrual history are also important points of history.

5. Focused Examination

The physical examination of the foot consists of three different components: static observation (standing still), dynamic (moving) examination, and shoe wear. Do all foot examinations with and without shoes and socks. In static observation, observe the athlete both in the weight-bearing and in the non-weight-bearing phases. Are there any obvious deformities? Is there significant bowing of the Achilles tendon or significant flattening out of the arch with or without weight bearing? While looking at the skin, check to see if there is any callous formation indicating areas of excessive pressure. The dynamic examination includes gait, range of motion (ROM), and strength examinations. Analyze gait with and without shoes and socks with the patient walking in the hallway. Have the patient walk toward you and away from you, several times. Concentrate on only one part of the foot in each cycle. With continued observation and practice, it is often possible to be able to determine excessive degrees of supination or pronation (Figure 15.3) as well as other gait abnormalities. Next, assess the ROM of the various joints of the foot. Motion of the hindfoot, or subtalar joint, is assessed by cupping the heel in one hand and alternately inverting and everting it (Figure 15.5). Midfoot motion and motion at the midtarsal and tarsometatarsal joints is assessed by maintaining the hindfoot in neutral while inverting (Figure 15.6) and then everting (Figure 15.6) the forefoot. Motion in the forefoot is dorsiflexion or toes toward the ceiling (Figure 15.7A) and plantar flexion toes toward the floor (Figure 15.7B) at the metatarsophalangeal joints. Test both motion and strength in all of these joints.

5.1. Shoe Examination

Patients with lower leg problems should have their shoes examined. Be sure to examine all the shoes they wear including the ones used for work, around the house, and recreational activity. If the pain is more common during one time of the day or during a certain activity, ask for the shoes worn at that time. First, look for the point of excessive wear. Because the average foot strike is on the lateral heel and push-off is from the great toe, these areas typically show excessive wear (Figure 15.8). Individuals who have significant pronation may have a different wear pattern. Examine the shoes with them off the patient and then with the patient walking in them. This provides valuable information about the ability of the shoe to limit abnormal motion or how not wearing a shoe may exaggerate an abnormal motion.

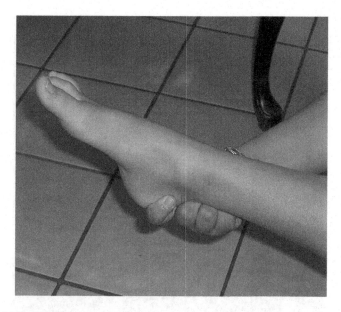

FIGURE 15.5. Hindfoot examination.

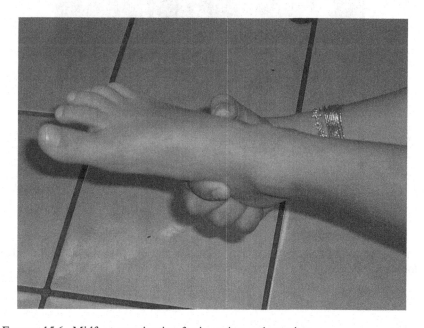

FIGURE 15.6. Midfoot examination for inversion and eversion.

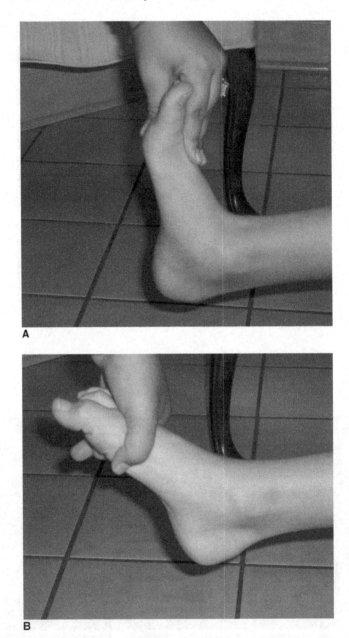

FIGURE 15.7. (A) Forefoot examination for dorsiflexion. (B) Forefoot examination for plantar flexion.

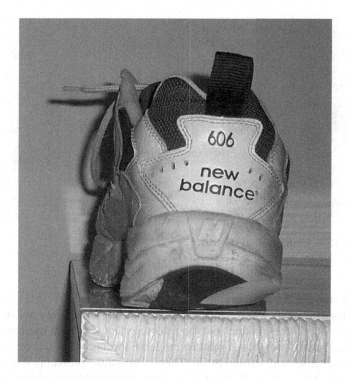

FIGURE 15.8. Shoe wear from heel strike.

The longevity of a running shoe is determined by how long the sole maintains its cushioning. This usually is between 350 and 500 miles, depending on the weight of the runner and the quality of the shoe. Some extension of the life of a shoe can be gained by using a liquid rubber solution (usually obtainable at sporting goods stores) to build up the areas of early sole wear. Suggest to runners that they change shoes regularly at 500 miles or sooner for heavier athletes. It is often best in aggressive distance runners to use several pairs of shoes simultaneously so that break-in can occur gradually.

5.2. Orthotics

Orthotics are inserts for the shoe designed to correct for an alignment or biomechanical abnormality of the foot. Figure 15.9 demonstrates arch supports for an orthotic that helps decrease pronation. In addition to helping with pronation, they help relieve pressure from other areas of the foot by coming in other shapes. Orthotics come in three basic groups: soft, semirigid, and rigid. Soft orthotics are made of felt or soft foam and are available over-the counter at pharmacies and sporting goods stores. Semirigid orthotics are custom-made from a moldable plastic, such as plastazote. Rigid orthotics are made

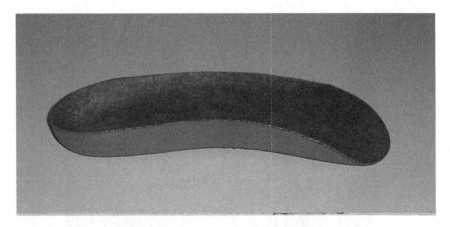

FIGURE 15.9. Orthotic arch support.

from hard plastic and usually require a casting of the foot. Semirigid orthotics are cheaper and somewhat easier to fabricate. They are more forgiving, so that the mold does not have to be perfect. They are used most commonly to relieve pressure in mild to moderate pronators. Rigid orthotics are more expensive and harder to fit. They often cause problems if used on a high-arched cavus foot. Rigid orthotics are best suited for moderate to severe pronators, when semirigid orthotics fail to alleviate the symptoms.

6. Hindfoot Injuries

This area includes the talus, calcaneus, plantar fascia, heel pad, and the tarsal tunnel. The peroneal as well as anterior and posterior tibial tendons traverse this area going to their more distal insertions. The hindfoot is the most common site of pain and injury for all these structures. Achilles tendonitis and rupture, a cause of pain in the hindfoot, is discussed in Chapter 13.

7. Case

7.1. History and Exam

A 36-year-old man presents to your office with left foot pain that is limiting his ability to run. He says the foot has been sore for several months, but he has been able to keep running by icing it and by stopping his running program for a few days when the pain increases. On the morning of the visit to his physician, he experienced severe foot pain 4 miles into his usual 7-mile run. He was unable to complete his run and walked with a limp back to his home. He was in the middle of a significant hill climb when the pain intensified. The patient has been a runner for about 10 years, and indicates that he had a stress fracture in the calcaneus of the left foot 8 years ago. He is wondering if the current pain is a return of his prior fracture. Prior to the recent event he noted the pain to be worse upon arising in the morning, especially when he first put his foot on the floor. The pain diminishes with continued ambulation and recurs with exercise. Pain occurs with running when the heel strikes the ground, and is increased when he pushes off. There is no history of numbness and tingling. Examination of his gait is normal with no pronation. He does have high-arched or pes cavus (Figure 15.4) feet. Palpation of the left heel over the medical tubercle of the calcaneus reveals significant tenderness (Figure 15.10). The pain is aggravated by dorsiflexion of the great toe and standing on the tips of his toes. There is no tenderness over the plantar surface of the foot or any of the joints. Dorsiflexion of the left foot is decreased compared with the right foot. Tapping over the area posterior to the medial malleolus does not produce any numbness or tingling (negative Tinel's sign). Strength is adequate and equal in both feet. An X-ray of the calcaneus was negative. He was diagnosed with plantar fasciitis and treated with NSAIDs, stretching, cross training on a stair master, and a splint to prevent plantar flexing during sleep. He responded to this treatment and within 3 months was able to return to his running program.

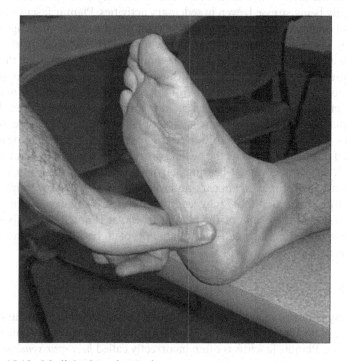

FIGURE 15.10. Medial tuberosity tenderness.

7.2. Thinking Process

Tarsal tunnel syndrome (compression of the posterior tibial nerve) would produce similar pain but the Tinel's sign is negative and he has no history of numbness or tingling. A recurrence of his calcaneal stress fracture is possible but ruled out by the negative X-ray and lack of persistence of the pain in between bouts of exercise. Gout or another type of inflammatory arthritis is not likely. Gout of the foot is most common in the first metotarsalphlangeal MTP joint of the big toe and both rheumatoid and osteoarthritis affect the subtalar joint. Heel pain that begins with the first few steps in the morning and reproduction of the pain by compression of the medial tubercle of the calcaneus is characteristic of plantar fasciitis. High-arched cavus feet predispose to plantar fasciitis. Decreased dorsiflexion indicates tightness of the gastrocnemius, and soleus (the calf muscles). This tightness can occur with a variety of lower leg problems but when combined with the above signs the diagnosis of plantar fasciitis is clinched.

8. Plantar Fasciitis

The plantar fascia is a thick band of connective tissue that originates at the bottom of the heel and progresses forward toward the ball of the foot. It helps maintain the arch of the foot. The tissue is not very well-vascularized and is constantly being stressed, even in sedentary activities. Plantar fasciitis is one of the most common foot problems seen in primary care. It is a challenge to treat and may take up to 12 months for complete recovery. It can occur in active or inactive individuals in all age groups. It seems to affect women more than men. The patient usually complains of burning electricity-like pain as soon as the foot touches the floor after arising from bed. Repetitive microtears and collagen degeneration of the plantar fascia at the medial tubercle of the calcaneus cause plantar fasciitis. The pain is worse in the morning because the foot assumes a plantar-flexed position during sleep and the microtears that occurred during the day start the healing process with the foot in plantar-flexed position. As soon as weight-bearing activity begins, the plantar fascia lengthens, microtears recur, pain appears, and what little was gained overnight is lost.

The stiff "high-arch foot" may lead to painful swelling because the force is concentrated at the origin of the plantar fascia, as is noted in the above case. Excessive pronation also causes the same problem because of increased torsional forces.

8.1. Imaging

An X-ray is not needed to diagnose plantar fasciitis. Some physicians like to obtain a plain film with plantar fasciitis to look for a heel spur. This leads to confusion. Plantar fasciitis is often incorrectly called *heel spur syndrome*. This terminology is incorrect because 15% to 25% of the general population without symptoms have heel spurs and many individuals with plantar fasciitis do not have a heel spur. Heel spurs play no part in the diagnosis or treatment of plantar fasciitis.

8.2. Treatment

Start by addressing mechanical problems and training errors. Good shoes that provide appropriate support are important. Shoes should be worn as often as possible (e.g., including a walk to the bathroom in the middle of the night) to decrease the strain on the fascia. The use of orthotics is appropriate for excessive pronation. A heel cup, particularly one that is soft and well-padded, can help plantar fasciitis in the high-arched foot. Heel cups are often of benefit in pain from the heel pad. Ice is helpful along with use of NSAIDs. With plantar fasciitis, the judicious injection of corticosteroid and local anesthesia may be of benefit. Corticosteroids may cause fat atrophy, and repetitive injections should be avoided.

Redeveloping the strength of the intrinsic muscles of the foot is important for rehabilitation in plantar fasciitis. Exercises such as towel stretches (see Figure 14.10) and walking on soft surfaces such as the sand or grass (once pain is diminished) can strengthen intrinsic muscles. The tight calf muscles must be addressed. Stretches like those demonstrated in the calf stretch (see Figure 14.12) are helpful. Stretching the plantar fascia with a cold water bottle as demonstrated in Figure 15.11 relieves pain and reduces edema. Telling an active person especially a runner to rest will not usually work. Relative rest is more likely to be an acceptable alternative. Cross training with a bike,

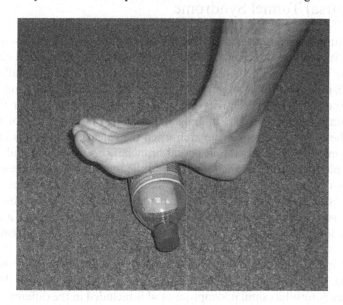

FIGURE 15.11. Frozen bottle roll.

swimming, or a stair master will work. Inform patients of the value of changing the exercise type and ask them to think about an alternative. The patient will choose no matter what you recommend.

Night splints or an ace wrap decreases the pain noted with arising and facilitates the healing process. The splints work by decreasing nighttime plantar flexion and facilitates the healing process in a neutral position. Night splints can be made or purchased from a supply house. For those patients who find the night splints uncomfortable an ace wrap is an acceptable alternative. The ace wrap is applied to limit night time plantar flexion.

9. Fat Pad Syndrome (Stone Bruise)

The fat pad of the heel is a specialized cushioning area, where there are thick fibrous septae dividing the pad into numerous compartments. This specialized area cushions heel strike. With aging, atrophy of the fat within these compartments may decrease the cushioning effect and lead to heel pain in the fat pad itself. Direct trauma may lead to bleeding into the fat pad. The problem is more common in older patients and in those who performed some type of activity that places a new and significant stress on the fat pad. One example is shoveling dirt that requires pushing hard with the heel. The syndrome is sometimes referred to as a "stone bruise." Once other entities are ruled out treat with extra padding or a heel cup. This usually provides symptom relief.

10. Tarsal Tunnel Syndrome

Tarsal tunnel syndrome is caused by pressure on the posterior tibial nerve, or one of it terminal branches (medial or lateral plantar nerves and calcaneal branch), at the level of the flexor retinaculum near the medial malleolus or more distally. Symptoms are often vague and intermittent. Symptoms include nighttime calf pain and activity-related pain in the heel or sole of the foot. The pain is accompanied by tingling and burning on the bottom of the foot at the heel and cramping at the arch when the calcaneal branch is involved. Involvement of the medial and lateral branches produces pain and tingling on the plantar surface of the foot down to the toes. Examination reveals tenderness over the tarsal tunnel below the medial malleolus (Figure 15.12). Compression with a finger for 30 s or percussion over the area (Tinel's sign) usually reproduces the numbness and tingling. An electromyogram and nerve conduction studies may be required to confirm this diagnosis. Treatment is usually a challenge. Try conservative measures like orthotics, NSAIDs, steroid injections, and proper shoe wear first. Surgery may help with some patients. Consider early referral for patients resistant to therapy. Posterior tibial tendonitis has similar symptoms and is included in the differential diagnosis. This entity is covered in Section 11.

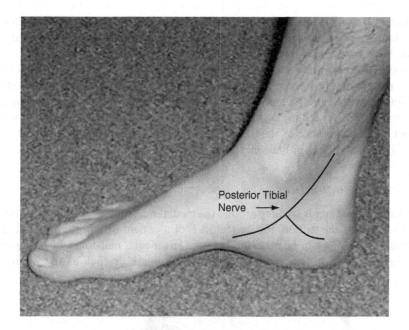

Posterior Tibial Nerve →

FIGURE 15.12. Tarsal tunnel area.

11. Tibialis Posterior Tenosynovitis/ Tibialis Posterior Dysfunction

This entity is not that common but when seen is a diagnostic and therapeutic challenge. It is in the differential diagnosis of tarsal tunnel syndrome and plantar fasciitis. It can be quiet disabling and the patient usually seeks medical attention. The patient is usually a runner who has had chronic discomfort and experiences an acute traumatic event. The symptoms are confined to the medial side of the ankle and foot. There is swelling and tenderness along the posterior portion of the medial malleolus down to the medial portion of the foot. This follows the anatomy of the posterior tibial muscle and tendon around the posterior malleolus to the insertion of the tendon onto the navicular bone.

Chronic tenosynovitis may render the tibialis posterior tendon insufficient to perform its tasks of plantar flexion, inversion and stabilization of the medial longitudinal arch. This description applies best to the weight-bearing posture of the foot, and the inability to perform each task varies in severity depending on the stage of tibialis posterior dysfunction.

There are three stages of tibialis posterior tendon insufficiency. Stage I is characterized by swelling, pain, inflammation, and often effusion within the tibialis posterior tendon sheath. Passive eversion of the foot produces discomfort along the course of the tibialis posterior tendon. There may be some mild weakness to resisted inversion but no unilateral flat foot deformity. The patient is able to invert the foot actively on a double-leg toe raise test and is able to perform a single-leg toe raise. Stage II disease is characterized by swelling, pain and inflammation, and the loss of function as indicated by an inability to perform a single-leg toe raise. In stage III disease, loss of function of the tibialis posterior tendon occurs. The asymmetrical pes planus (flat foot) now appears. Patients may report foot and ankle fatigue after limited activity and not feeling ankle support during ambulation. Shoes may wear out medially because of the foot rolling out. Pain occurs medially at first, but with long-standing pronation, the pain localizes laterally.

11.1. Examination

Examination reveals swelling around the medial malleolus and tenderness along the course of the tendon. Figure 15.13A is of a patient with posterior tibial tendonitis. Swelling can be observed over the left medial malleolus. Inverting and everting the foot may produce pain and a squeak or click as the inflamed

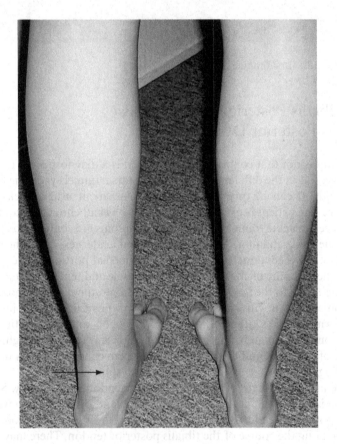

FIGURE 15.13A. Patient with posterior tibial tendonitis

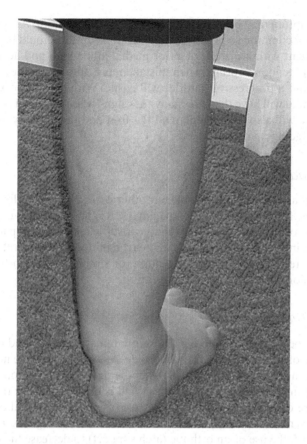

FIGURE 15.13B. Too many toes.

tendon glides over the medial malleolus. Observing the patient from behind may reveal some increased medial buckling and increased flattening of the foot. Observe for the number of toes visible laterally compared with the opposite side. If the tendon is ruptured or significantly dysfunctional there may be "too many toes" (Figure 15.13B) visible on the lateral side. Only one or two toes should be visible. Have the patient attempt to stand on the tiptoes to see if they invert, which is normal. Posterior tibial tendonitis and/or dysfunction decreases the ability of the foot to invert. Standing on the tiptoes may need to be repeated several times to tire out the tendon. An inability to rise on the toes indicates rupture or significant discomfort. Other entities can mimic the deformity of a foot with tibialis posterior tendon insufficiency. For example, degenerative arthritic deformities or a collapsed arch from neuropathic arthropathy like a diabetic Charcot joint produces similar-looking deformities. Tightness of the gastrosoleus complex frequently accompanies this condition early in the disease. In the late stages of the disease, contracture of the gastrosoleus complex occurs.

Acute rupture may be mistaken for a medial ankle sprain. As medial ankle sprain is not common so posterior tibial tendon rupture should be considered in any patient with a history of prior medial ankle pain and acute onset of pain. Acute tendon rupture, when mistaken as a sprain, will not improve as expected and a progressive flat foot will ensue. With rupture of the tendon, the individual will have the "too many toes sign" when observed from behind. The athlete will also have a unilateral flat foot and the inability to invert the foot when going up on the toes.

11.2. Imaging

Plain films are only helpful to rule out other cases of the pain like a fracture or arthritis. Magnetic resonance imaging (MRI) has become a useful tool in evaluation of tibialis posterior tendon insufficiency. If the patient has a swollen, painful tendon, MRI aids in the recognition of degenerative changes within the tendon, tearing of the tendon, or simply peritendinitis with synovial effusion without tendon degeneration.

11.3. Treatment

Treatment begins with nonsteroidal anti-inflammatory agents and relative rest. Some type of bracing device like a short leg walking cast may be needed if the patient cannot walk without pain. After the acute inflammation subsides, a stretching and strengthening program should begin. Treating the tightness and contracture of the gastrosoleus complex (see exercises at the end of the chapter) with exercises is vital for successful treatment. Preventing recurrence can be assisted with the use of an orthotic (arch support) to decrease the stress being placed on the tibialis posterior muscle and tendon unit. Obtain the help of a professional who can design a patient-specific orthotic. For traumatic rupture, early surgical repair is appropriate. Treatment for chronic rupture is the same as in tendinitis. Consider surgical treatment for resistant tendinitis, ruptures that remain symptomatic, and muscle contractures.

12. Calcaneal Fractures

The calcaneus is the largest bone in the foot and the most commonly fractured tarsal bone. It is also the most common location in the foot for a stress fracture. It articulates with the talus superiorly (forming the subtalar joint) and with the cuboid anterolaterally. The calcaneus provides a foundation for the transmission of the body's weight down through the tibia, ankle, and subtalar joints. Acute fractures are associated with falls and stress fractures are associated with running and jumping activities.

Patients with acute fractures typically present with a history of a fall resulting in a direct impact on the heel. Examination reveals pain, swelling, and

tenderness over the affected heel, and weight bearing on the hindfoot is usually impossible. Ecchymoses may extend over the entire sole. Stress fractures
are more likely to produce chronic heel pain that waxes and wanes with activity. Medial and lateral compression of the heel produces pain.

The key to diagnosis is imaging. The initial radiographs are usually negative
with calcaneal stress fractures. Repeat radiographs over time eventually show
the typical, often subtle, radiographic appearance. The fracture best seen on
the lateral standing radiograph usually occurs in the dorsal two-thirds of the
calcaneus. An MRI or technetium bone scan may be required to make the
diagnosis. In acute fractures, the diagnosis is usually clear on plain film.

12.1. Treatment

Treatment of stress fractures includes decreasing the quantity and intensity
of running, jumping or walking, wearing a heel pad, and NSAIDs. If conservative measures fail, crutches or cast immobilization may be necessary. It
may take 6 to 8 weeks for healing to occur. Fractures secondary to falls are
more problematic. Treatment is controversial and outcomes are not always
positive. An orthopedic surgeon should evaluate all acute calcaneal fractures.

13. Sever's Disease (Calcaneal Apophysitis)

Active prepubertal children 8 to 12 years of age can develop calcaneal
apophysitis. The cause is repetitive microtrauma to the calcaneal apophysis.
The symptoms are posterior heel pain and a limp. Examination reveals posterior heel tenderness. Radiographs are not necessary but commonly
obtained. The film will reveal the open apophysis with the typical appearance
of an unfused apophysis. Always obtain a view of the opposite heel to see if
there is a difference. The most important part of treatment is explaining to
the child and parents that this is a self-limited benign condition that will disappear as soon as the apophysis closes (usually at age 8 to 9 in girls and
2 years later in boys). A heel cup helps minimize the pain. If possible, activities that require jumping should be curtailed. Tylenol or ibuprofen can be
given on an as-needed basis. This problem is similar to Osgood–Schlatter's
disease of the tibial tuberosity.

14. Midfoot Injuries

The midfoot contains the navicular, three cuneiforms, and the cuboid bones
(Figure 15.1). Midfoot pain is not common but when it occurs, it frustrates
both the patient and the clinician. Two entities, Lisfranc ligament sprains and
navicular fractures, need to be understood for the clinician to evaluate and
treat midfoot pain.

14.1. Lisfranc Ligament Sprains

Strong transverse metatarsal ligaments connect the second through fifth metatarsals and provide stability. No similar ligament exists between the first and second metatarsals. Stability is provided by the Lisfranc ligament, which runs obliquely from the medial cuneiform to the second metatarsal base. Twisting of the planted foot, an axial load and rotation applied to the plantar-flexed foot (another person landing on the firmly planted heel), and a crush injury to the dorsal foot are mechanisms of spraining this ligament. The clinician should maintain a high index of suspicion for Lisfranc injury when evaluating active individuals with midfoot pain.

Patients with Lisfranc injuries will present with complaints of midfoot pain. They may not recall the specific event in which they were injured. More subtle injuries may reveal only point tenderness at the base of the first and second metatarsal (Figure 15.14). Acute injury signs include midfoot swelling and tenderness, followed by plantar ecchymosis. The patient may find it painful or impossible to perform single-leg toe rises, weight bearing, or cutting maneuvers.

Routine radiographs of the foot are obtained to look for a diastasis or greater space between the first and second metatarsal joint compared with the other foot. A small avulsion fracture at the base of the second metatarsal may be the only subtle finding of a more severe injury.

Treatment of midfoot sprains that have no diastasis or instability includes non-weight-bearing for 4 to 6 weeks with progressive weight bearing as

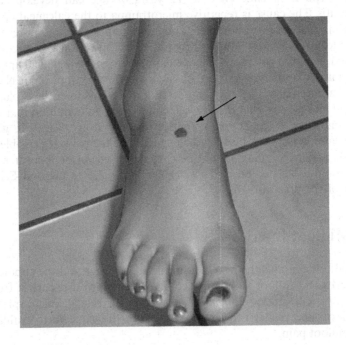

FIGURE 15.14. Lisfranc area.

tolerated in a short leg walking cast. Return to full activity takes longer than expected compared with sprains elsewhere. If diastasis or avulsion fracture is present, referral to an orthopedic surgeon is indicated for possible surgery.

14.2. Navicular Fractures

About 50% of acute navicular fractures occur when an eversion stress causes a bony avulsion of the medial deltoid ligaments from the navicular. Avulsion injury also occurs at the insertion of the tibialis posterior tendon. Consider these types of injury with medial ankle sprains and posterior tibial dysfunction. Fractures involving the body of the navicular are not as common but are more likely to lead to avascular necrosis.

Clinical presentation for acute fractures is usually straightforward. Acute midfoot pain after an eversion injury accompanied by difficulty bearing weight and tenderness over the navicular (Figure 15.15) is highly suggestive of navicular fracture. Plain film X-rays are usually diagnostic. A primary care clinician who is skilled in the care of fractures can manage acute fractures that do not involve the navicular body. Acute fractures of the navicular body and stress fractures are the ones that often lead to avascular necrosis.

Stress fractures, on the other hand, are more challenging to diagnose. Stress fractures of the navicular are typically seen in individuals involved in activities like basketball, volleyball, or running. Vague, poorly localized pain that is gradual in onset is common. The initial X-ray is usually negative. The diagnosis is usually delayed unless the clinician is suspicious of this possibility.

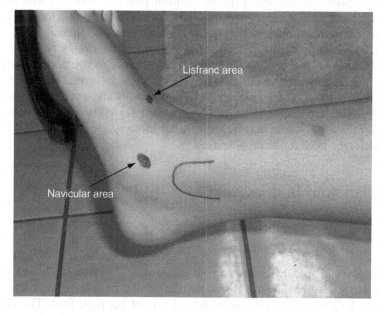

FIGURE 15.15. Navicular area.

Navicular stress fractures are the most difficult stress fractures of the foot and ankle to treat because of slow and recalcitrant healing. This process can be reversed by early diagnosis and non-weight-bearing treatment.

The routine three-view foot radiographic evaluation is adequate in acute eversion injuries but not always helpful in stress fractures. Computerized tomography scan is the study of choice for definitive diagnosis of navicular stress fractures. The location of the fracture line corresponds to a zone of avascularity. The blood supply enters from medial and lateral poles of the bone, and diminishes in the zone where the fracture occurs.

The role of the primary care clinician is to be highly suspicious for navicular stress fractures. If the plain films are positive, an orthopedic referral is appropriate. If the X-ray is negative, buy some time by encouraging the use of crutches and other forms of non-weight-bearing and reevaluating in 2 weeks. If the patient remains symptomatic after 2 weeks, a CT scan may help make the diagnosis. Be sure the patient understands that strict non-weight-bearing has a positive impact on healing of the fracture and stress fractures frequently require surgical intervention if the diagnosis is delayed.

14.3. Köhler's Disease

This condition affects children between 5 and 9 years of age. It is an idiopathic avascular necrosis or osteochondrosis that involves infarction, revascularization, resorption, and replacement of the navicular bone. It is similar to Sever's disease of the heel and Freiberg's disease of the head of the second metatarsal. Typically, only one foot is involved but both feet are involved in 25% of cases. Patients complain of midfoot pain that worsens with weight bearing, and may cause a limp. Physical examination reveals localized tenderness over the navicular midfoot area, swelling, and erythema.

Plain X-rays demonstrate increased sclerosis and narrowing of the navicular. The navicular can have an irregular appearance in the normal growing foot. Diagnosing Köhler's disease may be difficult, however, because an estimated 20% to 30% of males exhibit irregular ossification of the navicular.

Most children respond well to rest, ice, and NSAIDs. Immobilization or casting for 4 to 6 weeks may be required for more severe cases. Early diagnosis limits the need for immobilization.

15. Forefoot Injuries

15.1. Case

15.1.1. History and Exam

A 17-year-old student comes to your office with foot pain of 2-week duration. He has no past history of acute trauma and he is in good health. The pain is located on the outside or lateral side of his right foot. The pain is becoming worse and now causes him to limp. His summer job requires that he be on his feet for prolonged periods of time and go up and down the stairs several times daily. The last few days he has great difficulty performing any of these tasks. He does not experience electricity-like pain when he first places his foot on the ground in the morning, there is no numbness or tingling on his heel, or any decrease in his ability to dorsiflex or plantar-flex the foot. The pain increases in intensity as the day wears on. He has recently increased his running routine from 20 min three times a week to 1 h five times a week to attempt to lose weight.

The physical examination reveals a negative Thompson test (see Figure 13.9). Palpation of the medial calcaneal turbercle (Figure 15.10) reveals no tenderness. Tapping posterior (Tinel's test) to the midpoint of the medial malleolus (Figure 15.12) did not produce pain or tingling. No tenderness was noted when the tibia was palpated. Significant tenderness was noted about 1/2 in. distal to the tuberosity of the proximal fifth metatarsal (Figure 15.16).

15.1.2. Thinking Process

The lack of acute trauma, pain of 2-week duration now becoming worse, and a recent substantial increase in the amount of running is a common story for stress fractures. The location of the pain in the foot and not the tibia makes tibial stress fracture less likely. The absence of pain, numbness, and tingling along the medial side of the heel and a negative Tinel's test

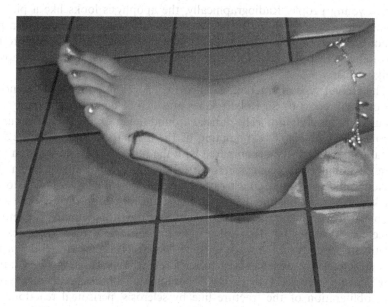

FIGURE 15.16. Fifth metatarsal area.

make tarsal tunnel syndrome unlikely. Lack of significant pain over the medial calcaneal tubercle and lack of pain when first placing weight on the foot in the morning makes plantar fasciitis less likely. A negative Thompson test rules out Achilles tendon rupture and Achilles tendonitis is not likely with absence of pain in the back of the heel. Pain over the fifth metatarsal on the lateral portion of the foot makes a fifth metatarsal stress fracture likely.

An X-ray was obtained and revealed a nondisplaced fracture about 1.5 cm distal to the tuberosity of the proximal fifth metatarsal. The fracture line was sharp with no widening and no sclerosis. This patient was diagnosed with a type I fifth metatarsal fracture and responded well to 6 weeks in a non-weight-bearing cast. He was advised to slowly increase the intensity of his running routine in the future.

16. Fifth Metatarsal Fractures

There are two types of fifth metatarsal fractures. The most common type is an acute tuberosity avulsion fracture and the other is a fracture of the shaft within 1.5 cm of the tuberosity. The avulsion fracture is also called "dancer's fracture." Acute inversion while the foot is plantar-flexed similar to ankle sprains is the usual mechanism of injury for this injury. Radiographically, the fracture is located on the tuberosity and perpendicular to the long axis of the fifth metatarsal. Remember there is an apophysis present in this area in girls aged 9 to 11 and boys aged 11 to 14. Apophysitis can occur in this area in very active young people. Radiographically, the apophysis looks like a piece of bone that is parallel to the turbercle of the fifth metatarsal and not a per-pendicular line. So in younger patients with pain in that area, be alert to this possibility. Treatment of choice for avulsion fractures is a wooden shoe or walking cast.

The second type of fracture is called the "Jones fracture," in reference to the original report by Sir Robert Jones in which he described the injury as it occurred in his own foot as he danced around the maypole. It is a fracture of the metaphyseal–diaphyseal junction of the metatarsal. It is located 1.5 cm distal to the tuberosity as compared with the tuberosity in the avulsion frac-ture. This injury can occur acutely or following repeated microtrauma. The radiographic appearance and treatment is the same for both. The history is the key to sorting out the diagnosis. Some authors think they are the same problem. It is an incomplete stress fracture of the fifth metatarsal. There are three classifications for the radiographic appearance of these fractures and treatment depends on the stage. In type I the fracture line is well-delineated and no sclerosis or perisoteal reaction is present. Type II has a widened frac-ture line and sclerosis. Type III is a nonunion with all the aspects of a type II plus obliteration of the fracture line by sclerosis, perisoteal reaction, and often displacement. Delayed diagnosis increases the chances of nonunion developing in types II and III.

16.1. Treatment

Initial treatment is conservative because a significant number of these fractures heal without surgery. In high-performance athletes, who need to return to high-stress activity sooner, internal fixation with an intramedullary screw may be indicated. Treatment of type I fractures consists of a non-weight-bearing cast or below-knee boot for at least 6 weeks and occasionally up to 20 weeks. Type II may also be treated nonsurgically but will take longer to heal. Competitive athletes are usually treated surgically to hasten their return to competition. All type III injuries are treated surgically.

Cessation of all weight-bearing exercise and choosing some type of alternative non-weight-bearing exercise like swimming or biking will help maintain conditioning. Physical therapy consultation may be beneficial. Altering training programs is important for treatment and prevention in the future

16.2. Imaging

An MRI is not needed if the diagnosis is clear with the plain film. Radiographic evidence of healing may take at least 3 months. If the patient does not respond clinically to conservative treatment an MRI may be indicted to evaluate response to treatment.

16.3. Other Metatarsal Stress Fractures

Stress fractures of the other metatarsals are common, especially in younger persons engaging in new activities such as running or aerobics. Older patients also experience these types of fatigue fractures from activities such as long walks in uncushioned footwear. The symptoms include mild to moderate swelling of the forefoot and redness. Usually the pain is localized to one or two metatarsal shafts dorsally. Early radiographs are usually negative. Plain films become positive approximately 2 weeks after the injury. Bone scans will be positive early. The examination will reveal a palpable painful bony prominence, on the dorsum of the affected metatarsal. Treatment should begin with a discontinuance of the recreational activities and substituting a non-weight-bearing activity. Ice, rest, elevation, and NSAIDs also help. A stiffer shoe should be used until symptoms have resolved. Crutches are usually not required, and the patient can return to work if walking can be limited. Stress fractures respond quickly to these measures, with symptoms resolving within a few weeks. Strenuous activities are generally avoided for 4 to 6 weeks.

17. Freiberg's Infraction

Freiberg's infraction is an osteonecrosis of the metatarsal head similar to Köhler's disease that appears in active adolescents especially females. It occurs most commonly in the heads of the second or third metatarsal.

Symptoms include a gradual onset of pain in the forefoot that worsens with weight bearing and activity. Examination reveals focal pain and tenderness over the affected metatarsal head. Initially, X-rays demonstrate widening of the metatarsophalangeal joint space, followed by collapse and sclerosis of the articular surface of the metatarsal head. The metatarsal head reossifies within 2 to 3 years. Similar to Köhler's disease, treatment consists of rest and immobilization. More severe cases may require casting for 6 to 12 weeks. Surgical intervention may be needed if conservative measures fail.

18. Metatarsalgia

Metatarsalgia is a nonspecific term used to describe pain on the bottom (plantar aspect) of the foot in the region of the metatarsal heads, typically concentrated under the second and third metatarsals. It may be a primary or secondary condition and the problem may be acute or chronic. Primary metatarsalgia is usually due to biomechanical reasons, such as excessive foot pronation, wearing high-heeled or pointed shoes, or shoes with poor padding. Secondary metatarsalgia may be due to other conditions such as gout, rheumatoid arthritis, sesamoiditis, trauma, stress fractures, or Morton's neuroma. The onset is gradual with no precipitating cause, associated with prolonged weight bearing and often described as "walking with a pebble in the shoe."

The examination will reveal the primary or secondary associated conditions that may be causing the metatarsalgia. Thorough evaluation of the foot facilitates making the diagnosis. Both non-weight-bearing positions and weight-bearing positions are included in the examination. In a non-weight-bearing position, inspect for swelling, masses, and calluses. Calluses are a response to abnormal weight bearing and good markers of abnormal stress and pressure. Weight bearing may reveal collapse of the arches (excessive pronation). Observing the length and shape of the toes may reveal other causes of the problem. A relatively long second toe with a short first toe may result in increased loading of the second metatarsal head. Hammer or claw toes may be indicative of a collapsed transverse arch. Palpate for calluses (that may not be obvious to inspection), swelling, and masses. Pain with foot compression test may indicate irritation of a Morton's neuroma (see Section 19). Pain with palpation under the first metatarsal head may be due to sesamoiditis (see Section 19). Test for tightness of the Achilles tendon (heel cord). A short tight heel cord increases forefoot area load and may contribute to metatarsal stress and discomfort.

Many of these patients end up with X-rays because of the difficulty in making a specific diagnosis. The X-ray is more helpful in discovering other diagnosis like a stress fracture. The treatment of metatarsalgia includes NSAIDs, correction of the tendency toward hyperpronation with improved footwear or orthotics, and heel cord stretching. The most common treatment is to use a metatarsal pad in the shoes. This will distribute the forces to a wider area and relieve the symptoms. A custom orthotic may need to be made for some patients.

19. Morton's Neuroma

These injuries are seen in running, walking, dancing, and aerobics. Women have a higher prevalence rate than men. The problem is not a true neuroma but a fibrosis secondary to the pinching of the digital nerves between the metatarsal heads. The most common location is between the third and fourth toes. Between the second and third toes is the next most common sight. Tight shoes that compress the toes are the most common cause of the neuromas.

The usual symptoms are pain and numbness in between the toes that are aggravated by wearing tight shoes during an activity. Sometimes the patient can feel a "mass" between the metatarsal heads. Compressing the metatarsal heads between the examiner's thumb and fifth digit (Figure 15.17) will accentuate the pain and make the diagnosis. Long-standing cases will have decreased sensation in the web space. Treatment first begins with avoiding tight-fitting shoes. This is a challenge in some patients who like the pointed toes tight-shoes

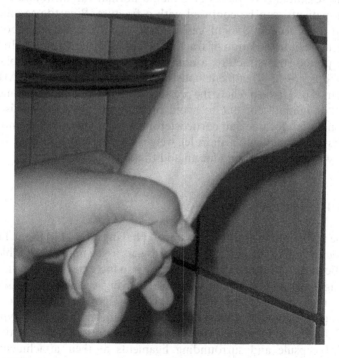

FIGURE 15.17. Compression testing for Morton's neuroma.

look. They believe that any other type of shoe is not cosmetically acceptable. If they continue to wear tight shoes nothing else will be of much help. Other treatment options include a metatarsal pad, NSAIDs, injection with a mixture of lidocaine and corticosteroids, and surgery. If an injection is given, it should be given dorsally (top of the foot) so that it is less painful. Intractable pain may require surgical removal. Because surgery leads to a permanent sensory deficit between the involved toes, a long trial of a conservative approach is well worth it.

20. Sesamoiditis Versus Sesamoid Stress Fractures

The sesamoids are small bones located on the plantar surface of the foot near the first metatarsophalangeal joint in the tendons of the flexor hallucis brevis (moves the big toe toward the floor). This area can be exposed to repetitive microtrauma in dancing, jumping sports, running, and prolonged walking. Sesamoiditis and stress fractures can occur with this overload. Patients will complain of pain under the great toe particularly when they push the foot off from the floor. Examination will reveal palpable tenderness, either medial or lateral to the first metatarsal head, that is made worse with dorsiflexion of the great toe. X-rays are a challenge to interpret because bipartite sesamoid (two pieces of bone), a normal variant found in 10% to 30% of patients, can be confused with a fracture. Bipartite sesamoids are bilateral (both feet) in 85% of cases. An X-ray of the opposite foot can be helpful in the differentiation of fracture versus bipartite sesamoid. In the case of a suspected stress fracture, a bone scan can be of help if the plain films are not diagnostic. Treatment consists of relative rest, ice, NSAIDs, and a metatarsal pad to help relieve the pressure on the sesamoids. Sometimes a pad, with a "doughnut" cut out to avoid pressure on the sesamoid is helpful. Injection with lidocaine and corticosteroids is of no benefit. Sesamoid stress fractures are treated with a short leg weight-bearing cast for 4 to 6 weeks followed by protective padding for an additional 6 weeks.

21. Turf Toe

Turf toe is a sprain of the first metatarsal phalangeal (MTP) joint. The name "turf toe" is due to the association of this soft tissue injury with athletic play on artificial turf. Multiple factors are known to increase the risk of this injury including hard and unyielding artificial playing surfaces, increased shoe–surface traction, limited MTP motion, type of sport and player position, as well as age, weight, and prior injury. The mechanism of injury is hyperextension of the first MTP joint. The hyperextension stresses and potentially tears the joint capsule and surrounding ligaments at their attachment to the metatarsal neck. Extreme hyperextension can also result in a compression injury of the dorsal articular surface.

Injuries to the big toe can be quiet disabling. The big toe supports 40% to 60% of body weight during walking, with significantly greater forces during running and jumping activities. Hyperextension injuries can limit all of these activities depending on their severity.

A grading system is used to classify the severity and clinical findings of turf toe injury. Mild grade I stretch injuries exhibit localized tenderness, minimal swelling, and ecchymosis. Range of motion (compare with other toe to establish normal for each patient) is minimally restricted and the patient is able to continue activities with minimal disability. Grade II injuries are partial ligamentous tears with more intense and diffuse tenderness, swelling, and ecchymosis. Range of motion is moderately limited with painful weight bearing. Symptoms, initially not severe, increase in the first 24 h. The patient has difficulty returning to activity and seeks medical attention. This is the most common type of patient who will seek care from the primary care clinician. Grade III injuries include a complete tear of the capsuloligamentous complex and a dorsal chondral impaction injury. There may be evidence of a fracture. These patients are unable to bear weight and have significant pain, swelling, and restricted ROM immediately. X-rays are indicated to rule out fractures if you suspect a grade III injury.

Treatment begins by determining the severity of injury. Grade I injury can be treated with restricted hyperextension of the big toe. Treatment for grade II injuries includes relative rest, ice, elevation, NSAIDs, a hard sole shoe, and other devices to limit hyperextension. Gradual resumption of first MTP ROM should begin in the first week. Vigorous activity should be avoided until symptoms subside. Some of these injures tend to linger because patients resume their activity without proper protection of recurrence. The trainer at your local high school can usually provide some good tips on how to treat turf toes. Grade III injury requires crutches and cast immobilization to promote soft tissue healing. These patients will require extensive time and rehabilitation. At a minimum, involve the physical therapist with all grade III injuries. Consultation with the orthopedic surgeon or someone in your community that commonly cares for athletes may be indicated. Grade III and some grade II injuries take a long time to heal. The length of time it takes for healing can be very frustrating to both the clinician and the patient.

Return to full activity is determined by not only resolution of symptoms but also the ability to extend and flex the injured big toe by an amount equal to the noninjured toe. Gait and running should also be normal and the patient should not be compensating by running or walking on the lateral aspect of the foot. The patient's shoe wear can be modified by replacing the flexible insole with a stiff steel or graphite plate in the forefoot. Taping the big toe to the adjacent toe helps restrict dorsiflexion.

21.1. Ingrown Toenails

The big toe is frequently the site of ingrown toenails. They are quite uncomfortable and can limit activity. Symptoms include pain, redness, and swelling at the edge of the toe. Soaks in warm water and oral antibiotics are the first line of treatment. Other popular treatments including packing cotton under the edge of the nail to limit its growth into the skin sometimes works. Removing a portion of the ingrown nail usually works. Good foot hygiene and proper fitting shoes need to be worn after removal to hasten healing and prevent recurrence. Adolescents experiencing a growth spurt are more susceptible because they experience frequent changes in shoe size. They may be wearing shoes that are too tight soon after they purchase them. Not cutting the nails too close to the skin and wearing properly fitted shoes prevents ingrown nails..

22. Advice to Patients About Purchase of Shoes

1. Always choose your shoe by how it fits. The size listed on the inside of the shoe can vary with brand name and style.
2. Your foot is bigger at the end of the day, so purchase your shoes then.
3. The size of your foot changes as you grow older, so expect a change in shoe size.
4. Measure both feet. One is usually bigger than the other. Purchase shoes based on the largest foot.
5. Stand during the fitting process. The foot lengthens and may become wider with standing as the two arches change shape. A fit in the sitting position may not be as comfortable with standing and walking.
6. Be sure you can place one finger between the end of the large toe and the end of the shoe. Less distance will result in too tight a fit and more distance would be a loose fit.
7. The heel and ball of the foot should fit snugly but not be too loose or tight. Walk around with both shoes on to access the fit before purchase.

23. Foot Exercises

Tell the patient to repeat each of the following exercises two times a day. Rotate from one exercise to the other. Do one set of one exercise and then rotate to another exercise and do a set. Do not exercise past the point of pain. Pain means stop. (Figures for all the foot exercises except exercise 7 (Figure 15.11) are located in Chapter 14.)

1. **Towel stretch (see Figure 14.10)**: Sit with your injured leg stretched out in front of you. Loop a towel around the ball of your foot and pull the towel toward your body keeping your knee straight. Hold this position for 10 s, then relax. Repeat five times.

2. **Standing calf stretch (see Figure 14.12)**: Face a wall, and put your hands against the wall at about eye level. Keep the injured leg back, the uninjured leg forward, and the heel of your injured leg on the floor. Slowly lean into the wall until you feel a stretch in the back of your calf. Hold for 15 to 30 s. Repeat three times. Do these exercises several times each day.

3. **Anterior leg muscle stretch (see Figure 14.13)**: Stand next to a chair or the kitchen counter and grasp one of them with your hand to maintain balance. Bend your knee and grab the front of your foot on your injured leg. Bend the front of the foot toward your heel. You should feel a stretch in the front of your shin. Hold for 10 to 15 s. Repeat five times. Do the exercise two times a day.

4. **Heel raises (see Figure 14.15)**: Stand behind a chair or counter to balance yourself. With your feet straight, raise your heels by standing on the tips of the toes for 5 s. Do this 20 times and repeat two times a day.

5. **Heel raises on the stairs (see Figure 14.17)**: Stand on a stair (grab a banister for support) and support your body weight on the tips of your toes. Raise up on your toes for 5 s and then lower the heel down below the toes to increase dorsiflexion for 5 s. Work up to achieving 10 repetitions three times a day. The ankle will be stiff and hard to dorsiflex initially but will become more flexible with increased repetitions. Once the degree of dorsiflexion in the injured ankle is the same as the uninjured ankle, activity-specific training can begin.

6. **Standing toe raises (see Figure 14.18)**: Stand with your feet flat on the floor, rock back onto your heels, and lift your toes off the floor. Hold this for 5 s. Repeat the exercise 10 times and do it two times a day.

7. **Frozen can/bottle roll (Figure 15.11)**: Roll your bare injured foot back and forth from your heel to your midarch over a frozen juice can or frozen bottle of water. Repeat the movement for 2 to 3 min. Do the exercise two to three times a day. Doing it the first thing in the morning is very helpful in plantar fasciitis.

8. **Proprioceptive training**: Once all the above exercises are performed without pain start this training. Walk on an uneven surfaces heel to toe for 50 ft slowly. Once you are able to do this with no difficulty, close your eyes and repeat the process. Initially, only close your eyes for few steps then gradually increase the time with your eyes closed. Have a partner with you when you walk with your eyes closed.

9. **Activity-specific training**: If you will be involved in a recreational activity or competitive sport, gradually acclimatize your ankle to the routines and stress of this activity. Start with a combined walk–jog–run that is characteristic of this activity/sport. The running–jogging component should gradually increase and replace the walking. Gradually increase the distance and add figures of eight and backward walking–jogging to the routine. The last routine attempted should be sharp cutting movement after coming to a stop.

A trainer, physical therapist, or coach may be able to help you with all of the above exercises.

Suggested Readings

Strayer SM, Reece SG, Petrizzi MJ. Fractures of the fifth metatarsal. *Am Fam Physician.* 1999;59(9):2516–2522.
Simons SM, Foot injuries in the runner. In: O'Connor FG, Wilder RP, eds. *Textbook of Running Medicine.* New York: McGraw-Hill; 2001:213–226.

Index

Page numbers followed by f and t indicate figures and tables, respectively.

A

Abduction, 92, 223
AC, *see* Adhesive capsulitis
Acanthosis nigricans, 31
Achilles tendinitis, 283–285
  treatment of, 285
Achilles tendon disorders, *see* Achilles
  tendinitis
AC joint separation, *see* Joint
  acromioclavicular separation
  history and examination, 66–68
  imaging, 68
  mechanism of injury and anatomy,
    65, 66
  treatment, 69
ACL tears, diagnosis of, 238
Acromioclavicular joint arthritis, 69
AC separation, 66
Activities of daily living (ADL), 93
Activity-specific training, 288, 307
Acute bursitis, 105–107
Acute compartment syndrome (ACS),
  277
Acute mountain sickness (AMS), 35–38
Acute trauma, 214–217
Adduction, 223
Adequate fluid content, 29
Adhesive capsulitis (AC), 83–86
Advice to patients about purchase of
  shoes, 340
AMS, *see* Acute mountain sickness
  prevention, 37, 38
  treatment of, 37
Anatomic risks, 10
Anatomy of ankle, 289–291
Anatomy of foot, 310, 311, 312f
Angina, 160, 173
Ankle, anatomy, 289–291
  exercises, 303–309
  fractures, 302
  injection, 303

Ankle problems,
  a case study, 296, 297
  examination, 292–295
  test, 295
Ankle sprains, 297, 298
  classification, 297, 298
  evaluation, 298, 299
  mechanism, 298
  medial, 291
  treatment, 300–302
Ankle stability, medial, 290
Ankylosing spondylitis (AS), 173, 194
Anterior dislocations, 72
Anterior drawer test tests, 295
Anterior inferior iliac spine (AIIS),
  avulsion of, 221
Anterior leg muscle stretch exercise,
  288, 305f
Anterior superior iliac spine (ASIS), 211
Anterior talofibular ligament (ATFL),
  289, 290
Anteroposterior (AP), 100, 171, 245,
  299, 302
Antidepressants, 170
Apley grind test, 242
Apley scratch tests, 84
Arthritis of shoulder, 87
AS, *see* Ankylosing spondylitis
ASIS, *see* Anterior superior iliac spine
Aspiration, for bursitis treatment, 106,
  107
Athletic footwear, construction of, 315
Atrophy, 55
Avascular necrosis (AVN), 208
  of the femoral head, 210–212
AVN, *see* Avascular necrosis
Avulsion, 109
  fracture, 334
  injuries 221
Axial loading test, 161, 166f
Axillary nerve deficit, 72

B

Back exercises, 195–198
Back hygiene, 198–200
Back problems, *see* Low back pain
Backward extension, 89–92, 223
Baker's cyst, 286, 287
Barotitis, 41; *see also* Ear barotrauma
Barotrauma, 41, 42
Benefits of exercise, 14t
Bennett's fracture, 146
Bimalleolar fractures, 302
Biomechanics of foot, 312, 314, 315
Bipartite sesamoids, 338
Blood, 301
Blood vessel, endothelial lining of, 16
Bouchard's nodes of PIP, 154
Boutonnière deformity, at PIP joint,
    148–150
Boxer's fracture, *see* Metacarpal
    fractures
Buddy taping, 143, 148
Bursitis, 253–256

C

CAD, *see* Coronary artery disease
Calcaneal fractures, 328, 329
    treatment, 329
Calcaneus, 328
Calluses, 336
Carbohydrates, 29
Cardiac output per beat, *see* Stroke
    volume
Cardiovascular disease, 9
Cardiovascular disease and exercise,
    16, 17
Cardiovascular fitness, 14
Cardiovascular respiratory response to
    exercise, 14–16
Carpal tunnel syndrome, case study,
    119–128
    symptoms of, 122
    treatment of, 126–128
Cauda equina (CE) syndrome, 180,
    192, 193
Cervical canal stenosis, *see* Spondylosis
Cervical collars, 168, 169
Cervical disk herniation, case study,
    170–172
Cervical pillows, 168

Cervical root compression, signs and
    symptoms of, 171t
Cervical spondylosis, *see* Spondylosis
Cervical strain, treatment of, 168
Cervical vertebral fractures, 168
Chilblains, 46
Childhood obesity, 32
Chronic bursitis, 105–107
Chronic microtrauma, 254
Chronic neck pain, 169, 170
Chronic obstructive pulmonary disease
    (COPD), 40
CKC, *see* Closed kinetic chain
Clinician obstacles to exercise, 23
Closed kinetic chain (CKC), 6
Coaches finger, *see* PIP joint dislocations
Cold injury, 45–47
Collateral ligament injury, 150
Compartment syndrome, 273, 278f;
    see also Exertional compartment
    syndrome
Computerized tomography (CT) scan, 5
Contemplation, 12
COPD, *see* Chronic obstructive
    pulmonary disease
Coronary artery disease (CAD), 16, 20
Corticosteroids, 323
Counterforce bracing, for lateral
    epicondylitis, 105
Cubital tunnel syndrome, *see* Ulnar
    nerve injury

D

Dancer's fracture, *see* Avulsion fracture
DCS, *see* Decompression sickness
DCS, prevention, 43
Decompression illness, 43
Decompression sickness (DCS), 42, 43
Degenerative diseases, of spine, *see*
    Disk herniation; Spondylosis
Deltoid ligament, 290
De Quervain's tenosynovitis, diagnosis
    and treatment of, 128, 129
    symptoms of, 122–124, 130
Diastole, 14
DIP, *see* Distal interphalangeal joint
    joint injury, 151–153
    case study, 152, 153
    treatment of, 153

Disease-modifying antirheumatic drugs
    (DMARD), 134
Disk herniation, symptoms and factors
    of, 171
Dislocation of MCP joint, 142–144
Dislocation of the elbow, 99, 101
Distal interphalangeal (DIP) joints,
    138f, 140f, 142, 150, 218
Distracting straight leg-raising test, 185
DMARD, see Disease-modifying
    antirheumatic drugs
    for hand problems, 156

E
Ear barotrauma, 41, 42
ECS, see Exertional compartment
    syndrome
    diagnostic studies of, 278
    treatment options of, 279
Ejection fraction, 14, 15
Elbow dislocations, 99, 101
Elbow exercises, 112–117
Elbow flexion and extension, 114, 116f
Elbow fractures, 99
Elbow pain, case study, 99, 100
Elbow problems, classification of, 94t
    focused history for, 94
    focused physical
        examination for, 95–99
Elbow splints, 101
Endothelium-derived NO, 17
Environmental problems, classification
    of, 36t
Erosive inflammatory osteoarthritis,
    155
Exercise, cardiovascular response, 15t
    and cancer, 20
    as medication, 13, 14
    precautions, 26, 27
    prescription, 9, 24–26
Exercises, for back pain, 195–198
    elbow problems, 112–117
    lower leg, 287, 288
    neck pain, 174–177
    wrist problems, 134, 135
    foot, 340, 341
Exertional compartment syndrome
    (ECS), 277–279
Extensor injury, 151, 152

External and Internal rotation 1, 2,
    88, 89
"External rotation test," 299

F
FABER test, 187
Facial barotrauma, 42
Fatigue fractures, see Tibial stress
    fractures
Fat Pad Syndrome, 324
Fever, in back pain, 193
Fifth metatarsal fractures, 334, 335
    imaging, 335
    treatment, 335
Finkelstein's test, 124, 125f
Flexion, 223
Flexor tendon, 152, 153
Foot, biomechanics, 312, 314, 315
    dynamic examination, 316
    physical examination, 316
    anatomy, 310, 311, 312f
    exercises, 340, 341
    extensors, 311
Foot problems, classification, 311t
    focused examination, 316, 317, 318f,
        319, 320
    focused history, 315, 316
Forefoot, 310, 311
    injuries, a case study, 332–334
Forward flexion, 89
Fractured clavicle, 58–64
Fractured proximal humeral head, 69, 70
Fractures, see specific fractures
Fractures of tibia and fibula, 285, 286;
        see also Tibial stress fractures
Freiberg's infraction, 335, 336
Frostbite, 46, 47
"Frostnip," 46
Frozen shoulder, see Adhesive
    capsulitis

G
Gait cycle, 312, 313f, 314, 315
Gallstone disease, 31
Gas principles, barotrauma, 41
Gastrocnemius tears, 279–282
    case study, 279, 280
    imaging of, 281
    treatment of, 281, 282

Genetic disease of insulin resistance,
18; *see also* Type 2 diabetes
Glenohumeral joint dislocations, 71–75
Glenoid labrum, 77
Glucosamine, 258
Golfer's elbow, *see* Medial
epicondylitis
Goniometer, 95, 96f
Gout, 112, 322

H

Hamstring strains, 216
Hamstring tightness pain, 179
Hand injuries, 136
organizational steps to overcome fear
and frustration for, 136
Hand problems, case study, 138–142
classification of, 137
focused history of, 137, 138
focused physical examination for, 138
HAPE, *see* High-altitude pulmonary
edema
HDL, *see* High-density lipoprotein
Heat cramps, 44
Heat exhaustion, 44, 45
Heat illness, 43–45
Heatstroke, 45
Heat syncope, *see* Heat cramps
Heberden's nodes, 256, 292
Heberden's nodes of the DIP, 154
Heel cups, 323
Heel raises on the stairs exercise, 288,
308f
Heel rises A exercise, 287, 305f
Heel rises B exercise, 288, 306f
Heel rises C exercise, 288, 307f
Heel spurs, 322, 323
Heel spur syndrome, *see* Plantar
fasciitis, imaging; Plantar fasciitis,
treatment
Henry's law, 41
Herniated disks, *see* Herniated
intervertebral disks
Herniated intervertebral disks, 180,
190–192; *see also* Disk herniation
imaging of, 191
treatment of, 191, 192
High-altitude pulmonary edema, 38
High-altitude sickness, 35–40

High-calorie sample meal plan, 30t
High carbohydrate content, 28
High-density lipoprotein (HDL), 9
Hill–Sachs lesions, 75
Hindfoot injuries, a case study,
320–322
Hip, 4
Hip and thigh problems, case
histories, 208–210, 218–220,
222, 223
focused history, 204
focused physical examination,
204–208
organizational steps, 203
Hip exercises, 223–226
Hip pointer, 218
Hip problems, 204
Humeral neck fracture, 99
Hyperlordosis, 194
Hypertension, 17
Hypoperfusion, 45

I

Ice, 6
Idiopathic avascular necrosis, 332
Iliotibial band (ITB), 212, 248
Iliotibial band stretching, 226
Immobilization, 6, 7
Inflammation and exercise, 20
Inflammatory arthritis, 87, 222
Infrapatellar tendonitis, 252, 253
Ingrown toenails, 339, 340
Injury rehabilitation, 3
Insulin resistance, 18, 19
Interosseous membrane, 269
Intervertebral disk herniation, *see* Disk
herniation
Inversion injury, 292
ITB, *see* Iliotibial band
ITBS, *see* Iliotibial band syndrome

J

Jersey finger, 152, 153
Joint acromioclavicular separation,
65–69
Joint mouse, *see* Loose bodies
Jones fracture, 334
Jumper's knee, *see* Infrapatellar
tendonitis

K

Knee exercises, 262–267
Knee extension, 6
Knee extension and flexion, 264
Knee immobilizer, 244
Knee problems, case studies, 235–239,
   246–252, 256–261
   common, 229
   history, 230
   organizational steps, 228
   physical examination, 230–235
   physical factors, 261, 262
Köhler's disease, 332

L

Labrum injury, patients with, 78
Labrum tears, 77, 78, 81
Lachman test, 237
Large-bore needle, 255
Lateral elbow pain, 93, 102–105
   case study, 102–105
Lateral epicondylitis, 104
   case study, see Lateral elbow pain,
      case study
Lateral subluxation, 245
Laxity testing, 238
LBP, see Low back pain
   case study, 187–189
   focused examination of, 180–187
   focused history of, 179, 180
LDL, see Low-density lipoprotein
Lidocaine, for elbow dislocations,
   101
Lidocaine, for MCP dislocations,
   143
   injection of, in joints, 69
Ligaments and muscles, anatomy and
   function of, 54
Limb symptoms, 43
Limping, 222
Lipids and exercise, 19, 20
Lisfranc ligament, 330
   sprains, 330, 331
Little leaguer's shoulder, 87, 88
Liver toxicity, risk of, 11
Localized tenderness over the
   spine, 193
Loose bodies, 245
Low-altitude illness, 41–43

Low back pain, mechanical, 189, 190
   associated with red flags, 193
Low back pain (LBP), 178–189
   problems, classification of, 179t
Low bulk or low fiber content, 29
Low-density lipoprotein (LDL), 9
Lower leg, anatomy of, 269–271
   exercises, 287, 288
   pain, 268
   case study of left, 272–274
   focused history of, 271
   focused physical
      examination of, 271
   medical problems of, 286, 287
   problems, classification of, 269
Low fat and low protein content, 29
Low salt content, 29
L5 root compression, 185
Lumbago, see Sciatica
Lying down hamstring stretch,
   264–267

M

Magnetic resonance imaging (MRI),
   5, 210, 240, 243
Magnetic resonance imaging (MRI),
   for disk herniation, 171, 172
Maisonneuve's fracture, 285, 286
Mallet finger, see Extensor injury
Malrotation of the bone, 142
MCL, see Medial collateral ligament
McMurray test, 242
MCP, see Metacarpal phalangeal joint
MCP dislocation and relocation, 143f,
   144f
MCP joint dislocations, 142–144
MCP joint problem, case study, 144–146
Meal plan for losing weight, 33t
Mechanical back pain, 179, 180; see
   also Mechanical low back pain
Mechanical low back pain, 189, 190
   diagnostic imaging of, 189, 190
   treatment of, 190
Medial ankle sprains, 291
Medial collateral ligament injuries,
   treatment of, 241
Medial collateral ligament (MCL), 238,
   240, 241
   tear, 240, 241

Medial epicondyle traction apophysitis
(META), case study, 107–110
Medial epicondylitis, 105
Medial tennis elbow, see Medial
epicondylitis
Medial tibial stress syndrome (MTSS),
274
Medical education programs, 23
Medical problems in wrist, 133, 134
Medical of elbow, 112
Medical of hand, 154–156
Medications for relief of pain, 10, 11
Meningitis, 159
Meniscal/cartilage injuries, 241–244
Meniscal injuries, treatment of, 243
Meniscus, tears in, 241
Metacarpal fractures, 142
Metacarpal phalangeal (MCP) joint,
138f, 142–146, 152
Metatarsalgia, 336, 337
Metatarsal phalangeal (MTP) joint, 338
stress fractures, 335
Microtrauma, 75
Midfoot, 310
injuries, 329–332
MONO, see Mononucleosis
Mononucleosis (MONO), 4, 12
Morton's neuroma, 337, 338
MRI, see Magnetic resonance imaging
for herniated disk, 191
for OCD, 111
for spondylosis, 173
MTSS, see Medial tibial stress
syndrome
Muscle fatigue, 44
Musculoskeletal benefits of exercise, 21
Musculoskeletal (MS) problems,
treatment of, 3–6
Myocardial infarction pain, 160

N
Navicular fractures, 331, 332
Neck exercises, 174–177
Neck extension exercise, 174, 175f
Neck flexion exercise, 174
Neck lateral rotation exercise, 175,
176f
Neck pain, case study, 167, 168
case study of radiating, 170–172

Neck pain, case study (Cont.)
factors for, 159
medical causes, 173
organizational steps for
caring for, 159, 160
Neck problems, common, 160t
focused history of, 160, 161
focused physical examination
for, 161
Neck side bend exercise, 175, 176f
Nifedipine, 39
Nighttime back pain, 193
Nondisplaced scaphoid fractures, 132
Nonsteroidal anti-inflammatory drug
(NSAID), 5, 6, 8, 9, 11
for elbow problems, 100, 104–106,
109, 111, 128
NSAID, see Nonsteroidal anti-
inflammatory drugs
for neck pain, 168, 169
Numbness, 46
Nursemaids' elbow, 101, 102
Nutrient-dense carbohydrate
foods, 29

O
OA, see Osteoarthritis
in elbow, 112
Ober's test, 249–251
Obesity, 31
Obesity-induced hypertension, 31
OD, see Osteochondritis dissecans
OKC, see Open kinetic chain
Olecrenon bursitis, 105–107
Open kinetic chain (OKC), 6
Orthotics, 319, 320
Osgood-Schlatter's disease, 253, 261,
329
Osteoarthritis, symptoms, 303
Osteoarthritis (OA), 5, 6, 8, 9, 303
in hand, 154–156
Osteochondritis dissecans (OD),
111, 245
Osteochondrosis, 332
Osteomyelitis, 180
Osteoporosis, 21
Ottawa ankle rules, 299
Outpatient musculoskeletal medicine,
principles of, 4–12

P

Pain, 87
Palpation, 246
Panner's disease, 107, 111
Partial curl exercise, 197, 198f
Patellar compression test, 246
Patellar dislocation and subluxation, 244, 245
Patellar femoral pain syndrome (PFPS), 245
Patellar femoral tracking syndrome (PFTS), 314
Patient obstacles to exercise, 22, 23
Patients, WAD, 169
Peak bone mass, 21
Pediatric hip problems, 220–222
Pelvic tilt exercise, 195–197, 197f
Pendulum exercises, 88
Pes planus, 326
PF, *see* Plantar fasciitis
Phalen's test, 122, 124f
PIP, *see* Proximal interphalangeal joint
PIP joint, boutonnière deformity at, 148–150
   treatment of, 148
   dislocations, 147
   problem, case study, 146–148
   swelling, 155
   volar plate injury, 150
Pitching techniques, for medial elbow pain, 110
Plantar fascia, 322
Plantar fasciitis, imaging, 322, 323
   treatment, 323, 324
Plantar fasciitis (PF), 5, 322–324
Plastazote, 319
Popliteal cyst, *see* Baker's cyst
Popliteus tendonitis, 282, 283
   treatment of, 283
Posterior ischial apophysis avulsion, 221
Posterior talofibular ligament (PTFL), 289
Posterior thigh, palpation of, 215
Precautions, exercise, 26, 27
Precontemplation, 22
Prepatellar bursa, 254
Proinflammatory agent, 301
Pronation, 10, 271, 273

Pronation (*Cont.*)
   and supination of the forearm, 115, 117f
Proprioceptive training, 307
Provocative tests, 161
Proximal humerus, physis of, *see* Little leaguer's shoulder
   fractures, 70
Proximal interphalangeal (PIP) joint, 138f, 140f, 146–148
Pseudogout, 112
Psychological well-being and exercise, 20

Q

Quadriceps contusion, 217
Quadriceps exercises, 243
Quadriceps (Q) angle, 247
Quadriceps strengthening exercises, 257
Quadriceps stretch, 262
Quebec classification of WAD injury, 169

R

Radial head fractures, 99
   types of, 100
Radial head pathology, 100, 104
Radiating neck pain, 170–172
Range of motion (ROM), 55, 93, 231
Rearfoot, 310, 311
Recurrent patella subluxation, 244
Rehabilitation for injury, 3
Repeated trauma, 106
Resistance exercises, for lateral elbow pain, 104
Respiratory response to exercise, 16
Rest, ice, compression, and elevation (RICE), 300
Retrocalcaneal bursitis, 283
Rheumatoid arthritis of elbow, 112
Rheumatoid arthritis of hand, 155, 156
Rheumatoid arthritis of wrist, 133, 134
Rheumatoid arthritis (RA), 219, 292, 302, 303
Rheumatoid nodules, 303
ROM, *see* Range of motion
Rotator cuff disease, 80–82
   treatment, 76, 77
Rotator cuff tears, 75–77

Rubberized cast, 146
Running gait, phases of, 313f

S

Sacroiliac joint stretch exercise, 197,
    198f
SC, *see* Sickle cell disease
Scaphoid fractures, 129–132
Scapholunate ligamentous disruption
    (SLLD), 129, 130, 132, 133
Sciatica, 179
Sedentary lifestyle, 13, 17
Self-reduction technique, 73
Septic bursitis, 106, 107
Septic joint, 257
Sesamoids, 338
    bipartite, 338
Shin splints syndrome, *see* Medial tibial
    stress syndrome
Shoe examination, 314, 316
Shoes, advice to patients about
    purchase of, 340
Shoulder anatomy, 4
Shoulder exercises, 88–92
Shoulder problem, case studies, 64, 65,
    70, 71, 79, 80
    classifications, 52
    focused physical, 55–64
    inspection of, 55
    organizational steps for, 51
    palpation of, 55
    provocative tests, 58–64
    resistance testing, 58
Shoulder shrugs exercise, 175, 177f
Sickle cell (SC) disease, 40
Sinding–Larsen–Johansson syndrome,
    260
Sinus barotrauma, 42
Skin abnormalities, 31
Sleep apnea, 31
SLLD, *see* Scapholunate ligamentous
    disruption
Spinal stenosis, 180, 192, 271, 287
Spine problem, *see* Low back pain;
    Neck pain
Splinting, for extensor injury treatment,
    151
Spondylolisthesis, 194
Spondylolysis, 194

Spondylosis, 170
Sports drinks, 44
Spurling's test, 161, 166f
"Squat" test, 242
Standing calf stretch exercise, 287,
    304f
Standing hamstring stretch, 264
    exercise, 195, 196f
Standing toe raises exercise, 288, 308f
Steroid injections, 104
    for wrist problems, 126, 127
Stone Bruise, *see* Fat Pad Syndrome
Stork test, 194, 195f
Straight leg raise, 262–264
Stress fractures, 7, 8, 209
    of tibial, 274–277
Stroke volume, 14
Structures of knee, anatomy and
    function of, 229t
Subluxation, 81
    of the annular ligament, *see*
    Nursemaids' elbow
Superior labrum anterior posterior
    (SLAP), 77
Suppurative bursitis, *see* Septic
    bursitis
Supracondylar fractures, 100
Supraspinatus strengthening, 89
Surgical decompression, 112
    intervention, 221

T

Talar dome fractures, 299
Talus, 289
Tarsal tunnel syndrome, 322, 324
Tears, types of, 241
Teens, weight control issues for,
    32–34
Tendonitis, 129
Tension fractures, 209
"The bends," 43; *see also*
    Decompression sickness
Thenar muscle strength test, 122, 123f
Thompson test, 284
Thumb, Bennett's fracture of, 146
    carpal metacarpal joint arthritis, 154
    metacarpal fractures, *see* Bennett's
    fracture
    spica cast, 132, 146

Tibialis Posterior Tenosynovitis,
    stages of tendon insufficiency,
    325, 326
Tibialis Posterior Tenosynovitis/ Tibialis
    Posterior Dysfunction, 325–328
    examination, 326–328
    imaging, 328
    treatment, 328
Tibial plateau fractures, 238
Tibial stress fractures, 274–277
    imaging in, 275, 276
    treatment of, 276, 277
Tinel's test, 122, 123f, 333, 334
Torticollis, 173
Towel stretch exercise for leg, 287, 301f
Training errors, 7, 10
Trench foot, 46
Tricyclic antidepressants, 190
Trochanteric bursitis, 212–214, 219
Tuning fork test, 271
Turf toe, 338–340
Tylenol, 219, 258
Tylenol, for neck pain, 168, 169
Type 2 diabetes, 18, 19

U
UCL, *see* Ulnar collateral ligament
    injury
Ulnar collateral ligament (UCL) injury,
    110
Ulnar nerve injury, 110, 111
Ulnar nerves, 110, 111
Ultrasound, 7
Undisplaced fractures, 100
Unhealthy eating, consequences of, 31, 32
Upper respiratory infection (URI), 4

V
Valgus instability, 110
Valgus stress, 238
    testing, 253

Varus force, 98, 99
Vasodilator, *see* Endothelium-derived
    NO
Vastus medialis obliquus (VMO),
    230
Volar plate injury of PIP, 150
Volar scapholunate, 132
VO$_2$max, 25

W
WAD, *see* Whiplash-associated disorder
WAD injury, quebec classification of,
    169
Wall slide, 262
Watson test, 130, 131f
Whiplash-associated disorder (WAD),
    169
Wrist, medical problems in, 133, 134
    arthritis, 133
    exercises, 134, 135
Wrist extension exercise, for elbow
    pain, 113, 115f
    for wrist pain, 135
Wrist extension stretch exercise, for
    elbow pain, 112, 114f
    for wrist pain, 135
Wrist flexion exercise, for elbow pain,
    113, 115f
    for wrist pain, 135
Wrist flexion stretch, for wrist pain, 134
    exercise, for elbow pain, 112, 114f
Wrist injury, 118
    organizational steps for overcoming
    fear and frustration for, 118
Wrist pain, case study, 119–131
Wrist problems, classification of, 119
    focused history of, 119
    focused physical examination for,
    119
Wrist splints, 126
    sprain, 133